Margin of Error
The Ethics of Mistakes in the Practice of Medicine

Ethics in Clinical Medicine Series

Margin of Error

The Ethics of Mistakes in the Practice of Medicine

Edited by

Susan B. Rubin
and Laurie Zoloth

University Publishing Group
Hagerstown, Maryland

University Publishing Group, Inc.
Hagerstown, Maryland 21740
1-800-654-8188

ISBN (paper):   1-55572-053-6

To my family, for making it all have meaning.
—Susan B. Rubin

To my parents, Helen and Arthur Zoloth,
for love in an uncertain world.
—Laurie Zoloth

Contents

Part 3: *Error in Ethics Consultation*

Acknowledgments

Over the years in our work together as clinical ethicists we have had countless conversations about the meaning and power of mistakes. We have engaged numerous clinical colleagues and ethics committees in discussion and have learned from their wisdom and insightful perspectives. In a workshop we presented at a joint meetings of the Society for Bioethics Consultation and the Society for Health and Human Values, we had the opportunity to explore with valued colleagues in the field of bioethics an area of particular interest to us—the possibility and nature of mistakes in bioethics consultation. We are indebted to all of the individuals who have shared their insights and wisdom with us and who have helped to shape our own perspectives on the problem of mistakes in medicine and bioethics consultation.

In particular, we want to thank each of our colleagues who so generously contributed chapters to this book. Many of them participated in our workshop on error, challenging us, agreeing with us, and revealing their stories to us. We were grateful then, and continue to be grateful for their spirit of collaboration. We asked many of these same colleagues to join us in delving deeper into the questions we raised, and received a warm and enthusiastic response from each of them. We know how busy our peers are. In an emerging field, there are many calls on one's time, many articles to write, and many compelling and competing moral appeals. We are thankful for the attention, skill, and thoughtfulness each of the authors brought to their chapters. Work of this sort is more than standard academic fare. It requires a willingness to pursue uncharted terrain and a commitment to honest self-reflection. Turning the critical gaze on one's own practice is never a facile matter. By their courage in doing so, our co-authors in this volume have taught us much in answer to our original question and have done much to advance the discourse on mistakes. We thank them.

Secondly, we want to thank Leslie LeBlanc and April McNamee at University Publishing Group for their early faith in the project and for their patient midwifery of the process. They have been enthusiastic supporters from the outset and dedicated to bringing the issues at stake in this book to a broader audience. Thanks go too to Rebecca Brown for assisting in research, editing, and technical advice—her work was invaluable.

Finally, we both want to thank our families and friends who were supportive throughout and who remind us always of the real-life significance of the questions posed in this book and in our work.

Introduction:
In the Margins of the Margin

Susan B. Rubin and Laurie Zoloth

This book has its roots in our long-standing fascination with the phenomenon of mistakes in medicine. In the course of our work as clinical ethicists, as well as in our roles as patients and family members, we have encountered a range of medical mistakes—some of seeming little consequence and some of great import. With each encounter with mistakes, we have been struck by the fragility of the human gesture of healing, by the multiple and breathtaking opportunities that exist for erroneous medical assessments and interventions, and by the painful and irrefutable fact that far less is certain or within our absolute control than the routinized practice of medicine would suggest.

Our initial pursuit of this inquiry focused on the nature, meaning, and significance of mistakes. We considered the epistemological challenges of identifying mistaken actions and judgments and the implications of mistakes for our understanding of medical truth, knowledge, and certainty. We worried about the normative implications of mistakes, and in particular the significance of harm, intentionality, accountability, truth-telling, and moral agency. We followed with interest developments in the literature on mistakes, and noticed the way in which our acute awareness of the possibility of mistakes shaped our approach to ethics consultation. Our skepticism about the certainty of medical knowledge was heightened each time the diagnostic and prognostic judgments on which we had relied were revealed in retrospect to have been mistaken. On more than one occasion, we found ourselves shaken by the reality of how error prone the practice of medicine is.

As our practice as ethics consultants evolved, we began to increasingly wonder: if mistakes are such an endemic and significant feature of medicine, what is the meaning and ramification of this truth for our own work? We first formally explored these questions in a workshop we presented at a joint annual meeting of the Society for Health and Human Values and the Society for Bioethics Consultation several years ago.[1] We began the session by asking a crowded room of colleagues whether they had ever made a mistake in bioethics consultation and what it would mean to make a mistake in such a context. The dynamic discussion that followed confirmed the need to pursue these questions further and served ultimately as the impetus for this book.

Margin of Error builds on the lively conversation that has evolved across disciplines about the nature, meaning, and importance of error in medicine. Theorists have noted that the problem of error in medicine is related to the essential and unavoidable features of the clinical world: temporality, creaturely limits, and an ever-expanding and changing knowledge base. It is perhaps the seeming unstoppable nature of mistakes in clinical medicine and the ways in which the practice of medicine stands as the *locus classicus* of the potential for human error that led Marianne Paget to introduce the notion of medicine as an "error-ridden" activity in her groundbreaking books[2] on the subject. As Paget and others have argued, there is an inevitability to the mistakes that arise in medicine due to medicine's inherent uncertainty, imperfect predictability, and unavoidable temporality. To complicate matters, all of medicine is a theoretical abstraction, and so the facticity of the real body will naturally undermine our claims of knowledge and certainty. In all pursuits, not only medical ones, the ability to understand—or control—the future is limited by the epistemic horizon that renders many potential outcomes out of view. Applied to medicine this means that, at both the level of the individual encounter and the level of standards of practice, the specter of possible mistakes looms large. We know this to be true and need look no further than the popular press accounts of egregious incidents of mistakes in drug dosages or amputations of the wrong limbs, recent findings about the real etiology of peptic ulcers, and reports of the inappropriate habitual use of such interventions as sodium bicarbonate in emergency resuscitation codes or Swan-Ganz catheters to appreciate the significance and gravity of this field of study.

As discourse on mistakes in medicine has expanded, attention has increasingly been focused on a systems approach to error detection and prevention, with an emphasis on establishing constructive measures of accountability and correction. But despite recent trends, there has been a need for renewed reflective consideration on the foundational questions that surround any approach to mistakes. What is the experience of making a mistake? What is the definition and measure of a mistake? Against what standards will mistakes be identified? What meaning will we make of mistakes? How ought we respond to mistakes, both prospectively and retrospectively?

And what of the rich literature on medical mistakes might be applicable to bioethics consultation? It is striking how little attention has been paid to the fact that the inevitability of error is as much an intrinsic part of ethics consultation as it is of medicine. To a significant degree, the very context and structure of ethics consultation, like the nature of medicine, makes error inevitable. In analyzing a case and offering recommendations, we rely unavoidably on an expanding and changing knowledge base, rooted in scientific claims that inevitably shift their ground beneath us. In addition, bioethics is often a kind of "secondary text" work, in that the ethicist comes to know the details and contours of each case through the frequently divergent perspectives of those involved in the dilemma. Because each participant inevitably sees the case in a different way and may highlight certain features as salient while discounting others, a large part of the ethicist's work is interpretive and therefore highly error prone. Furthermore, the field of ethics is itself always evolving, with central tenets challenged and modified over time. What bearing does this have on the meaning of mistakes in ethics consultation?

One way to begin addressing this question is to appeal to the etymology of the word *mistake,* which directs us toward the normative meaning of "taking the wrong path." In this way we see that the framing of the question as one of "mistakes" and "errors" relies on a number of significant and contested metaphysical and epistemological assumptions—most importantly, that there is an appropriate and correct approach to any given case, and that we can reliably identify and judge acts of clinical ethics consultation against that standard. Embedded in the very concept of mistakes is knowledge or intuition about their opposite, about the contrasting reality of things going as they should or as they were intended and designed. Ironically, clinical ethics consultation is rooted in the broader discipline of ethics, a field in which there is no uniform agreement about the universal "right" and "good." How to come to terms with this paradox, in light of many ethics consultants' intuitive sense that they at times have "taken the wrong path," is one of the questions this book explores. It is our goal that *Margin of Error* serve as a springboard for lively conversation in considering this broad range of questions, offering new approaches to the understanding of mistakes in medicine, and setting the stage for a new line of inquiry with respect to the study of mistakes in ethics consultation.

In bringing together some of the most thoughtful and engaging scholars in the field, it is our intention to advance the discourse on mistakes and to stimulate a new line of critical inquiry about the possibility of mistakes in ethics consultation. It is an inquiry that we hope will not only deepen the literature on mistakes, but will help set the agenda for the range of issues in need of our collective attention as the discipline of bioethics evolves.

We have invited colleagues from a range of disciplines including philosophy, history, sociology, medicine, law, and literature to think aloud about the concept of error from the perspective of their respective disciplines. The book begins with a series of essays focused on the conception and perception of error itself in which contributors offer reflections on the nature, meaning, and significance of mistakes. Drawing on this theoretical framework, the next section focuses on the problem of mistakes in medicine, in which contributors consider both how we have, and how we should, respond to mistakes in clinical practice. The final section introduces a new line of inquiry by taking on the parallel problem of mistakes in ethics consultation, probing what it might mean to make a mistake in such work and how we ought to respond when mistakes occur. Here is a guide to our partners in pursuing this conversation:

THE CONCEPTION AND PERCEPTION OF ERROR

Tod Chambers (chapter 1) begins by inviting us to consider the way in which discussions of medical mistakes have been traditionally structured. He examines systematically the way in which the literature on medical mistakes has framed the problem. He reveals that, far from being neutral, the standard description of mistakes found throughout the literature rhetorically supports particular philosophical positions. Drawing upon the work of literary critic Kenneth Burke, Chambers analyzes the various ways ethicists explain, teach, and frame the presence of mistakes by constructing and emphasizing distinct features of these dramas. In the end he argues that descriptions of mistakes are not mere objective presentations but rather are didactic representations that support specific moral frameworks.

Kenneth De Ville and Carl Elliott (chapter 2) take a broad perspective as well, noting that the concept of medical error is inescapably dependent upon cultural context and a product of specific intellectual and historical developments. They describe how medical error is socially and culturally constructed in that individuals must be predisposed to seek mechanistic, tangible reasons for error when they see human suffering and medical misfortune rather than assuming that such physical misfortune is a result, say, of bad luck, fate, or a punishment from a supreme being. Under this construct, errors are perceived not as events, but as human actions. In analyzing our prevailing conceptions of medical error, De Ville and Elliott trace the degree to which technological advances have led paradoxically both to heightened (and frequently excessive) expectations and to greater opportunities for mistakes at the hand of human actors.

Rita Charon (chapter 3) draws on literary theory to deconstruct the nature and structure of a particular kind of mistake—a mistake rooted fundamentally in an error of interpretation. As she explains, interpretation is a central feature of the human condition; as members of interpretive communities, we are all continually engaging in a process of interpreting the world around us. To understand fully the anatomy of a mistake, we must begin by uncovering and examining the underlying interpretive apparatus at work. Drawing on an analysis of two texts, Henry James's short story "The Beast in the Jungle" and an actual patient chart, Charon shows how interpretive mistakes emerge and spread, and how their recognition may be postponed.

Judith Andre (chapter 4) turns our attention to the importance of virtue, particularly the virtue of humility, in the practice of medicine and the response to error. Drawing on virtue theory, feminist theory, Christianity, and Buddhism, she offers an account of the kind of humility she envisions as a necessary part of clinical practice. Turning her attention to the context within which medicine is practiced, she considers the kind of institutional structures that encourage and discourage the development and exercise of the virtue of humility.

John D. Lantos and Martha Montello (chapter 5) draw on *The Adventures of Huckleberry Finn, The Remains of the Day,* and *The House of God* to explore the role that context has in framing what counts as good or mistaken behavior. Noting that deviance or problematic behavior is defined exclusively with respect to existing standards and expectations, they ask whether some of the current practices in medicine might be wrong in ways that practitioners within the system do not see and question. They suggest that making what might be defined as an error according to existing standards may in fact represent a higher moral response to human dilemmas than the achievement of what is currently defined as technical perfection.

ERROR IN MEDICAL PRACTICE

David Hilfiker (chapter 6) offers one of the most candid and powerful first-hand accounts of the experience of making devastating medical mistakes. Drawing on his own clinical experience as a family practice physician, he demonstrates how routinely mistakes can be made and how damaging their cumulative effect can be not only for patients and families, but for the practicing clinician as well. Noting the absence of any real opportunities for confession or restitution, Hilfiker calls for and models a different approach to medical mistakes, one that would grant physicians permission to recognize, face, and honestly discuss mistakes and their consequences.

Lucian L. Leape (chapter 7), in this classic article, proposes a systems approach to the identification of and response to medical error. Echoing some of Hilfiker's sentiments, he argues that our traditional approach to medical error is impoverished and, with its emphasis on infallibility and blame, doomed to fail. He draws first on the field of human factors research and cognitive psychology and offers an alternative vision of how to address medical mistakes. Arguing that we must fundamentally change the way we think about errors and why they occur if we are to succeed in reducing their occurrence, he calls for a dramatic shift in the culture of medicine; a recognition that mistakes are an inevitable but manageable part of everyday practice; and an understanding that errors are evidence not of character flaws, but of system flaws that can be strategically corrected.

Joel E. Frader (chapter 8) offers a searing account of two errors he has made as a practicing physician, one in the course of his training and one later in his career as an attending physician. Given the complexity, uncertainty, and imperfect information that surrounds any medical encounter, he notes how difficult the simple act of defining and categorizing errors can be. These factors, coupled with the powerful force of the culture of medicine, make it difficult to even broach the subject of mistakes in a forthright way. Reflecting on his own experience in this context, Frader considers the moral cost of covering up mistakes. He joins the call for reform so that uncertainty can be acknowledged with humility, and errors can be responded to more clearly and honestly.

Rosa Lynn Pinkus (chapter 9) offers an historical account of one profession's approach to the occurrence of mistakes. Drawing on case reports and journal articles, she reveals that, contrary to current practice, early in the development of neurosurgery it was commonplace for mistakes to be openly published and widely discussed. Pinkus suggests that, because this practice of honest public disclosure took place at a time when the boundaries for what counted as acceptable practice were being set, it offers a unique entry into the discussion of how professions define and attempt to prevent mistakes. Tracing the developments in neurosurgery, she reveals that roughly 30 years after the inception of the subspecialty, open and frank discussion of mistakes went underground, becoming the private business of the profession. Offering a useful reference point for our contemporary discussion, Pinkus describes how societal changes in law, medicine, and public reaction influenced the disappearance of frank public discourse about mistakes in neurosurgery.

James Lindemann Nelson (chapter 10) calls for a redirection of our focus on efforts to detect and respond to mistakes in clinical medicine. Noting the overwhelming popularity of a systems-based approach, he worries that such a model used alone might actually lead to clinicians' making more mistakes because clinical evidence and outcomes data are used not to supplement but to supplant clinical judgment. After analyzing the epistemological assumptions at stake in the application of clinical knowledge to particular patients, he recommends against simply replacing clinical judgment with an outcomes-based approach and encourages more systematic study of the nature and structure of clinical judgment, with particular emphasis on how it can be improved.

Edmund G. Howe (chapter 11) examines the normative implications of an ethics consultant's knowledge that a medical error has occurred. He explores the question of how ethics consultants should respond to the mistakes of their colleagues and suggests that it might be a mistake to insist on disclosure and truth-telling in all instances. He suggests that mistakes come in a variety of forms and that, in certain circumstances, particularly those in which a mistake is questionable or not verifiable, it might be a mistake for an ethics consultant to disclose the error to the patient. Reflecting on a mistake he made as a medical student, he considers whether blind allegiance to truth-telling is always the most humane response or whether it might actually be an act of indulgent self-righteousness.

Virginia A. Sharpe (chapter 12) offers a philosophical analysis of the concept of medical mistakes, noting the implications of adopting a retrospective versus prospective approach to the identification and response to mistakes. She suggests that the prospective models of continuous quality improvement (CQI) and the doctrine of no-fault liability are powerful and constructive frameworks for approaching medical error prevention, unlike retrospective approaches such as quality assurance (QA) and medical malpractice, which focus blame on individuals for poor results. Sharpe argues that CQI and no-fault liability more accurately reflect the nature and etiology of the majority of medical mistakes and offer more meaningful opportunities for prevention and correction than do retrospective models.

ERROR IN ETHICS CONSULTATION

Susan B. Rubin and Laurie Zoloth (chapter 13) introduce a new line of inquiry by asking what it would mean to make a mistake in ethics consultation. Reflecting on their intuitive sense that it is possible and perhaps inevitable to make a mistake in ethics consultation, they struggle with the challenge of defining precisely what might constitute a mistake in this field of work. They acknowledge the challenge of pursuing such a discussion given the lack of clearly established standards, according to which consultants are expected to function and against which they can be judged. Noting both the difficulty and importance of raising questions about mistakes at this stage in the field's development, they consider the possibility of both substantive and procedural mistakes and outline some of the central considerations that might be used in recognizing and responding to mistakes. Above all, they call for greater self-reflection and more collective discourse about the occurrence of mistakes in ethics consultation.

George C. Webster and Françoise E. Baylis (chapter 14) offer a rich account of our "experience of the ethical," an experience they describe as being fraught with moral uncertainty and moral distress. They suggest that in some instances it is not clear to the ethics consultant how to approach a moral dilemma, or there is inconsistency between the ethics consultant's beliefs and actions. In such situations, ethics consultants may experience compromised integrity and what the authors call "moral residue"—that which we carry with us from those times in our lives when in the face of moral distress we have allowed ourselves to be seriously compromised. Such failure to pursue what we believe to be the right course of action can be rooted in errors in judgment, personal failings, or institutional constraints. Although the resultant moral residue we experience might lead to greater clarity about our personal commitments and moral boundaries, it can also lead to significant errors such as denial, trivialization, or unreflective acceptance of the inconsistency between our beliefs and actions. To address the challenges of integrity, compromise, and moral distress constructively, the authors call for more honest self-reflection and greater attention to these issues in our workplaces.

Paul J. Reitemeier (chapter 15) offers a comprehensive philosophical overview of the issues at stake in identifying, understanding, and responding to errors that may arise in the practice of bioethics consultation. Beginning with the premise that truth and error are meaningful concepts in moral judgment, Reitemeier struggles to identify standards of practice against which we might recognize and evaluate errors in bioethics consultation. Noting the distinctive nature of bioethics, a pursuit that he claims has not yet achieved the stature of a "profession" per se, he offers a taxonomy of possible errors that can be made in ethics consultation. He joins the call for more focused consideration and investigation of these issues by practitioners in the field.

Ellen W. Bernal (chapter 16) suggests that it may not be possible to specify in advance a clear path or set of correct actions that an ethics consultant should pursue in any particular situation. Drawing on the work of Michael Polanyi, Bernal proposes instead that ethics consultation is a complex skilled performance that unfolds over time. The ethicist frequently must engage in creative innovation or pioneering; under such circumstances, and especially when consultants enter "unfamiliar territory," mistakes may be more likely to occur. Bernal shares the results of an ethnographic study she conducted in which she queried ethics consultants about mistakes they had made in their practice. She concludes that there is need for more conversation about mistakes, errors, and midcourse corrections as a source of learning and in the service of developing of what we might all consider expert practice.

Charles L. Bosk (chapter 17) draws from his seminal work on the sociology of mistakes in medicine and medical education to consider the implications of his findings for the practice of bioethics consultation. He reviews the standard sociological accounts of error and considers their application to the fields of medicine and bioethics consultation. He concludes that, given the current state of the field of ethics consultation, in which the structural and cognitive features that would support a shared collective understanding of mistakes are lacking, individual clinical ethicists or ethics committees cannot make a mistake. This is because the features that allow for public identification of mistakes in other occupational segments simply do not exist in the world of clinical bioethics. Bosk offers a framework for understanding what would need to change in order for the concept of mistakes to have meaning in the field of ethics consultation. To establish a collective understanding of mistakes in ethics consultation, he suggests that the following elements would be necessary: regular case review, agreement on outcomes and a means for assessing them, and some systematic data that compare different approaches to ethics consultation. In conclusion he calls on the community of practitioners in ethics consultation to devote attention to these concerns.

Robert S. Olick (chapter 18) considers the problem of mistakes in ethics consultation from the perspective of the law. Noting the trend toward the development of standards in ethics consultation, he asks whether it would be possible for an ethics consultant to commit malpractice and he considers the legal significance that existing standards might have in a potential lawsuit. After providing a primer of the traditional medical malpractice model, he asks whether it would ever make sense by analogy to hold that an ethics consultant had a legal obligation to act as a reasonable consultant would under the circumstances, and what it would mean to understand the consultant's role in this way. He notes that the growth of clinical ethics consultation and the movement toward professionalization lay the groundwork for the emergence of legal accountability and for the development of a legal standard of care for ethics consultation.

Bruce E. Zawacki and William May (chapter 19) propose the use of a CQI approach to address what they call "problems in ethics consultation." They note that CQI has succeeded in producing measurable, sustained results in improving hospital medical care and suggest that such an approach can be applied with success to the process of ethics consultation by hospital ethics committees. To that end, they outline in some detail what the process of CQI would look like and offer concrete suggestions for ways that hospital ethics committees can structure and apply a CQI model. They offer the example of one institution's experience using CQI to improve the ethics committee's process and encourage other ethics committees to adopt a similar approach.

Giles R. Scofield (chapter 20) offers a provocative essay in which he calls attention to what he sees as a fundamental error in the underlying assumptions as well as the structure of the practice of ethics consultation. Locating the central problem in a distinction between "uncertainty" and "Uncertainty," he asserts that the ethics consultant's fatal error has been the practice of being generous with the former and parsimonious with the latter. Tracing the evolution of the field of bioethics, Scofield points out the mistake of not taking more seriously and disclosing more forthrightly the metaethics critique of normative ethics—that is, that there are no objective grounds for ethical judgments or methods for resolving disputes. He argues that the corrective lies not in eliminating Uncertainty, but in changing our response to it. Rather than persisting in promoting the illusion that Uncertainty is not a problem, he advocates clearer acknowledgment by ethics consultants that Uncertainty is inevitable and unavoidable.

John C. Fletcher, Robert J. Boyle, and Edward M. Spencer (chapter 21) offer an overview of the history of ethics consultation and review in detail the evolution, content, and implications of the current standards for ethics consultation recommended by the Joint Task Force of the Society for Bioethics Consultation and the Society for Health and Human Values. The authors suggest that the most serious mistakes currently being made in ethics consultation have as their source confusion about the nature of the consultation process, lack of consensus about standards of consultation, and the error of "taking sides" in serious moral conflicts. To illustrate their points, they include concrete examples of many of these mistakes, drawing on their own clinical experience and on cases that have been reported in the literature.

We are grateful to our colleagues for joining us in this endeavor, and for sharing their rich and diverse perspectives on the problem of mistakes in medicine and bioethics consultation. It is our sincere hope that this book will stimulate lively discussion and debate about the issues that the authors have helped us to outline. They are issues in need of our active collective attention—as scholars, as practitioners, as patients, and as citizens.

NOTES

1. S.B. Rubin and L. Zoloth, "Dead Wrong: Error in Clinical Ethics Consultation," (Workshop presented at the Joint Meeting of the Society for Health and Human Values and the Society for Bioethics Consultation, Cleveland, Ohio, October 1996).

2. M.A. Paget, *The Utility of Mistakes: A Phenomenological Interpretation of Medical Work* (Philadelphia: Temple University Press, 1988); M.A. Paget, *A Complex Sorrow: Reflections on Cancer and an Abbreviated Life* (Philadelphia: Temple University Press, 1993).

Part 1

The Conception and Perception of Error

1

Framing Our Mistakes

Tod Chambers

What is involved, when we say what people are doing and why they are doing it? —Kenneth Burke, *A Grammar of Motives*

INTRODUCTION

In a study titled "Do House Officers Learn from Their Mistakes?" Albert Wu and colleagues observe that residents who blamed mistakes on "job overload" were less likely to learn from these mistakes than residents who took personal responsibility for them; the authors conclude that "house officers should be encouraged to accept responsibility for their mistakes."[1] Their recommendation follows from the assumption that the cause of the mistakes was primarily the residents' ignorance. But what if the residents who indicated the work environment as the cause were actually correct in their observations? What if the residents who took personal responsibility were blaming themselves for external causes? Would we not judge the authors' recommendation as absurd? Why would one desire individuals to take responsibility for that which they are not responsible? The study's authors seem to direct their attention toward the actors rather than the environment in which the acts occurred. Because the authors are concerned with how house officers learn from errors, their focus on the actors is perhaps not so surprising, for how could one provide recommendations for teaching residents if one focused on the environment in which residents work?

The literary critic Kenneth Burke argued that in order to describe human action we need to take into account five terms: act, agent, purpose, scene, and agency. Burke referred to these five terms taken as a whole as a *pentad,* and he believed that to make a complete statement of human action, a speaker must "offer *some kind of* answer to these five questions: what was done (act), when or where it was done (scene), who did it (agent), how he [or she] did it (agency), and why (purpose)."[2] By systematically identifying how a speaker describes an action through these terms, we can gain insight into how the speaker perceives the world. One cannot view the world without a frame, so speakers inevitably reveal their worldview through the emphasis of one of the terms in the pentad. For example, in the study by Wu and colleagues cited above, the authors emphasize the agent of the action and discount the importance of scene. This decision to emphasize agent over scene is crucial in terms of the authors' final recommendation for helping residents to learn from their mistakes. Through pentadic analysis, Burke contended, one can systematically analyze the rhetoric of speakers, such as the authors of this study.

Pentadic analysis entails identifying the five terms in a speaker's description and then comparing what Burke referred to as the various "ratios." For instance, in the ratio of agent to scene, one analyzes how the agent identified by the speaker determines or conditions the scene. If in medical decision making one portrays physicians as the sole agents—as opposed to, for instance, including third-party payers—then the scene portrayed will tend to be restricted to the hospital environment. In some descriptions, specific ratios are more notable than in others. Once one has looked at all the relevant ratios, Burke claimed that one of the terms in the description can be identified as having more influence over the others, and this featured term then can be related to the speaker's way of seeing the world. The featuring of certain terms, Burke contended, can be linked to particular philosophical worldviews. Speakers who emphasize the *act* are often motivated by the philosophy of realism. Those who emphasize *agent* incline toward idealism. When *agency* is the featured term then the corresponding worldview is one of pragmatism. The tendency to emphasize *purpose* indicates a mystical worldview. And when the speaker highlights the *scene* of the act then he or she is generally motivated by materialism. Every act of emphasizing one term is also an act of undervaluing other terms. According to Burke, human beings "do not use the full range of all the possible terms in giving meaning to events" and, consequently, Burke's pentad becomes a way of critiquing descriptions for how the term selected "is a reduction of reality, a way of seeing that is partial."[3]

This essay examines four descriptions of medical mistakes using Burke's pentad in order to uncover the philosophic ramifications for emphasizing terms and ratios. By viewing medical mistakes through specific terms in the pentad, authors are able to promote their worldviews while they seem to be simply describing the world. This essay also draws upon another methodological tool of Burke's known as *cluster analysis;* Burke held that speakers often cluster particular terms with other terms, and this also reveals how they implicitly see the world.[4] Each of the descriptions of medical mistakes examines how some of these clusters relate to the featured term. Pentadic analysis offers a useful tool to reveal not only the featured terms but also the undervalued terms in our description of medical error. The significance of this tool is perhaps best seen in terms of the solutions proposed, for each of the terms featured allows the authors to suggest particular responses or policies to mistakes in medical practice. The featured term is not only a way of seeing the world but also a call to change it.

It is important to note a basic bias in analyzing mistakes through Burke's pentad: the tool cannot be used to understand how people explain *unintended* acts. Burke was concerned with how a speaker's worldview affects the framing and understanding of human action in the world. Some critics have noted that the limitations of Burke's work is that it is confined to human action, for the pentad does not provide a "way to discuss natural things except as scenic material."[5] This is perhaps best illustrated by viewing the term *purpose*. From a contemporary Western worldview, for instance, one would be thought odd to ascribe purpose to the acts of a tornado; a person could view a tornado as an act of God, but this would be appealing to an outside, supernatural agent. In an analogous manner, we assume that no one intends to cause a mistake; if anything, medical mistakes are not actions but accidents because they lack purpose. Aristotle observed in his *Nicomachean Ethics* that for an action to be involuntary (as I assume all mistakes to be) there must be an "ignorance of the particulars"—that is, "(1) who is doing it; (2) what he is doing; (3) about what or to what he is doing it; (4) sometimes also what he is doing it with, e.g., the instrument; (5) for what result, e.g., safety; (6) in what way, e.g., gently or hard."[6] Now certainly someone could not be ignorant of *all* of these unless he were mad.

One should view a pentadic analysis of medical mistakes as an examination of how the authors view medical acts in general and how they, in turn, see one of the terms going astray toward an ignorance of a particular. Each of the authors examined in this essay argues that there is an ignorance of one of these particulars. In Wu and his colleagues' study, some of the residents believed that it was not their knowledge of medical acts that was at fault but the scene in which they acted; from the residents' perspective, if the scene were altered these mistakes would not have happened. In other words, mistakes are always due to an unintended aberration of one of the terms.

THE FALLEN AGENT

David Hilfiker's "Facing Our Mistakes" is a seminal work on the issue of medical mistakes, in which the author recounts several of his own mistakes.[7] [This classic article is reprinted as chapter 6 of this book—ED.] The first mistake Hilfiker describes concerns his care for a woman during her second pregnancy. Following a series of tests, Hilfiker diagnosed her with a missed abortion and scheduled a dilation and curettage. Afterwards he discovered that he had aborted a living fetus. Hilfiker reflects on the response that physicians tend to have when faced with such an incident. "As physicians our automatic response to reading about such a tragedy is to try and discover what went wrong, to analyze why the mistakes occurred, and to institute corrective measures so that such things do not happen again. This response is important, indeed necessary, and I spent hours in such a review. But it is inadequate if it does not address our own emotional and spiritual experience of the events."[8]

Hilfiker's account and his subsequent argument about medical mistakes focus primarily upon the issue of the agent. In the above quote, he mentions that physicians' common response when faced by a mistake is to focus on agency. Hilfiker suggests, however, that this approach is fruitless and does not provide assistance to the practicing physician. Hilfiker also discounts in the article the importance of scene: "Our work in the intensive-care unit, in the emergency room, in the surgery suite, or in the delivery room offers us hundreds of opportunities daily to miscalculate, often with drastic consequences. And it is not only in these settings but also in the humdrum of routine daily care that a physician can blunder into tragedy."[9]

Hilfiker recalls another event in which, following a car accident, he examined an injured boy and decided the child simply had a dislocated foot. He told the patient and his mother that he could reduce the dislocation at the local hospital or they could travel to Duluth to see a specialist. The mother decided to go to Duluth, and Hilfiker states that he was "somewhat offended" at her decision. The next morning he received a call from the specialist who thanked him for the referral and informed him that the boy had "a severe posterior compartment syndrome, which had hyperflexed the foot, causing it to appear dislocated."[10] This condition necessitated surgery in order to save the muscles in the boy's leg. Hilfiker recalls, "I felt physically weak as I realized that this young man would have been permanently injured had his mother not decided on her own to take him to Duluth."[11] What is interesting about Hilfiker's choice of this event as significant is that it is a mistake of which only Hilfiker was aware. The final outcome was good, and according to some who write about medical mistakes, this should not be identified as a mistake because of this outcome. Hilfiker also gives examples where physicians as agents may never know whether there are mistakes but may still feel as if they caused mistakes. For instance, if a patient whose condition forces "almost continuous decision making on the part of the physician" dies, the physician "is left wondering whether the care provided was adequate."[12] In the agent-act ratio, Hilfiker features the agent as significant. It is his attitude toward the act that is significant, not the outcome of the act or the act itself.

After discounting act, scene, and agency, Hilfiker comes to what he considers the heart of the problem. "As practicing primary-care physicians . . . we work in an impossible situation. Each of the myriad decisions to be made every day has the potential for drastic consequences if it is not determined properly. And it is highly likely that sooner or later we will make the mistake that kills or seriously injures another person. How can we live with that knowledge? And after a serious mistake has been made, how can we continue a daily practice and expose ourselves again? How can we who see ourselves as healers deal with such guilt?"[13]

Hilfiker repeatedly states that he does not believe this has anything to do with problems in the way medical decisions are made but rather is simply part of the innate fallibility of being a person. He reiterates that we all make mistakes, but the difference between most people's mistakes and those of the physician is the extraordinary consequences of the physician's mistakes, to patient and to physician. In Hilfiker's rhetoric, the agent-purpose ratio is important; the purpose of being a healer comes in conflict with the inevitability of an agent's making mistakes, which results in the profound pain that physicians experience when facing their mistakes.

For Hilfiker it is not that physicians are inadequately trained; that is, it is not an issue of agency, but rather an issue of our nature as fallible human beings. When Hilfiker uses the term mistake, it is often clustered with terms such as tragedy, agony, sin, or guilt; this clustering suggests the linking he makes between medical errors and a particular vision of human nature. The solution to this problem thus is somehow to provide a forum for the expression of mistakes. In this, Hilfiker turns toward a Christian worldview in portraying mistakes as analogous to a sin that requires confession, restitution, and absolution. In his conclusion, Hilfiker argues that the real problem lies in a false concept of the agent in medical practice as "having to wear the yoke of perfection."[14] Hilfiker's rhetoric features the agent, for he views human beings as unavoidably flawed and limited and thus requiring redemption.

An examination of Hilfiker's other works reveals that he has continually featured agent. In *Not All of Us Are Saints*, a book that concerns his work among the poor in Washington, D.C., Hilfiker emphasizes agent over scene and agency; this is illustrated in such statements as: "This book is less about bold prescriptions for political or societal change than about what it's like to find oneself suddenly enmeshed in the crumbling relationship between government and the poor."[15] As mentioned above, Burke associated an emphasis upon agent with idealism. The philosophy of idealism argues that reality does not have an existence outside of the mind. Burke observed that idealists "think in terms of the 'ego,' the 'self,' the 'super-ego,' 'consciousness,' 'will,' the 'generalized I,' the 'subjective,' 'mind,' 'spirit,' the 'oversoul,' and any such 'super-persons.' "[16] Hilfiker's spiritual worldview becomes entangled in an idealistic philosophy that makes him react to medical mistakes in terms of the final reality for him, which is the self. It is his contention that this self is where we should focus our attention when considering medical mistakes, for it has a reality outside of the material world.

ACTS OF SCIENCE

Unlike Hilfiker's highly confessional, agent-centered account of medical mistakes, Samuel Gorovitz and Alasdair MacIntyre's "Toward a Theory of Medical Fallibility" emphasizes the act.[17] This is revealed in the first sentence of their essay: "No species of fallibility is more important or less understood than fallibility in medical practice." Medical mistakes in Gorovitz and MacIntyre's view are entities that can be grouped together with similar acts. In discussing the "basic data" of medical mistakes, Gorovitz and MacIntyre view them without any relationship to an agent, in a manner that makes them appear as if they are an entirely different issue from the problem Hilfiker describes. This approach is possible because of their tendency to employ the passive voice in their description of medical actions: "Those data [of medical fallibility] include the facts that medical error not only occurs but seems unavoidable; that some medical error seems innocent even when severely damaging, whereas other medical error seems culpable; that the harm that results from medical error seems sometimes but not always to warrant compensation; that the error that causes harm seems sometimes but not always to warrant sanctions; and finally, that the relationships among culpability, harm, compensation, and sanctions are obscure."[18]

In their account of medical mistakes, Gorovitz and MacIntyre focus on acts divorced from scene, agent, or purpose. The ratio of most importance to these authors is the act-agency ratio. This can be seen in the way that they wish to challenge traditional assumptions about medical fallibility that have focused on "medical responsibility." They believe that, to understand medical error, we should examine medicine not as a "profession" but as a "science."[19] In this challenge, these authors are concerned with medical acts rather than with the agents of those acts, which characterizes sociology's concern with medicine as a profession.

Gorovitz and MacIntyre begin their analysis by looking at internal and external norms in science. "Internal norms are those which derive from the essential character of scientific activity as a cognitive pursuit. External norms are those which govern motives either for participating in or making use of the results of scientific activity."[20] In Burkean terms, the internal norms are those that deal with act and agency, and the external norms come from agent, scene, and purpose. Consequently, issues of personal motivation, academic competition, and social utility are scientific factors, yet these features do not influence science's acts or agency. Gorovitz and MacIntyre claim that from the perspective of science, errors will occur either because of "the limitations of the present state of natural science" or because of "the willfulness or negligence of the natural scientist."[21] Science's practitioners believe that mistakes are caused by factors related to the agent; Gorovitz and MacIntyre counter that the problem lies not with the agent but with the act itself. In other words, the authors contend that error can exist within the application of science even if the internal norms are practiced correctly, for medical practice is not a *pure* science but instead a form of *applied* science.

Gorovitz and MacIntyre analyze an example of a surgical mistake. They claim that the traditional way of finding fault for the mistake is either the state of the art or the state of the surgeon's skill—that is, either agency or agent. The problem with this traditional explanation is that it does not take into account the nature of medical science to be concerned with particulars. Unlike pure science, applied science is the application of scientific principles to the world of particular entities. "Many particulars—salt marshes, hurricanes, and the higher primates, for example—cannot be understood solely as the sum total of the physical and chemical mechanisms that operate on them."[22] These types of individual entities cannot be contained by simple "lawlike generalizations," for we cannot know what factors may be relevant in the actions of a particular entity." What is important to the meteorologist, navigator, or veterinary surgeon is an understanding of particular, individual hurricanes, cloud formations, or cows, and thus what is *distinctive* about them as particulars is what is of crucial importance."[23] Because medical science is a science of particulars, its actions are always conditioned by the "necessary fallibility of our knowledge of particulars."[24] Gorovitz and MacIntyre claim that errors in medicine may be the result of scientific ignorance (agency) or negligence (agent), but they also may be the result of a third factor—the necessary fallibility of its practice (act).

Gorovitz and MacIntyre's focus on act influences their recommendations for policy decisions regarding bad outcomes in medicine. If medical science is a type of act that invariably is unpredictable, then malpractice law should not focus on the responsibility of the agent; instead we should create a social policy that responds to the inherent limitations of the medical act. Unlike Hilfiker, Gorovitz and MacIntyre do not perceive clinicians as fallen and fallible agents but as individuals performing acts that are inherently errant. These authors portray errors as simply occurring in the manner that natural events occur. Errors thus "occur," "arise," or "take place."

In their concluding paragraph, these two philosophers argue for the importance of philosophy in medical education. Although they do not discount the intrinsic rewards that the liberal arts have for students, they suggest that the true goal of philosophic study for medical students is an understanding of the nature of their acts. This conclusion becomes a parallel argument to their early discount of sociology's focus on the agent. Their conclusion implies that Hilfiker could have slept more easily at night if he had understood the philosophic fallibility of his acts. What Hilfiker needed was not a Bible but a copy of Kant's *Critique of Pure Reason*. According to Burke, these authors' emphasis upon the act indicates a philosophic system of realism. Realism holds that universal principles have a reality and thus can be studied in an empirical manner. Burke suggested that an emphasis on act results in treating "individuals as members of a group," and Gorovitz and MacIntyre tend to see mistakes as a necessary condition in this type of science.

THE SYSTEM OF AGENCY

According to Lucian Leape, "Errors must be accepted as evidence of systems flaws not character flaws. Until and unless that happens, it is unlikely that any substantial progress will be made in reducing medical errors."[25] These sentences, which conclude his "Error in Medicine," bring into sharp focus the key ratio of Leape's analysis of mistakes: the agency-agent. [Leape's classic article is reprinted as chapter 7 of this book—ED.]

Leape's article begins with an analysis of the relationship of act to agent in the creation of errors. He notes the way physicians are educated and socialized in their training to be infallible. The emphasis on a perfect agent places the blame for errors upon physicians. Consequently, when physicians are confronted with mistakes, they tend to think: "How can there be an error without negligence?"[26] Leape believes that it is absurd to associate the person who is responsible for someone's care with responsibility for errors, and he refers to the emotional impact of the discovery of mistakes on physicians. For Leape this results in an insoluble dilemma for physicians: they are taught to be perfect in doing work that invariably they cannot do perfectly.

This focus on agent, Leape believes, is the reason we have not been able to prevent errors in medicine. He refers to this agent-centered approach as the "perfectibility model." He notes that we try to achieve this perfectibility through training and punishment. However, responses to error in medicine that aim "toward preventing a recurrence of a similar error, often by attempting to prevent *that* individual from making a repeat error" do not address the "underlying causes" of these errors.[27] Healthcare professionals must rethink how they conceive of errors; they must focus not on personal perfection but on how medicine is practiced.

A significant part of Leape's article is the examination of a theory of human cognition and the mechanisms of cognitive errors. With emphasis upon agency rather than agent, Leape's argument relies on terms such as *process, system,* and *design.* He remarks on the potential usefulness of examining air travel, an activity that has highly trained professionals whose errors can result in devastating outcome; the difference between physicians and pilots is not the manner that the individuals are selected but rather the systems designed in aviation to anticipate errors.

Burke linked this emphasis upon agency with the philosophy of pragmatism, which is concerned with achieving an end and values the workability of an analysis. Leape's essay shifts the analysis of medical mistakes away from the agent and toward agency; his goal is the pragmatic end of preventing mistakes.

OUR MISTAKEN PURPOSE

Eric Cassell's article "Error in Medicine" is unique among discussions of medical mistakes in featuring purpose.[28] He begins his analysis of error by considering the basis for malpractice action, and he notes that the primary concern of malpractice law has been with technical mistakes. He argues that this concern with agency provides only a limited understanding of why medical mistakes take place. "Errors in medicine are not only technical, but also arise from the moral sphere, social or interpersonal interaction, and from problems of thought. It is in the nature of so complex an activity as medicine that these all interact."[29]

Cassell argues that attention to agency gives us only partial insight into the reason medical mistakes occur. He also criticizes medicine's tendency to emphasize the agent, for this "merely shows that medicine is a human activity and is thus subject to human weakness"; he believes that this "is hardly more illuminating than the opposite single-mindedness of malpractice law."[30]

Cassell argues that what we usually mean by error requires three factors: responsibility, causality, and injury. He contends that these three factors have objective and subjective qualities. The requirements of malpractice law deal primarily with the objective quality of a medical error, and we tend not to be aware "that the objective nature of responsibility, causality, and injury . . . are the societal expression of individual subjective sense of" these factors.[31] Our understanding of the objective qualities of medical mistakes is dependent upon our community's understanding of these factors as well as its "understanding of the nature and cure of illness and of the function of physicians."[32] Cassell points out, for example, that if one administered morphine for the relief of pain and this action led to a patient's death, then "the injury would not have come through error, but rather as an unavoidable consequence of mercy."[33] In his concern with the subjective quality of understanding medical mistakes, Cassell directs the reader's attention away from agency, act, and agent and toward the purpose of medical acts.

The purpose of medical intervention, Cassell believes, is revealed in the expectations by contemporary patients that medical treatment should always achieve a perfect outcome. This unrealistic purpose that we have assigned to medicine affects our thinking about responsibility, causality, and injury and thus medical mistakes. Since the purpose of medicine is a perfect outcome, we tend to believe that fate can be controlled; if a bad outcome occurs, then the physician must be responsible. Cassell argues that we are mistaken in our tendency to see the sources of error in terms of the agent. Cassell's focus on purpose is reflected in his selection of verbs that are linked to "error"; he frequently uses "understand," "comprehend," and "view." For Cassell, our problem in responding to medical error has to do with preconceived notions we bring to contemplating the practice of medicine.

As the title of his essay, "The Nature of Suffering and the Goals of Medicine" suggests, Cassell believes that the relief of suffering should be one of the primary goals of medical care.[34] This article echoes Cassell's focus on purpose when looking at medical issues. Burke associated the emphasis upon purpose with the philosophy of mysticism, for this philosophic worldview is characterized by the "unity of the individual with some *cosmic or universal purpose.*"[35] Burke observed that mysticism arises during periods of social confusion concerning the nature of human purpose. "Thus, precisely at such times of general hesitancy," Burke claimed, "the mystic can compensate for his own particular doubts about human purpose by submerging himself in some vision of a *universal* or *absolute* or *transcendent* purpose, with which he would identify himself."[36] This mystical tendency in Cassell's analysis (not to be confused, however, with some "religious" tendency) can be found in his conclusion, in which he criticizes thinkers such as Gorovitz and MacIntyre in their attempt to understand errors by "choosing this or that individual instance of disease as the conventional framework of reference." He goes on to argue that "diseases as we know them could conceivably be seen as entities, but they are not individuals in the Gorovitz-MacIntyre sense that salt marshes are, free standing and unique."[37]

Cassell argues that we should not try to understand the occurrence of medical mistakes by focusing on any individual unit but, rather, we should view mistakes within a larger vision of medical practice. In his concluding paragraph, he provides a final image that could have been drawn directly from Burke's own imagery: "Each case, whether error is present or not, is like a stage play. A setting, an audience, a disease whose story is told, and a set of actors. Only by examining that piece of theatre—medicine's individual—can one gain understanding of error—or even of cure or care."[38] This final paragraph does not include the term *purpose*, because it is so much a part of Cassell's worldview that it need not be mentioned.

CONCLUSION: THE PERFECTION OF OUR ERRORS

The notion of attempting to create a master system to explain and correct (or accept) mistakes in medical practice is a mistake. As Burke continually pointed out, we come to anything with screens that, by providing a way of framing the world, must exclude some things from our vision. Each of the authors discussed in this essay have brought their own lens to bear upon medical mistakes; they all attempt to explain perfectly why some particular aspect of human action is imperfect—fallible agent, fallible act, fallible agency, or fallible purpose. In order to make such arguments, each of these authors must argue against some other aspect of human action as salient. Each must in some manner downplay the other terms of the pentad in order to create an enclosed system. One way to highlight how featuring one term tends to hide other concepts is to see what happens if another term is featured in the pentad.

What does Hilfiker ignore by emphasizing the *agent* in his analysis? His dismissal of scene, for instance, is quite telling. He begins his account of caring for the pregnant woman by mentioning that he was looking forward to this appointment because he has "so much exposure to disease every day in [his] rural practice."[39] Following this, Hilfiker refers to the negative urine test and notes that in order to get an ultrasound the patient would have to go to Duluth, which is "110 miles away from our northern Minnesota village, and it is expensive."[40] Another observer might have told this story emphasizing *scene*. Hilfiker was a physician just out of medical school who entered into a scene that placed him under unusual pressure. His mistakes could have been recounted by focusing on events that can occur in a rural environment, where more specialized care exists a great distance away and where patients do not have the economic means to make the long trip to receive unnecessary care. Hilfiker does not mention how scene influences a judgment he made about a woman who asked him to examine her mother, who was suffering from chest pains. Hilfiker was very busy seeing to the delivery of a baby and said that he would see the woman later. The woman collapsed and died. Once again, one could argue that the significant factor here is the rural scene, which like many offices "was not equipped with the advanced life-support equipment necessary to handle the situation."[41]

Cassell's emphasis on *purpose* tends to lack an interest in how *agency* affects medical practice. Cassell begins his analysis by telling the story of a 90-year-old man whose successful operation was followed by mismanaged postoperative care; he died in intensive care. The internist had found that the morphine was causing the patient problems and had written an order in the chart to stop giving morphine. The morphine was not immediately stopped, and, then after it was stopped, was restarted. Cassell's subsequent analysis of this case does not take into account how the issue of agency (such as Leape portrays it) profoundly affected the man's care. He does not take into account why a relatively simple issue (stopping the morphine) seemed to cause such difficulty. Cassell does not address these errors (there were several in the case) in his analysis, for they are mistakes that truly do not concern the issue of purpose. His conclusion has essentially screened out the term *agency* from consideration.

Burke concluded his definition of the human animal by declaring that we are "rotten with perfection."[42] In this he meant that we are a symbol-using animal and need to create perfect systems that encompass everything. This perfectionist tendency leads us to ignore those elements of the world that do not fit within our self-constructed systems. Burke's analytical tools were attempts to engage in what Joseph Gusfield has dubbed the "systematic thinking about the limitations of systems."[43] Pentadic analysis—one of Burke's tools—provides a necessary corrective for our tendencies to see issues through limited and thus limiting perspectives. It can be applied not only to reveal the featured elements in others' descriptions but also to expand our own vision of the world.

NOTES

1. A. Wu et al., "Do House Officers Learn from Their Mistakes?" *Journal of the American Medical Association* 265, no. 16 (24 April 1991): 2093.

2. K. Burke, *A Grammar of Motives* (Berkeley: University of California Press, 1962), xv.

3. K. Burke as quoted in J.R. Gusfield, "Introduction," in *On Symbols and Society,* ed. J.R. Gusfield (Chicago: University of Chicago Press, 1989), 16.

4. K. Burke, *The Philosophy of Literary Form,* 3rd ed. (Berkeley: University of California Press, 1973).

5. W. Rueckert, "Some of the Many Kenneth Burkes," in *Representing Kenneth Burke,* ed. H. White and M. Brose (Baltimore: Johns Hopkins University Press, 1982), 11.

6. Aristotle, *Nicomachean Ethics,* trans. T. Irwin (Indianapolis: Hackett, 1985), 57.

7. D. Hilfiker, "Facing Our Mistakes," *New England Journal of Medicine* 310, no. 2 (12 January 1984): 118-22.

8. Ibid., 119.

9. Ibid., 120.

10. Ibid.

11. Ibid.

12. Ibid.

13. Ibid., 121.

14. Ibid., 122.

15. D. Hilfiker, *Not All of Us Are Saints* (New York: Hill and Wang, 1994), 15.

16. See note 2 above, p. 171.

17. S. Gorovitz and A. MacIntyre, "Toward a Theory of Medical Fallibility," *Journal of Medicine and Philosophy* 1, no. 1 (1976): 51.

18. Ibid., 51-52.

19. Ibid., 52.

20. Ibid.

21. Ibid., 54.

22. Ibid., 57.

23. Ibid., 59.

24. Ibid., 62.

25. L.L. Leape, "Error in Medicine," *Journal of the American Medical Association* 272, no. 23 (21 December 1994): 1857.

26. Ibid., 1851.

27. Ibid., 1852.

28. E.J. Cassell, "Error in Medicine," in *Knowledge, Value, and Belief,* ed. H.T. Engelhardt Jr. and D. Callahan (Hastings-on-Hudson, N.Y.: Hastings Center, 1977), 295-309.

29. Ibid., 299.

30. Ibid.

31. Ibid., 301.

32. Ibid.

33. Ibid.

34. E.J. Cassell, "The Nature of Suffering and the Goals of Medicine," *New England Journal of Medicine* 306, no. 18 (1982): 639-45.

35. See note 2 above, 288.

36. Ibid.

37. See note 28 above, 308.

38. Ibid.

39. See note 7 above, 118.

40. Ibid.

41. Ibid., 120.

42. K. Burke, "Definition of Man," in *Language as Symbolic Action* (Berkeley: University of California Press, 1966), 3-24.

43. See note 3 above, p. 7.

2

To Err Is Human: American Culture, History, and Medical Error

Kenneth De Ville and Carl Elliott

INTRODUCTION

In *Witchcraft, Oracles and Magic Among the Azande*, Evans-Pritchard writes of a Azande villager who unintentionally destroyed his hut.[1] The villager was examining the beer he had stored there for the next day's mortuary feast and, because it was dark, he lit a handful of straw. When he raised the straw above his head, he ignited the thatch hut and burned it to the ground. An unfortunate mistake—we might think, and so does Evans-Pritchard—but the Azande disagree. The culprit, explains the hut's owner, is witchcraft.

Another of Evans-Pritchard's informants, a man named Kisanga, is an expert woodcarver—a maker of stools and bowls. Occasionally a bowl he is making splits, even though he has been very careful and selected only the hardest wood. Human error? "No," Kisanga explains, "it's witchcraft." His neighbors are spiteful and jealous. Could he be mistaken, questions Evans-Pritchard, who points out that the neighbors seem well disposed toward him. "No," Kisanga replies, holding the bowl out as evidence. "How do you account for this split bowl," he asks, "if I am not bewitched?"

Occasionally in Zandeland an old granary collapses. The wood decays over time, and termites decimate the granary support beams. People often sit under such granaries during the heat of the day and, if one collapses, the people sitting under it are sometimes injured. Chance? Perhaps, but it is more likely that a witch is to blame. For if witchcraft were not involved, the Azande want to know, why would people be sitting under the granary at the precise time when it collapses?

We should not be deceived into thinking that the Azande fail to see the causes of misfortune, Evans-Pritchard points out. The Azande can see as well as

Evans-Pritchard can that people holding torches burn down huts, that brittle wood may split, that sometimes termites eat through the beams of a granary and cause it to collapse. What the Azande want to know is why did the event occur now, in this situation, and not in others? Hundreds of Azande inspect their beer in thatched huts every year and light up torches to do it. Why is it that this particular man ignited his hut on this particular occasion? Kisanga has made many bowls successfully. He is an expert woodcarver. Why did one particular bowl split, and not others? Witchcraft supplies the missing link between the universal and the particular, between the explanation of why thatched huts burn and why a particular one burned. When Evans-Pritchard remarks to his Azande companions that he is feeling sick and speculates that it must have been the bananas he has eaten, he is told, "No, people eat bananas all the time. Bananas don't make you sick no matter how many you have eaten unless, that is, you are bewitched."

In pointing to witchcraft as the cause of misfortune, the Azande are simply selecting the cause they believe to be *socially* relevant and ignoring the other causes. If an elephant kills a man and witchcraft is involved, the Azande say the elephant is the first spear, witchcraft the second. But the elephant one can do nothing about and witchcraft one can, because witchcraft involves a human being who can be brought to justice. The Azande speak of witchcraft as the cause of death, says Evans-Pritchard, "because it is the ideological pivot around which swings the lengthy social procedure from death to vengeance."[2]

As for the Azande, so also for Americans. How one explains particular instances of misfortune will inevitably be tied to one's judgment of the socially relevant facts, which are in turn dependent on one's understanding of the way the universe works. To explain an unfortunate event as carelessness, as mechanistically determined, as witchcraft, or as the will of God is to say something about the way one sees the world. It reveals notions about blame and responsibility, about what might have happened but did not, about the gap between what was expected and what was done. When an individual conceptualizes an unfortunate event as an error, he or she also, inescapably, makes an important statement about his or her cosmology.

Many Americans believe that we are currently experiencing a plague of medical errors. A recent article in the *New York Times* compared the rate of error in American hospitals to three jumbo jets crashing every two days. "If the airlines killed that many people annually," the writer argues, "public outrage would close them overnight."[3] The perception that medical error is a widespread cause of patient injury seems to be confirmed in the academic literature.[4] In 1991, for example, investigators in the Harvard Medical Practice Study reported that 4 percent of hospital patients suffered iatrogenic injuries,[5] 69 percent of which were due to medical error.[6] According to Lucian Leape, error studies report high rates of missed diagnoses, mistaken treatments, medication errors, and a wide range of other mistakes in patient management.[7]

The common-sense explanation for all this apparent mayhem is that healthcare workers are being careless or reckless or, for those who are more charitable, that mistakes are an inevitable product of inherent human fallibility. Either way, the implication is that the current plague is a consequence of something that humans *do*—they are behaving carelessly, they are designing faulty systems, they are being pressured to work too hard, and so forth. All true enough, perhaps, but it is not the whole story. For Americans, as for the Azande, particular unfortunate events require explanation. But unlike the Azande, Americans typically look to ordinary human beings for explanations, and not to witches.

This essay connects the way that Americans explain medical misfortune to two changes that have occurred in American culture over the past several centuries. First, the weakening of providential views of the world has led Americans to explain misfortune as the result of actions or inactions on the part of human agents, rather than as the work of God. In Anglo-American culture, the gradual secularization of society and the transformation of society's view of God's role on earth has gradually led people to search for human agents of misfortune. When God no longer ordains specific social and physical ills, and temporal solutions for misfortune are apparently available, it becomes acceptable to search for human culprits and assign responsibility. Second, while medicine has developed more sophisticated technological approaches to illness and injury, these new approaches have generated higher expectations about what is possible— expectations that sometimes cannot be met. In addition, because these new approaches often require a greater degree of skill, care, and learning than the procedures they replace, they carry with them a greater susceptibility to human fallibility, carelessness, and ignorance.

The distinction between culpable and nonculpable error is important morally, professionally, and legally. An individual may act mistakenly—he or she may be wrong—and that error may not be blameworthy. But this essay does not attempt to differentiate between these two types of error. Instead, it explores the factors that induce individuals to view undesirable outcomes as error.

A PUNISHMENT ORDAINED BY SIN?

As late as the 17th and 18th centuries, many American Protestants subscribed to the doctrine of direct, or specific, divine providence. Providence theory reflected the prevalent 17th-century belief that nothing in heaven or earth occurred merely by chance. God sustained the earth from moment to moment. God might punish sinners on earth and reward saints, or he might will misfortune on the holy to test or teach them.[8] Many American Protestants followed the Calvinist Westminister Confession, which proclaimed: "God the great creator of all things, doth uphold, direct, and dispose, and govern all creatures, actions and things from the greatest even to the least by his most wise and holy Providence."[9]

As historian Keith Thomas has suggested, supernatural explanations in the 16th and 17th centuries may also have helped believers accept unfathomable physical misfortunes.[10] Providential intervention might include lightning, bad crops, earthquakes, epidemics, a sick horse, or the death of a child.[11] John Winthrop, who helped found and govern 17th-century Massachusetts, noted in his journals dozens of examples of colonists who were punished or rewarded by "a special providence of God." The "righteous hand of God" spared or smote individuals with fire, drowning, Indian attacks, accidental injury, smallpox, and birth defects.[12]

This view of providence affected the way individuals reacted to physical misfortune when it occurred. A believer who assumed that the wise hand of God lay behind his or her misfortune would be unlikely to look for other origins or to blame others. Humans could not possibly expect to understand God's plan, and faith demanded that they believe that the Lord ultimately worked only to good ends. Although Americans in the 18th century began to shift their views of the direct impact of the hand of God on human affairs, providential sentiments remained strong through the early 19th century.[13] For example, during a 1793 yellow fever epidemic in Philadelphia, one inhabitant reported: "most, if not all were convinced it was a judgment sent by the immediate hand of God."[14] Cholera swept through many large U.S. cities in the early 1830s, most ministers and laypersons viewed the epidemic as "a rod in the hand of God"— even though most physicians had begun to look for scientific causes.[15] In an 1823 article entitled "The Doctrine of Providence Vindicated," a writer declared that providence "extends to all beings that have existed, or ever will exist; to all events that have occurred or ever will occur. . . . the humble Christian will discern in them all the hand of a wise and holy God."[16] Another writer in the same magazine proclaimed that "without [God's] permission, no power can harm, no ill can befall us, and every afflicting stroke is meant for our good."[17]

An 1824 incident illustrates the persistent belief in the relationship between providence and physical misfortune and the notion of medical error. Dr. Gerald Bancker was hired by New York City to provide smallpox vaccinations for residents of an assigned urban district. Eight days after Bancker had vaccinated the four-year-old son of Michael O'Neil, the boy became dreadfully ill with what appeared to be smallpox. Over the next four months the child went blind, he lost his hair and teeth, his lower jaw disintegrated, and he developed an ulcerous hole through his neck and into his throat. Finally, he died. O'Neil sued Bancker for medical malpractice. Medical witnesses claimed that the physician had mistakenly drawn material from a smallpox sore rather than a cowpox sore, thus inoculating instead of vaccinating the boy and subjecting him to the risk of the disease.[18] In fact, the doctor may have made an even more substantial error. Blindness, jaw necrosis, and tooth and hair loss are classic symptoms of poisoning by mercury-based calomel—an ubiquitous remedy of the period. Thus, human error in this case probably included not only the unintentional infection with smallpox, but also the excessive and possibly fatal use of calomel.[19]

Although the father of the dead child clearly considered his son's death a consequence of an act of a human being rather than of God, the notion of providence still carried much social influence. In his argument to the jury, the physician's lawyer argued that the child's disease was nothing short of miraculous. No other child had been so affected, and there was no instance in all of medical history of such horrendous symptoms following any inoculation. Providence, the defense attorney claimed, was responsible for the tragedy. "In a word," the attorney explained, "we expect to prove the child died of smallpox, proceeding from the visitation of God, and not from any negligence or any want of skill on the part of the defendant."[20] The jury retired after the testimony and found in favor of the physician.

The defense attorney's use of a divine explanation for the disease, and its apparent success, suggests that at least some of American society still accepted the notion of a specific or direct providence as late as the 1820s. But change was already well under way. Social and theological debates of the 1820s and 1830s centered on the apparent contradiction between human free will and God's providential control. Some writers attacked the notion of direct providence, claiming that it undermined the responsibility of the individual. Others noted that providential ideas necessarily left the status quo untouched and encouraged the passive acceptance of remediable ills. Theologians who saw God's direct intervention in every sparrow's fall lost ground during the first half of the 19th century. Instead, a growing proportion of society began to believe that God worked in the world through universal, natural laws and influenced world events only on a grand, historical scale, creating an environment for the unfolding of his will.[21]

This trend varied from person to person, denomination to denomination, and region to region; but as the 19th century progressed fewer Americans viewed social and physical ills as purely God's will. Once again, attitudes toward epidemic diseases serve as an important gauge. Where Americans once saw yellow fever and cholera as moral retribution, they now began to explain such diseases in scientific terms. By the time of the cholera epidemics of the 1860s, the majority of Americans had abandoned the idea of direct divine intervention and embraced scientific explanations and solutions. The work of John Snow in the 1850s had demonstrated that cholera was transmitted through contaminated water. Physicians and government officials used statistical surveys to demonstrate that clean streets, ventilated houses, and pure water were more effective than prayers and fasting in preventing the epidemics.[22]

Secular interpretations of specific misfortunes, such as cholera, frequently started with scientists and physicians and then were embraced by broader segments of society. American intellectuals and theologians were also influenced by European philosophers such as John Stuart Mill and Auguste Comte. As historian Charles Cashdollar has explained, these writers' conception of God "forced man away from a pietistic or providential to a naturalistic view of social problems, from prayer to human action."[23] Thus, what had before been viewed as divinely ordained burdens or punishments for sin, came to be seen as potentially remediable ills. Samuel Gross, one of the most important and revered surgeons in 19th century America, declared in his 1887 autobiography that "God cannot be said ever to have killed or willfully afflicted any human being."[24] On the contrary, individuals suffer and "die by and through natural laws, none by and through God's interposition or direct agency; and the same is true whether life is destroyed by disease or by accident."[25]

Religious attitudes have continued to change through the 20th century, of course. Even more Americans have replaced their acceptance of providence with a faith in progress[26] and their acceptance of divine will with a search for earthly causation. Thus, physical misfortune can now often be comfortably described as medical error.

TECHNOLOGICAL ADVANCEMENT
AND THE PROLIFERATION OF ERROR

While the move from divine to human explanation for misfortune helped bring about the widespread recognition of medical error, other forces have come into play as well. In several important ways, technological innovation and scientific advancement have created a larger space for medical error.

As Mark Grady has explained, medical innovation and technological advancement capture what was previously "natural risk" and transform it into "medical risk." Before the development of a given medical technique, people tend to accept physical misfortune as part of the known and expected sequelae of an injury.[27] But once people see the new medical technique as effective, they can also see its failure or its denial as a harm. The availability of the technique means that the patient may be denied a potential benefit, and the patient may see the absence of the expected benefit as an error.

Again, an historical example is illustrative. In 1800, the conventional treatment for compound fractures was amputation, a procedure that frequently resulted in death. Despite this horrendous result, amputations generated few claims of incompetence or malpractice. Individuals who had severely fractured limbs could expect death and/or amputation. Stated another way, amputation or death was the "natural risk" of serious orthopedic injury. During the first half of the 19th century, however, the medical profession developed a dazzling array of techniques that allowed physicians to save rather than amputate limbs. Amputations rapidly became less acceptable, and by 1850, preserving limbs in severe orthopedic injuries had become the norm. This revolution in orthopedic care understandably fostered excitement and inflated expectations in both the profession and the lay public. Medical treatises frequently referred to treatment of fractures as a relatively mechanical procedure in which patients could expect nearly perfect cures. Those hopes and claims, of course, were unfounded. Although physicians could more frequently save rather than amputate badly injured limbs, fractures and dislocations usually yielded permanent injuries—shortened or deformed limbs, frozen joints, and complications associated with long recovery periods. Yet physicians and the lay public frequently viewed these side effects of successful fracture treatment as "medical error" rather than as a less severe, "natural" consequence or risk of suffering a compound fracture. Consequently, severe fractures were the single most important source of medical malpractice litigation from the mid-19th century through the first third of the 20th century.[28]

Medical advancement influenced the perception of medical error in other important respects. New medical procedures often require greater skill, learning, and attention than the procedures they replace, and so they may carry greater opportunity for accidents, ignorance, or lapses of attention.[29] For example, the new orthopedic procedures of the mid-19th century were very complex and required more technical proficiency and knowledge than did amputations. Thus, surgeons who eschewed amputation and saved limbs were more likely to make mistakes. Rapidly advancing medical treatments can also create a form of error associated with technology lag, in which physicians favor one technique over another because they have not kept current on evolving practices.

Human error is recognized as a cause of misfortune when medical science appears to promise results. When those results are not achieved, it is easier to point to lapses in skill, care, and knowledge—which are often required in progressively higher quantities as medical science advances. Only if the physical misfortune is seen as medical risk rather than natural risk is it attributed to human agency. Primitive medical procedures promised little and they required relatively low levels of physician vigilance, knowledge, and skill.[30] Moreover, they were often iatrogenically benign. So if human "errors" occurred, they often went unrecognized. In contrast, when a medical advancement commands the attention of the medical profession and the public, expectations increase and so do the opportunities for oversights and lapses of attention.

Medical error is not typically associated with a particular illness, injury, or procedure until medical breakthroughs encourage the public and the profession to believe that there is an available medical remedy that generates predictable results and significant benefit. There were relatively few such medical procedures for much of medical history. Since the 19th century, however, medical practice has seemed to offer patients much more. As medical practice boasted advancements in a broad number of areas, lay and professional expectations increased. Technical and intellectual demands on practitioners multiplied, and success or failure appeared to rest on human performance and knowledge rather than on the vagaries of a poorly understood medical problem or God's will.[31]

Consider the field of general surgery. Before the 1880s, when a patient died of peritonitis or an intestinal blockage, the death was usually not viewed as a medical error.[32] Instead, it was viewed as the result of a poorly understood medical condition or as an illness for which no effective treatment had been developed. Neither conceptualization can generate claims of error. These views persisted even after the prevalence of surgical procedures increased, albeit with very mixed success, in the early 20th century.[33] It was not until the early 1930s—and the advent of sulfa drugs, transfusions, and surgical residency programs; the refinement of aseptic practices; and the development of more sophisticated surgical instruments—that surgeons were able to boast more noteworthy, numerous, and regular successes.[34] It was only then that "surgical intervention could be represented as the inevitable scientific solution to disease."[35] And it was only then that people started to apply claims of error and charges of malpractice to surgical shortcomings and surgically related maladies in large numbers. Surgery became the most common source of medical malpractice accusations in the early 1940s and, according to one study, represented 57 percent of the total malpractice claims between 1950 and 1971.[36]

Not only did the revolution in surgical procedures engender immoderate expectations, but surgeons of the post-1930s medical world had to monitor and manage shock, bleeding, and vital signs while performing complex and new procedures—demands unheard of in previous medical care. Researchers have found that complex medical-technological environments increase the likelihood of mistakes due to deficits in knowledge, skill, and attention.[37] The perceived cost of skill deficits and momentary lapses of concentration are greater in high-tech procedures such as surgery because the promise is greater, but also because the procedure is, itself, more dangerous.[38]

A similar tension exists in many other modern medical practices. For example, mechanical ventilation of neonates helps physicians save infants who otherwise would not have survived; however, positive pressure ventilation itself may lead to pneumothorax injuries and other complications. The perception of error in the administration of pharmaceutical remedies has also increased dramatically in recent decades, a period during which drug treatments have become more useful, more common, more sophisticated, and more complex. Consider, too, the development of obstetric care in the second half of the 20th century. Maternal and fetal risk remained high at mid-century, but by the 1970s new drugs, medical regimens, and technologies provided obstetricians "with an armament which is unsurpassed in the history of medical practice."[39] Yet at the same time, expectations have increased, contributing to the perception of error when the birth results in an injured or dead child. In surgery, drug therapy, obstetrics, and a wide range of other areas of medical practice, the knowledge, skill, and care that is required to perform responsibly in a late-20th-century medical environment has far outstripped that which would have been required of physicians at the end of the 1800s.[40]

It is true, of course, that some medical advancements are specifically designed to increase the safety of patients, and that they ostensibly prevent rather than increase medical errors. A great number of diagnostic technologies fall into this class of innovations. So do precautions such as warning buzzers, gauges, and padded bars on operating tables, and procedural precautions such as sponge counts and sterilization protocols.[41] Yet these innovations themselves play a dual role. Although they are designed to prevent error, they also represent a new source of potential error. It is, after all, a species of error to fail to complete a sponge count, to neglect to lock a guard rail into place, or to forget to ground a piece of electrical equipment in the operating theater.

In fact, diagnostic technologies are especially likely to serve as a double-edged sword when it comes to medical error. Diagnostic-imaging technologies are capable of preventing errors, of course: an x-ray might help physicians avoid misdiagnosing a fracture. But imaging technologies may also carry risks of their own, such as the risks associated with the use of contrast media. They have also increased expectations of lay persons and professionals and created the context for an entire new range of medical error—that of misinterpretation and the failure to diagnose an injury or illness.[42]

Diagnostic technologies also help increase the perception and discovery of error by providing a record of previously unseen and unrecorded information.

Such records provide evidence that error has occurred. This is clearly the case with x-rays, but it has also been true with more recent innovations such as electronic fetal monitors. Physicians have quite reasonably viewed electronic fetal monitoring as an improvement in care, a means to allow intervention when the fetus is in distress. Yet while this diagnostic technology is beneficial in many cases, it may simultaneously increase the risk of perceived error following the birth of an injured infant by providing a retrospective record of the fetal heart rate.[43] Similar observations might be drawn from the use and implications of many of the vast array of diagnostic technologies that have entered conventional medical practice in the latter half of the 20th century. These technologies may decrease medical error of some types and contribute to patients' well-being, while at the same time creating the perception of new classes and varieties of error.

CONCLUSION

The apparent rise in medical error in the United States must be seen not merely as a product of human action or inaction, but as a product of our culture and history. The interpretation of misfortune as error is as much dependent on a cosmology as it is on the actions and decisions of healthcare institutions and physicians. It is also contingent on particular social circumstances, such as the ease with which a particular physical misfortune can be explained in scientific terms or the particular type of technologies that have been developed as remedies. The opportunity for medical error may be intensified by the iatrogenic dangers of the particular therapeutic or diagnostic procedure in question, and by the skill, care, and knowledge the procedure requires of the physician.

Although misfortune may be explained in differing ways that are culturally and historically contingent, it would be a mistake to think that one way of interpreting misfortune excludes all others. As Evans-Pritchard explains, "Azande belief in witchcraft in no way contradicts empirical knowledge of cause and effect."[44] Just as the Azande may see a death as caused both by an elephant and by witchcraft, an American may view a hospital death both as the will of God and as an error by a doctor. He or she may see it as scientifically explainable, yet also as a matter of carelessness. One explanation does not always rule out other explanations, and explanations are not always tidy and consistent. Medical error, like disease itself, continues to be an amalgam of physiological explanation and social definition.[45] The relationship between scientific progress and a particular view of the cosmos is complex, and it is not simply the acceptance of available scientific explanations and remedies over and above religion, fate, or magic. Although the notion of divine providence has been altered and profoundly diluted in American culture, it continues to play some role in this and other societies. As a result, the way in which medical misfortune is interpreted varies—not only from one culture to another, but from one individual to another and from one physical ailment to another. One need only consider the degree to which many Americans viewed the appearance of the human immunodeficiency virus (HIV) as a punishment from God to recognize the role that a particular cosmology can still play in conceptualizing the causal origins of physical maladies.[46]

If we take seriously the idea that the interpretation of misfortune as error is contingent on broad cultural and historical developments, it would be misguided to think that current rates of medical error can be adequately addressed without paying heed to the role of those developments. It may well be that the perception of error is too closely linked to our American views of medical innovation to be very easily dislodged. Given our faith in progress, our high expectations of medical innovation, and the fact that most of us look to human agency as an explanation for misfortune, the perception that we are experiencing high rates of medical error may be, if not unavoidable, at least unremarkable. But, the model set out here may help explain why medical error has seemingly increased in the United States in the 20th century at the same time that medical professionals have almost certainly become better educated, more skillful, and more careful than their historical counterparts.

NOTES

1. E.E. Evans-Pritchard, *Witchcraft, Oracles and Magic Among the Azande* (Oxford, England: Oxford University Press, 1937), 63-83; see also C. Geertz, "Common Sense as a Cultural System," in *Local Knowledge: Further Essays in Interpretative Anthropology* (New York: Basic Books, 1983), 73-93.

2. Evans-Pritchard, *Witchcraft*, see note 1 above, p. 73.

3. M.M. Weinstein, "Checking Medicine's Vital Signs," *New York Times Magazine*, 19 April 1998.

4. L.L. Leape, "The Preventability of Medical Injury," in *Human Error in Medicine*, ed. M.S. Bogner (Hillsdale, N.J.: Lawrence Erlbaum, 1994), 13-52, p. 13; and E.M. Schimmel, "The Hazards of Hospitalization," *Annals of Internal Medicine* 60 (1964): 100-10.

5. L.L. Leape et al., "The Nature of Adverse Events in Hospitalized Patients: Results of the Harvard Medical Practice Study II," *New England Journal of Medicine* 324 (1991): 377-84.

6. L.L. Leape et al., "Preventing Medical Injury," *Quality Review Bulletin* 81 (1993): 144-9.

7. L.L. Leape, "Error in Medicine," *Journal of the American Medical Association* 272, no. 23 (1994): 1851-7. [Leape's article is reprinted as chapter 7 of this book—ED.]

8. P. Miller, *The New England Mind: The Seventeenth Century* (Cambridge, Mass: Harvard University Press, 1939), 14-7.

9. H.F. May, "The Decline of Providence?" in *Ideas, Faiths and Feelings: Essays on American Intellectual and Religious History*, ed. H.F. May (New York: Oxford University Press, 1983), 136.

10. K. Thomas, *Religion and the Decline of Magic: Studies in Popular Beliefs in the Sixteenth and Seventeenth Centuries in England* (London: Weidenfeld, 1971), 5-7, 651-63.

11. P. Miller, *The New England Mind: From Colony to Province* (Cambridge, Mass.: Harvard University Press, 1953), 345-66; E.M. Tilton, "Lighting Rods and the Earthquake of 1775," *New England Quarterly* 13 (March 1940): 85-97; and C.E. Clark, "Science, Reason, and an Angry God: The Literature of an Earthquake," *New England Quarterly* 38 (1965): 340-62.

12. J. Winthrop, *Winthrop's Journal: History of New England, 1630-1649*, ed. J.K. Hosmer (N.Y.: Charles Schribner's Sons, 1908), 1: 4-9, 226, 270, 291; 2: 138, 141, 153-4, 209-10, 220, 354-5.

13. L.O. Saum, "Providence in the Popular Mind of Pre-Civil War America," *Indiana Magazine of History* 72 (1976): 341-2.

14. Quoted in W. Gribbein, "Divine Providence or Miasma? The Yellow Fever Epidemic of 1822," *New York History* 53 (1972): 287-9.

15. C. Rosenberg, *The Cholera Years: The United States in 1832, 1849, and 1866* (Chicago: University of Chicago Press, 1962), 43.

16. "The Doctrine of Providence Vindicated," *Christian Spectator* 5 (1823): 173-4.

17. "The Doctrine of a Particular Providence, *Christian Spectator* 8 (1836): 2.

18. *"Michael O'Neil v. Gerard Bancker,"* *New York Medical and Physical Journal* 6 (1827): 145-52.

19. Ibid.

20. Ibid., 150.

21. C.D. Cashdollar, "Social Implications of the Doctrine of Divine Providence: A Nineteenth Century Debate in American Theology," *Harvard Theological Review* 71 (1978): 265-84; K.A. De Ville, *Medical Malpractice in Nineteenth Century America: Origins and Legacy* (New York: New York University Press, 1990), 119-37.

22. See note 15 above, pp. 193-6.

23. C.D. Cashdollar, "European Positivism and American Unitarianism," *Church History* 45 (1976): 490-92.

24. S.D. Gross, *Autobiography of Samuel D. Gross* (Philadelphia: George Barrie, 1887; reprint, Manchester, N.H.: Ayer, 1972), 2:44, 202-3.

25. Ibid.

26. M. Marty, "From Providence to Progress: A New Theology," in *The Righteous Empire: The Protestant Experience in America* (New York: Dial, 1970), 188-9.

27. M.F. Grady, "Why Are People Negligent? Technology, Nondurable Precautions, and the Medical Malpractice Explosion," *Northwestern Law Review* 82 (1988): 293-334.

28. De Ville, see note 21 above, pp. 92-113.

29. See note 27 above; J. Rasmussen, "Afterword," in *Human Error in Medicine,* ed. M.S. Bogner (Hillsdale, N.J.: Lawrence Erlbaum, 1994), 385-93.

30. See note 27 above.

31. K.A. De Ville, "Medical Malpractice in Twentieth Century United States," *International Journal of Technology Assessment in Health Care* 14, no. 2 (1998): 197-211.

32. W.G. Rothstein, *American Physicians in the Nineteenth Century: From Sects to Science* (Baltimore: Johns Hopkins University Press, 1972).

33. G.H. Brieger, "From Conservative to Radical Surgery in Late Nineteenth Century America," in *Medical Theory, Surgical Practice: Studies in the History of Surgery,* ed. C. Lawrence (New York: Routledge, 1972), 216-31.

34. P.C. English, *Shock, Physiological Surgery, and George Washington Crile: Medical Innovation in the Progressive Era* (Westport, Conn.: Greenwood Publishing Group, 1980), 57-68; see note 31 above, pp. 201-3.

35. J.D. Howell, *Technology in the Hospital: Transforming Patient Care in the Early Twentieth Century* (Baltimore: Johns Hopkins University Press, 1995), 57.

36. A.A. Sandor, "The History of Professional Liability Suits in the United States," *Journal of the American Medical Association* 163 (1957): 459-66; U.S. Department of Health, Education, and Welfare, *Report of the Secretary's Commission on Medical Malpractice* (Washington, D.C.: U.S. Government Printing Office, 1973).

37. E.C. Lambert, *Modern Medical Mistakes* (Bloomington, Ind.: University of Indiana Press, 1978); see note 7 above.

38. See note 27 above.

39. M.D. Volk and M.D. Morgan, *Medical Malpractice: Handling Obstetric and Neonatal Cases* (New York: McGraw-Hill, 1986), vi.

40. De Ville, "Medical Malpractice," see note 20 above, pp. 205-6.

41. See note 27 above.

42. S.R. Reuter, "The Use of Conventional vs Low-Osmolar Contrast Agents: A Legal Analysis," *American Journal of Radiology* 151 (1988): 529-31; H. Van Cott, "Human Errors: Their Causes and Reduction," in *Human Error in Medicine,* ed. M.S. Bogner (Hillsdale, N.J.: Lawrence Erlbaum, 1994), 53-81 at 58; De Ville, see note 21 above, pp. 203-4.

43. M.G. Gilfix, "Electronic Fetal Monitoring: Physician Liability and Informed Consent," *American Journal of Law & Medicine* 10 (1985): 31-90; B.S. Schifrin, H. Weissman, and J. Wiley, "Electronic Fetal Monitoring and Obstetrical Malpractice," *Law, Medicine & Health Care* 13 (1985): 100-05; and C. Walter and E.P. Richards, "Engineering and the Law: How Effective Safety Devices Lead to Secondary Litigation" *IEEE Engineering in Medicine and Biology* 10 (June 1991): 66-7.

44. Evans-Pritchard, see note 1 above, p. 72.

45. See note 15 above, p. 5.

46. L.M. Kopelman, "The Punishment Concept of Disease," in *AIDS: Ethics and Public Policy,* ed. C. Pierce and D. VanDeveer (Belmont, Calif.: Wadsworth, 1988), 49-55.

3

The Life-Long Error, or John Marcher the Proleptic

Rita Charon

THE INTERPRETIVE ERROR

The conceptually interesting error in medical or bioethical practice is not the instrumental error (the intern called for 100 milliequivalents of potassium chloride instead of 10), the structural error (the confused patient who was allergic to penicillin was given penicillin because the medical records department could not locate her chart and the computer does not list allergies), or the error of slovenliness (the resident did not check the head computed tomography before doing the lumbar puncture), but rather the interpretive "error"—so distant conceptually from the other kinds that one must at first use quotation marks in writing about it. More failure than mistake, interpretive error results from a falling short of understanding, a paltriness in the face of conceptual challenge, an impoverishment of language and thought. Using a broad definition of *interpretation* helps to set the ground for a productive discussion of interpretive error, and literary scholar E.D. Hirsch's definition seems as helpful as it seems oceanic: "Interpretation is the central activity of cognition. . . . We always perceive (construct) something other than the language through which we know that thing. This constructive process is interpretation."[1] Not only the most interesting but also the most consequential kind of error, it occurs at profound levels in interpreter and situation, requires skill to commit, and—by virtue of its being irrevocably entwined with its singular setting—can only be committed once. What most distinguishes interpretive error from its less interesting cousins is the fact that it lives a long life.

Medical interpretive error results from misconception or misunderstanding, processes that start well before the hospital admission or the office visit of the patient. All humans undergo the process, however haphazard, of becoming interpreters of their world, and they rely on their interpretive apparatus to find their way to the grocery store, to vote, or to watch the New York Mets as well as to choose a profession, a religion, or someone to love. Deeply imbedded in the psychological and textual identity, the interpretive apparatus grows from a lifetime of assigning meaning to events and particular texts of all sorts, and reflexively is altered by the texts and events chosen for interpretation. Since the practices of deconstruction have widened the definition of text to include not only poetry and fiction but also graffiti and reality, skills of textual interpretation are relied upon and influenced whenever anyone tries to find the meaning of anything. According to Harold Bloom, "The strong reader . . . wishes to find his own original relation to truth, whether in texts or in reality (which he treats as texts anyway), but also wishes to open received texts to his own sufferings."[2] Making one's way in one's family, engaging in religious activities, reading books, following world events, and laughing at jokes contribute to and follow from an individual's singular path toward understanding what texts mean, the mingled predetermination and revisability of interpretation endowing it with both the prophesy of *a priori* and the memory of *a posteriori*.[3]

Once an interpreter assigns a meaning to a text or event, he or she will recognize its significance. According to Goldman, "The illumination of a meaningful structure constitutes a process of comprehending it [meaning]; while insertion of it into a vaster structure is to explain it [significance]."[4] Little Red Riding Hood pays a visit to her grandmother but is deceived by and set upon by the Big Bad Wolf dressed in grandma's clothing. Whether one reads Little Red Riding Hood as victim, dupe, or hero depends on one's history of childhood trauma, experience of betrayal, and fondness for forest smells. Abraham is prepared to sacrifice his only son upon the word of God. Whether one takes Abraham's and Isaac's brink to signify the courage that risks everything or the weakness that caves in to authority depends on one's relation to one's faith and the sense of protection afforded by one's own father. If "meaning is a principle of stability in an interpretation" and "significance embraces a principle of change," then a full-bodied interpretation engages the reader on a dialectic search toward a message at once universal and only one's own.[5] Individual interpretations of life and of text accrete to lend characteristic frames to a person's vision of the world, a vision that might be colored by guilt or fate, blurred by mastery or surrender, narrowed by suspicion or irony, or suffused with generosity or vengeance.

All interpreters become members of interpretive communities—the family dinner table, a seventh-grade English class, a church congregation, the Democratic Party. Within these communities, idiosyncratic readings can be informed by received and contesting readings, thereby rounding in outliers and challenging traditional interpretations. "Interpretive communities," according to Stanley Fish, "are made up of those who share interpretive strategies not for reading (in the conventional sense) but for writing texts, for constituting their properties and assigning their intentions. . . . These strategies exist prior to the act of reading and therefore determine the shape of what is read rather than, as is usually assumed, the other way around."[6] Because reading is always both a lone and a social practice, readers find their way toward the meanings of stories by testing their own interpretations against those of others, perceiving that no reading is ever the privileged one, experiencing both the terror of not understanding and the joy of the occasional transparency of text.[7]

Both medicine and clinical ethics, except for their most routinized practices, call forth and rely on wide-ranging and consequential interpretive acts on the part of their practitioners. (Sadly, it may be the case that students enter medicine and medical ethics because these fields seem, from the outside, devoid of the need for interpretation. That is to say, they seem to supply the answers and not just the questions. Consequently, these two fields may attract exactly the wrong trainees.) Understanding errors in medicine and bioethics, then, requires an examination of the underlying interpretive apparatus of the doctor who errs or the ethicist who errs. Short of psychoanalysis, one can begin to systematize attention to these professionals' impulses to find meaning by framing their clinical interpretive activities within the universe of readings. By placing clinical interpretive acts beside more conventionally recognized acts of reading, individual practitioners may come to understand that their professional decisions are inflected with all that inflects any act of reading. A fundamental rationale for the subdiscipline of literature and medicine, such framing of clinical acts as reading acts draws attention to the processes through which individual readers achieve meaning and significance in texts, granting not only exposure of their interpretive apparatus but—and here is the powerful dividend—a means to make them better readers, that is to say, readers who have the ability to examine their interpretations closely enough to gain the power to alter them.

Henry James's short story "The Beast in the Jungle" is a story about a life-long error.[8] As is true of any great story, it circles around what it is "about" by engaging the reader in considering its plot, its form, and its consequences. That is to say, "The Beast in the Jungle" transmits its message through the events narrated, the formal choices James made in deciding how to build the story—its narrative frame, its governing images, its temporal scaffold, its diction—and the experience undergone by its reader. A close reading of this short story provides a textual laboratory in which to examine the anatomy of a life-long error, the depth within the erring self from which such an error emerges, the waves of influence that may spread from it, and the local factors that may postpone its recognition. Such an exercise will also grant the reader the opportunity to brood on his or her own singular "reader-response" to a serious error—perhaps recognizing individually characteristic affective clues to the presence of error and characterologically inflected methods of judging the one who errs. Simultaneously and probably of the most moment, a close reading of this masterpiece demonstrates James's singular textual responses to the error of his protagonist, moves of thought and language that constitute a revolt against error, and a method to reverse it.

THE GIVEN STORY

John Marcher grows up with "the sense of being kept for something rare and strange, possibly prodigious and terrible, that was sooner or later to happen" (71). He tells May Bartram his secret that "[s]omething or other lay in wait for him, amid the twists and the turns of the months and the years, like a crouching beast in the jungle," and together they await "the inevitable spring of the creature" (79). Precluding marriage and conventional life, the secret of the beast organizes Marcher's life into a caricature of passive waiting. Bartram sees through Marcher's self-delusion early on but, for reasons over which critics clash, she opts to organize her life, too, around the futile wait for the imaginary beast.

Over time, Bartram seems to realize that the beast is but Marcher's excuse never to engage fully with life or with love. Marcher does not get her oblique hints about the self-delusive and protective nature of his belief in his beast, and he becomes inflamed with the impression that she seems to know something about his beast that he does not know. When Bartram becomes seriously ill, Marcher wonders whether the beast will end up to be his loss of her but drops the idea as "an abject anti-climax . . . a drop of dignity under the shadow of which his existence could only become the most grotesque of failures" (96). Bartram tries, during her slow death, to show Marcher his error and to offer herself for him to love, "The door isn't shut, the door's open. . . . It's never too late" (105). Finally, as she dies, she tells Marcher that the beast has already come, that "It's past. It's behind" (112). When Marcher objects that it cannot have passed if he has never felt it, Bartram tells him with the greatest clarity she can find, "You were to suffer your fate. That was not necessarily to know it" (113).

After Bartram's death, the beast abandons Marcher, leaving him bereft of a future. Tormented by the absence of "anything still to come," Marcher never fills the lack opened up by the dual loss of Bartram and of the beast (p. 117). Finally, at his friend's grave two years after her death, Marcher is stirred by the "deep ravage of the features" of a grieving man visiting a fresh grave in the cemetery (123). Looking at "the raw glare of his grief . . . with envy," Marcher wonders, "What had the man *had*, to make him by the loss of it so bleed and yet live?" (124). Marcher realizes—with great pain in a sudden epiphanic rush—the "sounded void of his life . . . Everything fell together, confessed, explained, overwhelmed; leaving him most of all stupefied at the blindness he had cherished. The fate he had been marked for he had met with a vengeance—he had emptied the cup to the lees; he had been the man of his time, *the* man, to whom nothing on earth was to have happened. . . . All the while he had waited the wait was itself his portion" (125). With the visitation of this certainty, the beast again appears to Marcher, and the story closes as Marcher throws himself onto Bartram's grave in an attempt to avoid the creature's lunge.

Wordlessly adding to the story's point, the climate of the story is described by various critics as a "vague airless unfurnished unpeopled medium,"[9] "a sealed-off formalized world,"[10] and "a bare space withdrawn from the social world."[11] Strictly an element of plot (although inflected by style, diction, and all the enunciating elements to be considered below), the atmosphere *carries* the sequence of events within a signifying capsule, clothing the bare plot elements with implication and innuendo. The reader responds to plot, character, and atmosphere while experiencing and interpreting this or any story. James's mastery is shown, in part, by his unerring ability to "place" his reader within the mysterious, intangible, permeating air of his situation.

A history of a life-long interpretive error, "The Beast in the Jungle" offers to the reader for inspection many stages of erring and many of erring's consequences. The reader does not witness the actual act of the committing of the mistake, as Marcher is presented as always having believed that he was being kept for something rare and prodigious. In fact, interpretive errors seldom have birthdates: they are not so much acts committed as they are accommodations, habituations, or the way one is built. The story does, however, document challenges to the mistake, by both a witness and the one who errs, providing opportunities to move away from the error if not to correct it entirely. Bartram tries, gently but persistently, to turn Marcher's eyes toward the futility of his belief, and yet Marcher does not have the courage or the vision to let her meaning penetrate. He is marooned in his point of view. And Marcher himself comes close to realizing his error before the end of the story but skitters away, as if in fear. Bartram might be seen to suffer the consequences of Marcher's error as much as does Marcher, but the key to the story, for those interested in interpretive error, will be not only who errs and who suffers, but how deep and wide and silent this error is.

Critics argue whether this story is a romantic morality tale with a cowardly protagonist and selfless heroine, a stern moralistic fable warning of the dangers of inflating one's expectations for the future, an embodiment of chronic homosexual panic, or one in a series of James's "melodramas of consciousness." (What could be more melodramatic than this story's governing image of a wild animal poised in the tropical underbrush, throughout the life of the man, ready to strike and altogether transform his life?)[12] A recent and welcome addition to the litany of conventional readings suggests that the story sits astride an oscillation between mastery and surrender, both Marcher and Bartram simultaneously powered by and victimized by one another's secrets and one another's prying. Acts of masochism alternate with acts of sadism, often within the same character.[13] In these interpretations, Marcher and Bartram take turns reading one another's "text," Bartram exacting mastery over Marcher's fate quite as much as does Marcher over Bartram's. "She is no angelic woman whose good love has no ambition but to save a man if it could. She is the passionate virgin who completely possessed another's consciousness and thus gave him all the being he has."[14] These readings give play to such themes as domination, deception, and bondage that are central to the examination of error and failure in medicine and bioethics. Another strong reading of this story might take light from Emmanuel Levinas's thinking about passivity and duration, on the one hand, and the "ethics of the face," on the other, to figure Marcher's error to have been an inability to move freely in and out of a prereflective self-consciousness and, therefore, a failure to sustain contact with the face of the Other.[15] However, to "choose" among these many contradicting readings of James's story, one has to move beyond the plot to examine the formal characteristics of the story, called by some the enunciating situation—not what is told but how goes the telling.[16]

THE ENUNCIATING SITUATION

Combining the voice, frame, images, and style through which a story is told, the enunciating situation embodies the *how* of telling. Who tells and from what sources of knowledge? What metaphoric structures are adopted? What are the temporal dimensions of the tale? And what kind of language does the author choose?

"The Beast in the Jungle" is told by a courtly and judging speaker who sometimes has access to Marcher's or Bartram's thoughts and at other times voices his or her own biased appreciation of their predicament. The speaker's own hermetic insularity from the action of the story, such as it is, models Marcher's lack of contact with his own life. Speaking in the first person singular or plural, the narrator voices, from afar, Marcher's knowledge and more, inserting judgmental observations in ironic intercalations that are never hostile but that always pierce through Marcher's self-aggrandizing fog. "This was why, above all, he could regard himself, in a greedy world, as decently—as in fact perhaps even a little sublimely—unselfish. Our point is accordingly that he valued this character quite sufficiently to measure his present danger of letting it lapse" (p. 78). The narrator marks out potential paths of interpretation for the reader, beating down the grasses of Marcher's psychologically obfuscating jungle so that readers can see clearly to the horizon.

The story builds by way of a number of powerful governing images that accumulate both meaning and significance throughout the short story. Ten years after their initial introduction, John Marcher and Bartram meet in Weatherend, a mausoleum-like mansion filled with antiques. Through the equation of Bartram herself, who cares for both Marcher and Weatherend as an "unremunerated" keeper, Marcher is seen as a dead shell of a man (what is left once weather ends?) haunted by ghosts, perhaps, but not inhabited by life (pp. 63, 81, 78). Secrets, treasures, seeds destined never to germinate, and corpses are buried in tombs, sepulcres, and hiding places, waiting to be excavated in the future, their drumming presence in the tale intimating that knowledge is dead, fruition is past (pp. 66, 76, 118).

Although several other images common to James's fiction contribute to the story's sense, including images of the stream of life and the investment banking model of life, it is the image of the abyss that commands this story. "The day inevitably came for a further sounding of their depths. These depths, constantly bridged over by a structure firm enough in spite of its lightness and of its occasional oscillation in the somewhat vertiginous air, invited on occasion, in the interest of their nerves, a dropping of the plummet and a measurement of the abyss" (p. 92). The abyss around which the story is built is the nothingness of Marcher's life, the emptiness of his relationship with Bartram, and the absence of human meaning in his actions. A characteristic figure for James, especially in the short stories and novels written during the 1890s and early 1900s, the abyss "may be taken to stand for all the evacuated centers of meaning in [James's] fiction that nonetheless animate lives [and] determine quests for meaning."[17] This abyss, like many for James, marks an absence, as Tzvetan Todorov explains: "The Jamesian narrative is always based on *the quest for an absolute and absent cause*. . . . The tale consists of the search for, the pursuit of, this initial cause, this primal essence. . . . The cause is what, by its absence, brings the text into being."[18] By reading the tale, itself the "structure firm enough in spite of its lightness," the reader too must plummet into Marcher's abyss. Lacking what Levinas describes as "interiority" or "a presence at home with oneself," Marcher himself "stands for" the absence of the abyss; he is the human equivalent of the void.[19]

Time operates as both plot and form. That the protagonists are named after months of the year fuels the reader's conviction that this story is "about" time, seasons, and cycles—redemptive and unredemptive—of life. Almost no page of the story is bereft of a reference to the passage of time and the actions of remembering, reuniting, losing beginnings, having destinies, growing older, and the like. Precise and friable, the temporal scaffolding begins years after the protagonists meet as the story tells, in retrospect (or analepsis, as a structuralist would call the flashback), the tale—now mediated by Bartram's memory—of Marcher's youth. The story pivots on the tense of one verb. Bartram muses to Marcher that " 'the form and the way in your case were to have been—well, something so exceptional,' [and Marcher] . . . look[s] at her with suspicion. 'You say "were to *have* been," as if in your heart you had begun to doubt' " (p. 85). Hinging his story on one use of the past perfect subjective tense, James insists—rhetorically, formally, and thematically—that what is at stake here is the nature of time itself.

A man whose past is out of his reach, Marcher exists in pure suspensefulness or anteriority that he has replaced for life. Deprived of analeptic vision, Marcher is cursed with a terminal literary disease: he is a proleptic, fit to look only in one direction—the future—and thereby unable to find meaning in his life. Marcher's story stages James's very understanding of life. He wrote in 1895 in his notebook, ideas to which he returned in 1902 to write "The Beast in the Jungle," about "the idea of the *Too late*. . . . I mean too late in life altogether . . . the wasting of life is the implication of death."[20] Halfway through both the story and Marcher's life, Marcher and Bartram once again brood on the nature of his beast: "All they had thought, first and last, rolled over him; the past seemed to have been reduced to mere barren speculation. This in fact was what the place had just struck him as so full of—the simplification of everything but the state of suspense. That remained only by seeming to hang in the void surrounding it" (p. 87). Gathering up with powerful hand the image of the abyss and the passage of wasted time, James tells his reader, with urgency enough to break a heart, that life is but time passing, that each person must choose to fill it or to leave it blank, *and that the reading of this story is itself a redemptive act, a filling, if one chooses so to make of it, of the otherwise sounded void.*

The plot, governing images, and temporal dimension together create great weight; what offers a key to their meaning is the style adopted by James in writing this late tale. The sentences are long, punctuated by comments housed in parentheses and adverbial clauses set off by commas or long dashes. Almost any sentence in the story can serve as an example, "What did everything mean—what, that is, did *she* mean, she and her vain waiting and her probable death and the soundless admonition of it all—unless that, at this time of day, it was simply, it was overwhelmingly too late?" (p. 96). Prolonged, the train of thought of each sentence brings the reader through qualifying ruminations and forces him or her to consider last-minute amendations. "Because of the syntactic discontinuity of sentences," Jane Tompkins suggests, "the reader is constantly pausing to reflect on subtle distinctions, and must postpone the act of final apprehension until the last possible moment."[21] Although some readers, no doubt, experience impatience or *ennui* when trapped in an interminable sentence written by Henry James, those readers who can give themselves over to the tempo of his discerning, careful, questing mind achieve, as a dividend to the story itself, a vantage point on the world—and once gained, never lost—that grants rare conceptual freedom and moral vision.

ACTS OF INTERPRETATION

As one reads "The Beast in the Jungle," one is beset with the tragic and infuriating aspects of John Marcher's egotism and May Bartram's seeming collusion in his delusion. Skilled reading yields a multitude of meanings regarding passivity, cowardliness, being too late, and knowing one's fate, while honest reading moves in great arcs toward significance regarding age, gender, and intersubjectivity. Young readers are less likely to extend toward the pair the forgiving detachment that older readers have at their disposal. Women readers seem to judge both Marcher and Bartram far more harshly than do men readers. Those familiar with James's other fictions often place Marcher in the Jamesian lineage of passive male bachelors (Strether in *The Ambassadors,* Densher in *The Wings of the Dove,* and many such short-story protagonists as Mark Monteith in "A Round of Visits" and George Stransom in "The Altar of the Dead") who are unable to act toward other humans with agency or with passion, thereby giving some genetic clarity to the otherwise obtuse actions of Marcher. Indeed, the story might even be found, ultimately, to be not only about failure and time but also about how humans live around meaning and significance. Bartram understands all too well both the meaning and the significance of Marcher's life, while Marcher is blind to them both until the final scene of the graveside epiphany, suggesting that epiphany consists exactly in that sudden and simultaneous dawning of both meaning and significance.

One also—and it takes many readings to realize this—is stymied by the indeterminacy of the story itself. Time periods blur, events seem to recur, evenings at Bartram's house cannot be kept straight. After several baffled readings, one decides that the state of being baffled is exactly what James is trying for. Closer inspection confirms that bewilderment is indeed built into the plot and the form. The story is introduced by way of a series of opposites, poised as if in Calder-like balance. "They either mingled their sounds of ecstasy or melted into silences of even deeper import, so that there were aspects of the occasion that gave it for Marcher much the air of the 'look around,' previous to a sale highly advertised, that excites or quenches, as may be, the dream of acquisition" (p. 62). The sentence balances precariously the sounds of ecstasy against the silences of deeper import, on the one hand, and then balances those two opposites against the imaged opposition between the excitation and quenching of desire. Several lines below, Marcher is "disconcerted almost equally by the presence of those who knew too much and by that of those who knew nothing. The great rooms caused so much poetry and history to press upon him that he needed some straying apart to feel in a proper relation with them" (p. 62). In immediate succession, James gives us the cognitive opposition ("knew too much" versus "knew nothing") and the psychological opposition ("press upon" versus "straying apart"). It is as if James warns the reader, in his opening paragraph, that the story about to be told will rock between opposites, will confound thesis with antithesis, and will attempt, if anything, a dialectic balance.

Characteristically, James inserts into the text instructions for its use. By the second paragraph's "She hadn't lost [the thread of remembrance], but she wouldn't give it back to him" and again its "If [their past contact] had had no importance he scarcely knew why his actual impression of her should so seem to have so much" (p. 63), the reader himself or herself understands that this reading task amounts to mediation of conflict, reconciliation of opposites, and a Rhombergian drill of to-and-fro. Furthermore, it is the narrator who presents the textual model for the kind of reading required by this story, and he or she does so by virtue of the actual construction of the sentences. Thereby playing the part of the surrogate reader in providing the model for the actual reader, the narrator enacts James's "contemplation and judgment, vacillation and decision, analysis and passion" that "coexist within the syntactic framework of his sentences."[22] Marcher himself, by contrast, is not interested in the to-and-fro. Marcher's thoughts continue in the sentence quoted above: "He scarcely knew why his actual impression of her should so seem to have so much [importance]; the answer to which, however, was that in such a life as they all appeared to be leading for the moment one could but take things as they came. He was satisfied, without in the least being able to say why, that this young lady . . . was more or less a part of the establishment—almost a working, a remunerated part" (p. 63). Marcher's unexamined satisfaction that he had arrived at the correct interpretation of Bartram's station contrasts fundamentally with the narrator's incessant (some would say obsessive) examination of all his or her own interpretations. The reader has to choose between the narrator's quest for a dialectical balance powerful enough to accommodate ideas and their opposites and Marcher's more simplistic mode of getting through life with the first explanation that comes to hand. The story quite strongly demonstrates which of the two might be the more desirable.

As it turns out, the plot and form converge on the commanding opposition between past and future, situating Marcher (the irony of his name now comes into view) at a paralyzed still point between the two. Not the present but the voiding of the present is where Marcher's past and future intersect, because, suggests James, Marcher has had neither the vision to claim his past nor the courage to make room for his future. Substituting an empty space where his present ought to be, Marcher indeed is "*the* man, to whom nothing on earth was to have happened" (p. 125). James describes Marcher in the preface to volume 17 of *The Novels and Tales of Henry James: The New York Edition* as "a poor sensitive gentleman" who is "condemned to keep counting with the unreasoned prevision of some extraordinary fate. . . . As each item of experience comes, with its possibilities, into view, he can but dismiss it under this sterilising habit of the failure to find it good enough" (pp. ix-x). Sterilizing, paralyzing, "exempting" the life with which he comes into contact, "his career thus resolves itself into a great negative adventure" (p. x).[23] The adventure of reading about Marcher is, in the end, that one turns away from Marcher's mode of understanding and thereby, the reader hopes, against Marcher's fate. One turns—with the model of the narrator and the help of James himself close behind—toward a reading that increases one's capacity for dialectic resolution, one's realization of multiple contradictory aspects of any thought or reality, and one's ability to envision the world in terms complex enough to reveal some of its ambiguity and meaning and beauty.

Finally, reading this story forces the reader to plummet into not only Marcher's abyss, but his or her own abyss as well. When a story is written as masterfully as this one, the reader is brought, by hand, as it were, to the edge of the abyss poised at the center of his or her life, to confront not only the "stable" meaning of the work but also its shifting, shocking, personal significance. James understands human life well enough to speak across years, genders, and cultures to each person who picks up his works. (Those of us who read and write on James carry on extended conversations with him, and he answers us.) The force of a serious engagement with great literature is not only the turn outward toward the meaning of life imagined and represented but the simultaneous and reciprocal turn inward toward the significance of life found and lived. And to find that the experience of reading transforms the life lived is not sentimental or unduly exuberant. As Trilling puts it, modern literature "asks every question that is forbidden in polite society. . . . It asks us if we are content with ourselves, if we are saved or damned—more than with anything else, our literature is concerned with salvation."[24]

CLINICAL CORRELATIONS:
STORY AND ENUNCIATING SITUATION

In an attempt to bring home the salience of a literary method in looking for and at medical and ethical errors, this discussion now turns to a story about a man, a woman, and a death as told in a contemporary hospital chart.[25] Although there are vast generic differences between a melodramatic, high mimetic short fiction written by Henry James and an ordinary hospital chart of an unremarkable inpatient admission culminating in an expected death, the thematic and formal considerations of "The Beast in the Jungle"—personal failure, wasted time, a state of being baffled, a sense of being too late—make transparent elements of this hospitalization that are otherwise extremely opaque. In James's story, personal choices are based on psychological drives and temperamental needs, whereas in the story of the hospitalization, personal choices are based on those factors as well as on institutional policy, professional power asymmetry, and the structural imperatives inherent in being sick or being a health professional. Despite these differences, the dramas equally turn on mastery, surrender, secrecy, bondage, and passive waiting for that which is beyond intentionality.

Mr. Robert Dowling, a 73-year-old African-American man, was born in North Carolina and lived in New York City most of his life. He became ill during World War II of a poorly defined psychiatric condition and has been, on that account, disabled ever since. He lives with his wife in an apartment in upper Manhattan. Although Mr. Dowling has no children of his own, he helped to raise his wife's three children, one of whom, Violet, lives close by the Dowlings in New York City. His so-called social history is summarized in the chart by the medical resident:

Married lives w/wife. Has stepchildren, ō [no] children of own. Lives NY most of life, army service, born North Carolina [10/22/9X]

and by the intern:

2-3 ppd [packs per day] x 55 yrs, occ [occasional] scotch (2-3 weekends/month). Denies other drugs, although wife uses marijuana. Lives w/wife, has VNS [visiting nurse service]. WWII veteran [10/21/9X].

Mr. Dowling was physically healthy until developing a painful swelling on the left side of his face and neck in July 199X. Initially, the doctors at Presbyterian Hospital thought that he had a cancer of the head and neck, probably related to his heavy use of cigarettes and alcohol. On further evaluation, however, they discovered that the swelling in Mr. Dowling's face and neck represented distant spread of a cancer originating in the stomach. The stomach tumor was inoperable, and Mr. Dowling was advised to have radiation treatments to his face and neck to try to reduce the swelling and attendant pain.

From the beginning of Mr. Dowling's illness, his wife was not able to do all that needed to be done for his care. She could not bring him in for doctors' appointments or radiation treatments, and Mr. Dowling's facial and neck pain got worse. As reported by the radiation oncologist upon the patient's admission to the hospital:

Pt [patient] known to our dept. Pt was simulated but wife called to cancel RT [radiation therapy]. Pt never received RT. Pt is 73BG w/gastric and nasopharynx CA [cancer] (poorly ÷) unclear path. Pt now wants RT . . . Need to arrange for social worker to bring pt to clinic to receive RT [10/22/9X].

It was not Mrs. Dowling but the visiting nurse who decided that Mr. Dowling was ill enough to warrant a call to 911 for transport to the emergency room (ER):

To ER MD—Pt has digestive neoplasm, missed ENT [ear, nose, and throat specialist] appt 10/17. Next appt 10/24. Pt not eating well, getting weaker, wt loss. Had PEG [percutaneous endoscopic gastrostomy] installed but ō tube feedings ordered yet. Please evaluate [10/20/9X].

Once hospitalized, Mr. Dowling is found to be even more seriously ill than had been thought. The mass on his face is described by the medical resident:

Lg [large] infiltrative soft tissue mass; involving entire jaw, L [left] neck. Erythema [redness of the skin] ↑↑ wmth [increased warmth], lt green purulent disch [discharge] L ext [external auditory] canal w/whitish exudate ext canal interior, too painful to visualize [10/22/9X].

The patient's tumor is found to have spread to his bones and his brain. The medical teams urged him to undergo intensive radiation. According to the medical intern, the patient

wants RTX [radiation treatment], but there is an important question of whether pt's wife will assist him to get to/from treatments. Pt adamantly <u>wants</u> RTX. SW [social worker] to see pt re: poss HHA [home health aid] and VNS to help him get to/from appts. Given wife's h/o [history of] noncooperation [10/23/9X].

Two days later, the intern describes Mr. Dowling as follows:

complains of being v. anxious. When asked, pt said "I'm worried I have cancer." Pt dx [diagnosis] explained to him, and treatment goals as well. Pt became v. depressed when told he had gastric CA and said he felt "hopeless" and "wanted to end it all." When questioned about plan, he said he would jump out the window. φ [psychiatry] called. 1:1 PDA [private duty attendant] placed [10/25/9X].

A one-to-one observer (PDA) is assigned to sit at all times by the patient's bedside to prevent the patient from hurting himself, multiple psychiatric medications are given to Mr. Dowling, and regular visits from the psychiatrist are added to the medical, surgical, otolaryngological, gastrointestinal, oncologic, nutritional, chaplain, and social worker attention he receives. Meanwhile, he develops bleeding in the stomach, fluid in the lungs, metabolic disarray, and pressure on the windpipe from the growing neck mass. Nonetheless, he responds somewhat to treatment of his hopelessness, according to the psychiatrist.

Pt reports mood "better." Good night's sleep. Still quite depressed, "I don't have much time" + "There's no one" + "They just want my $" and passive SI [suicidal ideation]. ō psychosis. Tolerating Ambien, CPZ [Thorazine]. CT ⓟ [computed tomography pending] [10/26/9X].

All the while, Mrs. Dowling is only intermittently available for discussion and consultation, declining to give permission for most medical procedures because they are not guaranteed to save her husband's life. She poses a problem to the social worker and doctors by refusing to pay for either a nursing home or for nursing care at home, thereby precluding discharge from the hospital. Behaving like the representative of institutional virtue, the social worker chides her for her failure to assume responsibility for her husband's premorbid care:

Pt's spouse seems to have a poor understanding of pt's needs at home & the amount of assistance she can provide w/out help. Pt's wife refuses to pay privately for services despite SW & MD educating pt's spouse on the importance of pt having extensive care 24 hours a day 7 days a week. Pt's wife focused mainly on cost of services versus the pt's needs at home [11/10/9X].

While the medical team focuses on discharging the patient to a nursing home or hospice, the patient receives radiation treatment but does not seem to either get better or get worse. A new intern takes over Mr. Dowling's case, writing the following in the assessment and plan:

Pt is a 73 yo ♂ w/gastric adenocarcinoma w/mets [metastases] to the head, neck, bone, and brain pending XRT. Pt now c̄ ? [may have] pneumonia and + pulm [pulmonary] edema [11/2/9X].

On 11/4/9X, the same intern writes,

Pt is a 73 yo ♂ w/gastric adenocarcinoma metastatic to the head and neck. Pt admitted for ↓ po intake [decreased oral intake] and dehydration responding to treatment of a superinfection of the head/neck mass. Pt w/old bleeding, now persistent of an ulcerated gastric lesion. Pt threatened suicide and has 1:1 PDA. Pt now w/↓ SaO$_2$ [decreased arterial oxygen saturation] + pulm edema [11/4/9X].

Again on 11/9/97, the intern reports:

Pt is a 73 yo ♂ w/gastric AdenoCa, metastatic to the head, neck and brain on XRT now. Pt. admitted for ↓ po intake & dehydration requiring blood transfusions 2° [secondary] to bleeding from an ulcerated gastric lesion. Pt w/PDA 1:1 for safety (although was suicidal recently—no longer) and s/p 2u PRBC 2° ↓ Hct last pm [status post 2 units packed red blood cells secondary to drop in hematocrit] [11/9/9X].

Mr. Dowling's voice is heard occasionally in the hospital chart, mostly through the agency of the PDA and the psychiatrist. The PDA reports to the psychiatrist, who records in the chart the patient "speaks frequently of death and wish to suffer no more" and "that pt sang song about death all day 10/29 [10/28/9X, 10/30/9X]. Later that day, the psychiatrist notes the patient to be

moderately agitated, frustrated at that time. Said "I'm already dead." Denies SI at this time. c/o [complained of] being unable to walk, wife's absence [10/31/9X].

The patient directly tells another psychiatrist:

he is particularly concerned about his house "crumbling down" as he is not there to take care of it [11/1/9X].

The next day, the psychiatrist writes:

PDA states pt has been restless overnight w/occ attempts to get OOB [out of bed] though redirectable . . . Pt states "I want to get my life together" [11/2/9X].

And the next day, the psychiatrist notes:

PDA mentioned that he appeared depressed and mentioned feeling very depressed about the fact that he was going to die [11/3/9X].

Eventually, all treatment ceases. The radiation oncologist reports the following:

Pt and wife refuse further XRT. Plans for transfer to VA [Veterans Administration]. Wife states she knows this is not what he wants and does not want him to suffer further from potential side effects induced by RT [11/11/9X].

A medical ethics consultant is asked to comment because of the stand-off between Mrs. Dowling and the hospital staff, and the ethics consultant repeats that "Pt's wife very concerned about financial aspects of decision-making" [11/11/9X]. By 11/14/9X, the ethics consultant reports the following:

Ethical issues center around difficulty of crafting a D/C [discharge] plan that is acceptable to pt, his wife & health care team . . . Soc Wk, through exceptional problem-solving efforts, may be able to embellish pt's home care to 12 hrs/day, which is best option currently available . . . Situation reviewed with Dr. R (ethics committee chair) . . . All are in agreement that D/C home w/12 hrs/day of nursing care + existing PEG is best option for this pt. This plan optimizes pt autonomy, as pt has repeatedly expressed wish to receive care at home. He will receive hydration and nutrition through PEG, although Kcals may be somewhat less than optimal because of chronic slow gastric bleed. However, pt would receive exactly the same hydration/nutrition plan at hospice; this plan is best available overall for this terminally ill patient.

VNS will train pt's wife on 11/17 re suction etc, + if she attains adequate competency, pt will be $ home [patient will be discharged home] [11/14/9X].

Once this plan is accepted by all members of the healthcare team and the patient and his family, the patient initially becomes slightly more alert and more responsive. However, by the next day, Mr. Dowling is described as unresponsive. The repetitious intern states on November 17:

Pt is a 73 yo ♂ w/metastatic Gastric adeno Ca to the head, neck + brain. Pt has persistent bleeding from an ulcerated gastric lesion. Now w/poor SaO_2, receiving RXT. Pt stable. [11/17/9X].

And yet at 10:45 a.m. of that same day, the medical junior resident is called to see the patient. The resident records the following:

CTSP [called to see patient] found x̄ [without] respirations + pulseless by PDA + RN. Pt lying in bed w/NRFM [non-rebreather face mask] unresponsive to verbal/noxious stimuli. ō chest movements; on exam: ō heart sounds; ō air movements; ō pulses.
    Pt declared dead @ 10:39 a.m. today.

ACTS OF CLINICAL INTERPRETATION

Of what did Mr. Dowling die? Why did he die when he did? What did any of the doctors, nurses, and social workers taking care of him know of his predicament? One suspects that no one caring for the patient read the whole chart of this near-month-long hospitalization. The medical team duly comprehended the meanings of the biopsies and radiographic images to point to the pathology and anatomy of Mr. Dowling's tumor. But no one seems to have comprehended the meaning of the patient's moving and urgent statements about dying, about being uncared for, about wanting—when it was evidently too late—to "put his life together." An old man nears the end of his life unwanted, confused, in pain, and among strangers. No one seems to have grasped the significance of the man's lonely realization of his impending death or of the extraordinary level of conflict among Mr. Dowling, his wife, and the health professionals. What does Mr. Dowling's predicament tell us about dying in America, about existential anguish, about this man's marriage and this man's wife, about the responsibilities of his doctors and nurses, about the doctors' and nurses' fates?

The chart, it must be noted, represents only one dimension of knowledge about the patient. Not everything thought or said about a patient is written in this legal document, a document read by many readers for reasons other than the clinical or personal care of the patient. Certainly, there are conversations about patients on rounds or thoughts deep in the hearts of doctors and nurses and social workers that are not recorded in the chart. However, when a patient is attended by many health professionals from many different departments or services, the chart—as the only method of communication among all members of the scattered team—must convey all that is clinically salient about the patient's care. What is given in the hospital chart is the "public truth" about a patient—a public truth which, although partial, must represent a patient's predicament accurately enough that fitting actions can be undertaken on his or her behalf.

Putting this hospital chart beside "The Beast in the Jungle" suggests, first of all, that the chart—and the experiences it represents—constitutes a text and, as such, requires interpretation. As Hirsch notes, "the distinguishing characteristic of a text is that from it not just one but many disparate complexes of meaning can be construed."[26] If so, then one proceeds to examine such textual aspects as plot, form, and "intention" to construe and then to choose among rival meanings. Indeed, the two stories share a number of important features of plot—passive waiting in the face of a "beast" (unlike Mr. Marcher's beast, Mr. Dowling's has a name—widely metastatic gastric adenocarcinoma), a life companion accompanying a dying person until the end, a death that responds temporally to its context, and unredemptive human relations. More salient to this discussion, the frames placed around those events by the stories' authors resemble one another. Like Marcher's vision, prognosis is a proleptic activity. Both stories' frames obliterate the past. James elects to exclude (or opts not to imagine) information about Marcher's and Bartram's past; the multiple authors of Mr. Dowling's chart too elect to exclude (or opt not to learn) information about Mr. and Mrs. Dowling's past life together, even though knowledge about Mrs. Dowling's past ability to care for her chronically ill husband is salient to the decisions being contemplated during this hospitalization. The iterative intern repeats her sentence about Mr. Dowling every day as if her relation with him is devoid of memory. Both stories privilege the future, putting the balance of interest firmly on suspense and outcome, although James darkens and doubles his story through irony while the chart tells its equally tragic story with what amounts to single-stranded naïveté.

Both stories resolutely ignore the meaningful present. Marcher's inability to take seriously his relation to Bartram and his "sterilising habit of the failure to find [the present] good enough" empties him, ultimately, of human agency and life meaning. Mr. Dowling does give voice to his urgent, painful present: all along, he puts into words his premonition of near death, his awareness of the "crumbling" of his house and, as a metaphor for his life, his recognition of his wife's absence from his side, his fear of having been exploited and abandoned. He says that he "wishes to suffer no more," that he feels "already dead." He sings songs about death, heard by the PDA, the person with the least professional training but who may have the most profound human sense, who almost alone seems to understand the significance of what this man says. Why does the patient's suffering—clearly documented, evident for anyone who takes the time to read his story—not reach anyone urgently enough to grant him succor? Why does no one comfort him or acknowledge his fear or stand by him in his peril? If only someone had found out how to diminish his crushing sense of isolation, perhaps by engaging his family members in a true attempt to meet him near his end or by engaging the patient himself in authentic consideration of his life choices. Instead, the psychiatrist responds to the patient's suffering by changing the doses of antidepressants, antipsychotics, and anxiolytics. The intern is dutiful in the tasks of the body but seems deaf to needs of the man. The social worker disbelieves Mr. Dowling and scolds Mrs. Dowling for what is interpreted as selfishness, without wondering about the wife's own predicament or even eliciting an explanation for her behavior. The ethics consultant, with a task limited to the instrumental by institutional requirements, places autonomy on a level with kilocalories, hydration, and suctioning, finding no room for freedom or desire or dread. It might have been impossible to alter this man's slow and painful death, but if only we had tried.

If these stories' plots are similar, the methods required to understand them are also similar. The ward team of a teaching hospital is, or could be, an interpretive community, and yet its abilities to illuminate collectively the complex and ambiguous human stories of illness are rarely, if ever, used. This hospital chart demonstrates a discontinuity between the vigorous raising and weighing of conflicting explanations for clinical phenomena, as seen in the activities collectively referred to as the "differential diagnosis," on the one hand, and the paucity of such raising and weighing of possible explanations for personal phenomena, on the other. That is to say, the ward team already functions as a sophisticated interpretive community in its search for pathophysiological understandings of derangements of the body, interpretations that culminate in the ability to choose clinical actions on the basis of rigorous and disciplined collective thought. Perhaps a close reading of any chart might expose lacunae in the personal interpretations chosen by the community, and exposing these lacunae might prompt a more robust generating, testing, and provisional choosing of hypotheses not only about the corporeal types of events witnessed by the ward team but also about the personal, ethical, and existential ones.

The narrator of "The Beast in the Jungle" exemplifies the kind of conceptualizing, weighing, and considering of alternative interpretations that alone can first recognize and then make sense of a contradictory tangle of thesis and antithesis. The teller of this tale is one of a family of James's narrators who are "slightly personalized, right-minded, historian/biographer narrators who ambulate among various centers of consciousness but diligently refrain from ethical evaluation, leaving that up to the characters themselves and to the emotionally responsive reader."[27] Sadly, there is no such Jamesian narrator in Mr. Dowling's chart who attempts a similar weighing of opposites, imagining of provisional meanings, recognizing of conflicting interpretations. Full of the indeterminacy—is it pulmonary edema or pneumonia or pulmonary embolus?—around which all doctors live their lives, the chart has little sense of mystery. Oddly, in the face of an extraordinary clinical turn of events (it was on a routine biopsy during placement of the PEG that the primary gastric tumor was found), there is no sense of being baffled or thrown. If there is little sense of mystery about the physical elements of Mr. Dowling's illness, there is none about the Dowlings' personal behavior. Those who interpret Mr. and Mrs. Dowling's language and behavior act, instead, like Marcher, as if "in such a life as they all appeared to be leading for the moment one could but take things as they came" (p. 63). They all seem "satisfied, without in the least being able to say why" with their impoverished and unidimensional interpretations of this complex state of affairs (p. 63).

Putting this chart beside "The Beast in the Jungle" shows the nature of the errors committed in the care of Mr. and Mrs. Dowling. Not instrumental or structural or slovenly errors, these errors are long-lived failures to have developed rich, complex, nuanced, perilous interpretations of meaningful and significant human events. Not restricted to the care of this patient, the failures that become apparent in a close reading of this chart are to be found in any similarly complex clinical record. Not the outcomes of care—which here are reasonable and clinically appropriate—but its interior process calls for examination. No doubt many conversations took place among members of the healthcare team who anguished about his care. And yet, such knowledge is not reflected in the written traces of care and so is excluded from clinical deliberations. The failures are not clinical but textual in nature.

What is missing from this hospitalization is not sharp thinking or encyclopedic knowledge or decisive intervention, nor yet a professional commitment to the patient's welfare. What is missing is a mind large and resonant and dispassionate enough to behold these human events, not in instrumental terms (What does his upper-gastrointestinal bleeding require of me? How does his history of war-time psychosis change my treatment of his depression? How will we deal with her alleged lack of funds?) but in interpretive terms—What do these events mean? What, for Mr. and Mrs. Dowling, *and for us,* do they signify? Absent is the "principled realism" of a critical reading "which holds that no objective truths or transcendentally privileged perspective can be found but that we can understand enough about a situation or event to be able to act responsibly toward all persons involved."[28] Absent is the skilled reader who has learned, through his or her interactions with many texts of living, how to absorb another's world with enough accuracy and patience and generosity that what is said can be heard.

One attains the knowledge needed to reach these interpretations through intersubjective means. (Does Levinas not remind his readers of "the impossibility of *forgetting* the intersubjective experience," giving them an orientation to meaning?)[29] One sits near Mr. Dowling's bed and one engages in conversation with him, letting oneself be guided by one's curiosity, one's appreciation of the gravity of Mr. Dowling's predicament, and one's commitment to truth and freedom. One might do the same with Mrs. Dowling and Violet, with the social worker and the PDA, with the psychiatrist and the surgeon. One bathes oneself in the atmosphere of the situation, becoming permeable to each participant's intimations, reflections, and reach of language. The questions to be asked are not to be found in a textbook of medical interviewing or in a protocol for establishing capacity or in the mental status examination. Singular, the questions arise from one's depths, one's own living of a life, one's understanding of the large matters of moment that are found in living—pride, shame, pleasure, pain, love, dismissal, exaltation, humiliation. Realizing that one is in the presence of death, one understands something about the experience of the dying man, and one realizes that Mr. Dowling might say, "Death is a menace that approaches me as a mystery; its secrecy determines it—it approaches without being able to be assumed, such that the time that separates me from my death dwindles and dwindles without end. . . . The last part of the route will be crossed without me."[30] Although the culture of the tertiary-care medical center does not currently encourage its professionals to enter such intersubjective relations with patients, perhaps individuals might be supported in their efforts to come close enough to patients' experiences to offer witness, to behold the meaning and significance of that which occurs as patients die.

One must then find the ground upon which to stand (this is what James does so masterfully in creating his narrators), which affords a vision of the full situation, safety from inordinate personal involvement, and a means of triangulating or in other ways validating those tentative interpretations emitted by the situation and registered by the narrating presence. Levinas describes thought in terms that might apply to this ideal ambulatory narrator as "disinterested and self-sufficient," and as "a regal and as it were unconditioned activity, a sovereignty which is possible only as solitude."[31] Using such "disinterested" thought, this narrator will attempt to be faithful to that which has been intersubjectively revealed by the patient, not expropriating the patient's experience but, rather, trying to reflect it. The narrator realizes that "if one could possess, grasp, and know the other, it would not be other. Possessing, knowing, and grasping are synonyms of power." And so the teller of Mr. Dowling's tale will attempt to offer a principled rather than an authoritarian account of the events of the illness.[32]

The story about Marcher and Bartram, Millicent Bell suggests, "disproves the idea that negativity can be maintained. It suggests that there is always a story, that in not writing one one writes another."[33] And so, one writes down what one has learned, even that which is "too painful to visualize," not in technical jargon but in ordinary human language resonant with the conflict and uncertainty and brave imprecision born of a vision so fine that it cannot exclude that which contradicts, that which forces and obstructs choice, that which undermines the simplest action. Perhaps the so-called ethics consultation activity should be conceptualized as a skilled Jamesian narrating—this and this alone—of the story and its situation and its climate so as to make the full text available to all its readers. Perhaps one way to recuperate strong moral vision, in the delivery of ordinary healthcare, is to require oneself, as James suggests the reader should, "to lend himself, to project himself and steep himself, to feel and feel till he understands and to understand so well that he can say."[34] Only then will the narrator/witness see into the past and the future, avoiding the errors born of smallness of scale and time, to consider interpretations of oceanic scope and of singular truth. Only then will the interpretive community be provided with the texts that reflect all the ambiguity and risks of living. Only faced with such texts can the entire community join with each witness to collectively behold and then acknowledge the large and small and contradictory truths of our patients' lives. In medicine as in literature, human beings can find themselves on a course between prophesy and memory, stability and change, meaning and significance, all the while discovering not Marcher's negative adventure or Mr. Dowling's unexamined peril, but the fullness of time, the reach of the abyss, and the jungles and horizons of our lives.

NOTES

1. E.D. Hirsch Jr., "The Politics of Theories of Interpretation," *The Politics of Interpretation,* ed. W.J.T. Mitchell (Chicago: University of Chicago Press, 1983), 321-33, p. 322.

2. H. Bloom, *A Map of Misreading* (Oxford, England: Oxford University Press, 1975), 3-4. Bloom suggests parallels between poetic acts of reading and psychological acts of defense and growth. "How can a poet write in the shadow of an ancestor?" becomes the same question as "How can a child act in the shadow of his or her parent?" Bloom contributes to the effort of examining errors in medicine and ethics by suggesting that how we learn about texts is not unlike how we learn about actual events.

3. See note 1 above, p. 323.

4. L. Goldmann, "Genetic Structuralist Method in the History of Literature," in *Marxism and*

Art: Writings in Aesthetics and Criticism, ed. B. Lang and F. Williams, trans. F. Williams (New York: Longman, 1972), 249-50, as cited in E.D. Hirsch Jr., *The Aims of Interpretation* (Chicago: University of Chicago Press, 1976), 2.

5. Hirsch, *The Aims of Interpretation,* see note 4 above, p. 80.

6. S. Fish, *Is There a Text in This Class? The Authority of Interpretive Communities* (Cambridge, Mass.: Harvard University Press, 1980), 171.

7. L. Trilling, in his introduction to *Prefaces to the Experience of Literature* (New York: Harcourt Brace Jovanovich, 1967), vii-xi, makes a case for the communal nature of literature. "We find a pleasure that seems instinctual not only in the emotions that are aroused by what we read but also in communicating them to each other, in trying to understand why we feel as we do, in testing our emotions by those that others tell us that they have, in discovering what we might possibly feel beyond what we do feel. And discourse leads to dialectic" (ix).

8. H. James, "The Beast in the Jungle," in *The Novels and Tales of Henry James: New York Edition* (New York: Charles Scribner's Sons, 1909), 17: 61-127, p. 71. Page numbers in parenthesis in the text refer to this edition.

9. F.W. Dupee, *Henry James, The American Men of Letters Series* (New York: William Sloane Associates, 1951), 181.

10. D. Przybylowicz, *Desire and Repression: The Dialectic of Self and Other in the Late Works of Henry James* (University, Ala.: University of Alabama Press, 1986), 109.

11. M. Bell, *Meaning in Henry James* (Cambridge, Mass.: Harvard University Press, 1991), 270.

12. For a critique of "Beast in the Jungle" as a story about homosexual panic, see E. Kosofsky, *Epistemology of the Closet* (Berkeley, Calif.: University of California Press, 1990); for a depiction of this story as a melodrama of consciousness, see P. Brooks, *The Melodramatic Imagination: Balzac, Henry James, Melodrama, and the Mode of Excess* (New York: Columbia University Press, 1985).

13. M. Banta, *Henry James and the Occult; The Great Extension* (Bloomington, Ind.: Indiana University Press, 1972); G. Buelens, "In Possession of a Secret: Rhythms of Mastery and Surrender in 'The Beast in the Jungle,' " *Henry James Review* 19 (1998): 17-35.

14. Banta, *Henry James and the Occult,* see note 13 above, p. 211.

15. For an introduction to Levinas's theory of the face, see E. Levinas, *Ethics and Infinity,* trans. R.A. Cohen (Pittsburgh, Penn.: Duquesne University Press, 1985), 83-92. For a more extensive discussion of the theory of the face, see E. Levinas, "Exteriority and the Face," *Totality and Infinity: An Essay on Exteriority,* trans. A. Lingis (Pittsburgh, Penn.: Duquesne University Press, 1969), 187-247.

16. G. Genette, *Narrative Discourse: An Essay in Method,* trans. J.E. Lewin (Ithaca, N.Y.: Cornell University Press, 1980).

17. Brooks, *The Melodramatic Imagination,* see note 12 above, pp. 173-4.

18. T. Todorov, *The Poetics of Prose,* trans. R. Howard (Ithaca, N.Y.: Cornell University Press, 1977), 145. See also F. Kermode, *The Genesis of Secrecy: On the Interpretation of Narrative* (Cambridge, Mass.: Harvard University Press, 1979) for a wide-ranging and generative discussion of the secrets contained in narrative and the reader's responsibility to suspect them, to recognize them, and to delight in their inexhaustibility.

19. Levinas, *Totality and Infinity,* see note 15 above, p. 110.

20. H. James, *The Notebooks of Henry James,* ed. F.O. Matthiessen and K.B. Murdock (Chicago: University of Chicago Press, 1981), 182-3.

21. J.P. Tompkins, " 'The Beast in the Jungle': An Analysis of James's Late Style," *Modern Fiction Studies* 16 (1970): 185-91, pp. 186-7. See also Banta in *Henry James and the Occult* for a discussion of the implications of James's late style for the conveyance of his meaning (see note 13 above, pp. 200-1).

22. Tompkins, *An Analysis of James's Late Style,* see note 21 above, p. 190.

23. See note 20 above, p. 311.

24. L. Trilling, "On the Teaching of Modern Literature," in *Beyond Culture: Essays on Literature and Learning* (New York: Harcourt Brace Jovanovich, 1978), 3-27, pp. 7-8.

25. This textual study of hospital charts was approved by the Institutional Review Board of the College of Physicians and Surgeons of Columbia University on 1 June 1997. Permission was granted to reproduce and publish excerpts from hospital charts from which are deleted all identifying information about patients and caregivers. Accordingly, all names, telephone numbers, beeper numbers,

and other identifying data are changed in the excerpts from the transcribed chart printed here. The chart under study was transcribed by the author.

26. E.D. Hirsch, *Validity in Interpretation* (New Haven, Conn.: Yale University Press, 1967), 25.

27. M. Kearns, "Henry James, Principled Realism, and the Practice of Critical Reading," *College English* 56 (1994): 766-87, p. 770.

28. Ibid., 769.

29. Levinas, *Totality and Infinity,* see note 15 above, p. 53.

30. Ibid., 235.

31. E. Levinas, "Ethics as First Philosophy," *The Levinas Reader,* ed. S. Hand (Oxford, England: Blackwell, 1989), 75-87, p. 77.

32. E. Levinas, *Time and the Other,* trans. R.A. Cohen (Pittsburgh, Penn.: Duquesne University Press, 1987), 90.

33. Bell, *Meaning in Henry James,* see note 11 above, p. 272.

34. H. James, "Criticism," in *Selected Literary Criticism,* ed. M. Shapira (Cambridge, England: Cambridge University Press, 1981), 133-7, p. 136.

4

Humility Reconsidered

Judith Andre

INTRODUCTION

On the one hand, mistakes are inevitable. On the other hand, they are to be avoided; nothing counts as a mistake unless in some sense we could have done otherwise. This fundamental paradox creates the moral challenge of accepting our fallibility and at the same time struggling against it. Humility is crucial to both aspects of this task—a humility not of shame but of compassion toward oneself. At the heart of compassion is simple kindness, an attitude that is essential to clarity about oneself and to living with imperfection while striving mightily for something better.

This essay explores and defends the conception of humility presented above. Current philosophical treatments of it are inadequate; they are overly intellectual, tending to reduce the virtue to one of its consequences (understanding the truth about one's relative worth). Self-knowledge is a different kind of achievement than scientific knowledge; understanding this paves the way to understanding humility in its fullness—as a moral virtue rather than an intellectual one.

The essay begins with an overview of the works of Lucian L. Leape and David Hilfiker, two significant writers on mistakes in healthcare. Their work points implicitly toward the importance of this deeper understanding of humility. Virtues are learned within communities, and so the essay concludes with a description of a particularly interesting way of fostering humility in a medical school.

LEAPE'S AND HILFIKER'S PERSPECTIVES
ON MEDICAL MISTAKES

Two of the most important writers on mistakes in healthcare are Lucian L. Leape and David Hilfiker. Their perspectives are interestingly different. Leape is scientific. "In a generic sense, errors are but variations in processes. Total quality management also requires a culture in which errors and deviations are regarded not as human failures, but as opportunities to improve the system. Errors must be accepted as evidence of systems flaws not character flaws."[1]

The last sentence is important. In spite of it, Leape's work directs us to moral growth as well as to systems improvement. His work has been groundbreaking, giving practitioners new ways to understand and cope with their failures. He believes that there are far too many mistakes in healthcare today and argues that one reason is the culture of medicine, so insistent upon perfection that it allows no room to admit one's errors. As a result of this suppression, the causes of mistakes go unexamined. Another result is that doctors suffer in silent agony, unable to tell anyone when they have made mistakes. Leape offers concrete suggestions for reducing error, usually through changes in systems management. The approach he advocates, realistic and candid, may help transform medicine's now-crippling culture of silence.

David Hilfiker's concerns overlap with Leape's, but his purpose and voice are quite different. Hilfiker yearns for medical customs that would provide more emotional and spiritual solace for dealing with mistakes: "Many [doctors] cannot bear to face their mistakes directly. We either deny the misfortune altogether or blame the patient, the nurse, the laboratory, the physicians, the system, fate—anything to avoid our own guilt. Perhaps the only way to face our guilt is through confession, restitution, and absolution."[2]

On first reading, Hilfiker seems at odds with Leape. He describes "blaming the system" as a way of avoiding personal guilt. Where Leape's voice is objective and systematic, Hilfiker's is subjective and personal. Leape focuses on protecting patients, Hilfiker on healing physicians. (Each, of course, cares about both physicians and patients, but each has a different primary intent.) In an interesting way, however, the concerns of these two writers converge. Both argue that doctors should be more candid about their errors, and that they need help to do this. Candor, Leape argues, would help us identify the causes of error and so help reduce them. Candor, Hilfiker argues, would make the experience of error less disabling for physicians. Both writers point implicitly to a central moral dimension of healthcare—the virtue that is referred to here as *humility*—and each offers suggestions that would improve it. But neither names the virtue; this is particularly understandable since *humility* is a word with some unpleasant connotations. Part of the task of this essay is to offer a sense of the word that puts aside its darker interpretations.

Although most readers welcome Leape's work, occasionally someone responds with alarm, worried about his apparently amoral stance ("systems flaws, not character flaws"), concerned that reducing personal responsibility in medicine would undermine it.[3] Such critics argue that, without the strictest of internal taskmasters, doctors will perform less well. Part of Leape's point, of course, is that doctors' performance is not the whole story. What matters finally are outcomes, and systems are as important to these as individual attitudes and efforts. That is, the efforts of the best doctors will be lost if the system is bad enough, and mediocrity does less damage in an excellent system. But the doubters may be pointing, even if unconsciously, to something different from outcomes—something of special importance to the moral life. Is it intrinsically improper to lessen a doctor's dread of mistakes? Do approaches that emphasize sociology and systems analysis blur moral perspectives? I do not think so, but I think the questions are significant.

One's attitude toward one's own mistakes is central to the moral life, in a way that is as yet poorly articulated. That one must admit and take responsibility for one's mistakes is obvious and uncontroversial. What is more interesting is a set of questions that appears at the intersection of work by Hilfiker, Leape, and Leape's detractors. Leape's approach, in spite of its focus on systems rather than on individuals, is morally praiseworthy—obviously in the sense that it should reduce suffering, but also in less obvious ways. To understand the full moral value of Leape's approach, to appreciate the half-conscious concerns of those who resist him, and to probe Hilfiker's spiritual commitments, one needs to look at moral life from several perspectives. The moral dimensions of life concern not only choices but also ways of seeing and valuing the world and the relationships of which one is a part; all of this is seen not only in relation to others but also to oneself. Growth in these things demands more than instruction and effort. Like other kinds of growth, moral development is more likely to occur in the right environment—one that provides models, mentors, heroes, and antiheroes; support, guidance and correction; relevant experiences; and time for healing, reflection, and building.

This picture of a moral life draws from Aristotle, from contemporary virtue theorists, from feminist theory, and from Christianity and Buddhism. Not all of those sources are made explicit here. Instead my hope is to draw a coherent picture that will have resonance for contemporary readers. Healthcare as Leape and Hilfiker envision it provides a richer medium for moral growth than does the silent and individualistic world of conventional healthcare. This essay focuses on one particular virtue—humility. This character trait is at once a relation to others and to oneself.

HUMILITY: PHILOSOPHICAL AND RELIGIOUS TREATMENTS

Humility is obviously important in facing and acknowledging one's mistakes. For most readers, perhaps, the word *humility* calls to mind stories of the arrogant being brought low. But arrogance—the unquestioned assumption of one's own superiority—is only one kind of failure in humility. Because arrogance is so offensive, the experiences that correct it make gratifying stories, and that phenomenon may explain our tendency to understand humility simply as humiliation. A morally desirable attitude toward one's fallibility, however, requires more than abandoning arrogance. Being brought low is at most one step, for some people, at some points in the journey. The deeper, subtler aspects of this virtue will be explored in a subsequent section of this essay.

As groundwork, this section summarizes current philosophical discussion of the issue. Probably not surprisingly, philosophers tend to intellectualize humility—to make it a matter of accurate self-assessment. Their secondary concern has been to focus on some apparent paradoxes, again intellectual: how can one honestly recognize one's own excellence and still be humble? Finally, philosophers have looked at the word's religious history, from which they try to extract what can be defended on secular grounds. Some of the problems in making sense out of humility are foreshadowed by David Hume, in his classic discussion of pride. "I believe no one, who has any practice of the world, and can penetrate into the inward sentiments of men, will assert, that the humility, which good-breeding and decency require of us, goes beyond the outside, or that a thorough sincerity in this particular is esteem'd a real part of our duty. On the contrary, we may observe, that a genuine and hearty pride, or self-esteem, if well conceal'd and well founded, is essential to the character of a man of honour."[4] The tension identified by Hume between self-respect and the apparent requirements of humility remains today.

The fullest recent philosophical examination of the question, Norvin Richards's *Humility,* manages to balance self-respect and humility quite well. Richards defines the virtue as "a matter of having oneself in perspective . . . [of] understanding oneself and what one has done too clearly to be inclined to exaggeration."[5] His attempt is reformative. He wants to release the word from its associations with a sense of worthlessness. Toward this end he describes humility as clarity about oneself, about one's strengths as well as one's weaknesses. Given human psychology, he believes, the more pressing danger is blindness to one's faults, and so it is natural that the word is associated with acknowledging shortcomings rather than with recognizing strengths. Richards's "having oneself in perspective" captures an important aspect of common understanding, but the idea that this includes one's strengths as well as one's weaknesses is foreign to many people. Cognates of the term *humility* emphasize that strangeness. The terms *humbled* and *humiliated,* for instance, refer solely to facing one's flaws. One cannot say, "I was humbled today. I learned how good my voice is." What Richards has done, however, is offer us a fuller, more consistent and defensible picture of a morally good attribute of self-assessment. This essay follows Richards in keeping the word *humility,* while recognizing its imperfect fit with ordinary language; it also follows him in endorsing the moral significance of seeing oneself clearly. It goes considerably beyond what Richards has done, however, in treating that vision as part of a virtue and not just as an intellectual attainment.

Others struggling to make moral sense of our intuitions sometimes choose the word *modesty* rather than *humility.* This allows them to stay closer to ordinary language, because modesty does not have the problematic association with a sense of inferiority. These philosophical attempts, however, are not fully successful. *Modesty* turns out to offer a milder version of the problems that *humility* does; each word seems to preclude a recognition of one's own worth. Can someone recognize his or her own excellence and yet remain modest? Two writers resolve the paradox by invoking *moral* equality: however well one can sing, one has no more moral worth than any other human being, and modesty is the recognition of that fact.[6]

Some of this is persuasive, some of it suggestive. The emphasis on the importance of clarity and perspective seems right. The argument that we honor humility because it displays an understanding of moral equality is less convincing. In 20th-century America we do have a foundational cultural commitment to the idea of equal moral worth. That commitment is also fundamental within moral philosophy, and within Judaism and Christianity. But surely one could attribute modesty or humility to someone without attributing moral egalitarianism. One could even attribute these virtues to someone taken to be one's own superior or inferior. Think, for instance, of slaves in the ancient world, who may have considered themselves intrinsically inferior to those they served. Could they not (occasionally) have thought of their masters and mistresses as humble or modest? Perhaps the modest or humble person is not so much committed to moral egalitarianism as disinterested in competitive rankings. This is an entirely different kind of character trait—not a commitment to the truth of some proposition, but an attitude, a way of being.

Several philosophers have looked to religious traditions for insight into this virtue; the world's major religions offer centuries of reflection about what makes life good. As one might expect, these traditions often resist the simplification sought by philosophers. Such untidiness, however, often provides a rich lode for exploration. Richards looks primarily at Christian sources, especially medieval writers such as Bernard of Clairvaux, Thomas Aquinas, and Ignatius Loyola. Richards summarizes what he found: "[In this tradition] nothing that is good about you is to your own personal credit: such things are only the particular gifts God chose to give you. On the other hand, everything that is bad about you is your own fault, a way in which you personally have failed. . . . To have a high opinion of yourself would always be to . . . take credit where none was due."[7]

Richards reforms this definition of humility by rejecting Christian metaphysics but retaining a commitment to accurate self-assessment.[8] He pays little attention, however, to what Christian thinkers have said about *acquiring* humility, and, as a result, fails to raise a fundamental question: since self-knowledge is so different from scientific knowledge, what are its necessary conditions?

In Judaism humility has a somewhat different cast. Ronald Green is one of the few philosophers who have tried to present a Judaic view of humility to a secular audience. He finds that humility's greatest importance in this tradition is with regard to relations with human beings rather than with God. "While the humble man is necessarily God-fearing . . . humility is believed important in other relations. It is an attitude held necessary to orient the self in all moral relations, and in some rabbinic discussions it is compared to salt in being required to lend savor to all moral deeds and dispositions."[9]

Green points out another element in the Judaic tradition. Since God is the exemplar of all virtue, "God's holiness must be interpreted to include as its central feature His humility"[10]—on the face of it, a difficult task. But "the humility of God is assumed to be shown by His solicitousness for human welfare,"[11] and especially a concern for the poor.[12] The idea is that God does not act in the way that rich and arrogant human beings do. "Accurate self-assessment" would seem to capture nothing of this; God's humility is not a matter of being correct about the Divine status, but of not being preoccupied by it. Divinity does not keep God from caring about those who are suffering, however lowly they may be. This development of humility's implications reinforces the thesis of this essay: clarity about oneself is a manifestation of humility rather than its essence.

One point needs to be emphasized. Although the word *humility* occurs in all these discussions, it does not mean exactly the same thing in each. The word has represented a variety of attitudes at different times and places, related to one another through what Wittgenstein would call family resemblance. It has meant self-abasement, a deep understanding of one's failings, a lack of preoccupation with one's status, concern for others, and service to the poor. Current, "everyday" secular speech retains only some of this, and not always those aspects we might wish. Humility continues to be contrasted with arrogance, to include respect for others, and to suggest lowliness and even abasement. It is not linked, at least in any obvious way, with concern for the poor. If there is a difference between traditional meanings of the word and current usage, there is also a difference between both of these and the discussions within moral philosophy. Richards, the others, and I are trying to identify the threads that, taken together, would make a coherent and attractive moral ideal. We are searching for a kernel hidden within the history of the word deeper than the superficial contradictions and unattractive connotations sometimes present. Although the word *humility* is retained for the trait explored below, this discussion emphasizes a moral ideal rather than an explication of general usage.[13]

The point of this essay is to argue that humility, described in a certain way, is a virtue of special help in living with fallibility while still struggling against it. What do these preliminary discussions tell us? They remind us that accurate self-assessment is a moral accomplishment and overestimation the more common form of failure. Obviously, seeing our mistakes clearly makes us more likely to correct them or to correct for them. In addition, the humble person as described here recognizes that other people can teach and assist him or her, another disposition that makes mistakes less likely.

But these characterizations of humility tend to make it an entirely instrumental good, and an entirely intellectual one. Humility becomes a matter of getting the facts right, useful in the way new glasses or a better microscope would be, rather than an essential quality of a fully moral human being. Most of these construals, in fact, do not treat humility as a *virtue* in a full Aristotelian sense. (The Jewish tradition may come closest to doing so.)[14] A virtue is a disposition toward doing the right thing, because one understands and is attracted by what is good. A virtuous person need not fight his or her feelings; on the contrary, a sign of the full possession of virtue is taking pleasure in doing the right thing. Virtues are acquired and practiced within a community. Exploring these points—the actions, emotions, and understandings that constitute humility, as well as the kind of community that supports it—will enrich our understanding of it. We will come to see it as a morally necessary stance toward human finitude, of which mistakes are one manifestation.

HUMILITY AS A VIRTUE: A DEEPER LOOK

If humility is a virtue, it is a richer object of study than the current philosophical discussion suggests. Humility is morally desirable in itself (as part of a harmonious self that is capable of flourishing) and also for its results (as are most virtues, as they contribute to the well-being of the individual, the household, or the broader community). In healthcare, as in other aspects of life, humility causes mistakes to occur less frequently, and their consequences to be less dire. For the purpose of this discussion, humility is defined as the ability to recognize and be at ease with one's flaws. What is obviously new in this definition is the phrase "be at ease," and it needs explanation. What may seem less new is the term *recognize*. In this context, however, the term *recognition* also needs attention. I turn to it first.

Recognizing truths about oneself is different from other kinds of knowledge. It is not like knowing algebra or being able to recognize quattrocento painting. Understanding human beings—subjects—is a different enterprise from understanding things that are only objects. Because this difference makes the social sciences markedly different from the physical sciences, it has been well explored.[15] Qualities of subjects—desires, intentions, emotions, knowledge, and so on—are intrinsically difficult to define, to describe, and to investigate. What counts as evidence for their existence is different than what counts as evidence about the physical world.

This is especially true in self-understanding. More precisely, understanding oneself is a different project from understanding other people. And the way that others help one acquire knowledge is different in learning about objects, learning about other persons, and learning about oneself. Knowledge of particular subjectivities cannot be attained just by instruction from an authority. In algebra or art history, a good teacher or book is essential. In the case of self-understanding, others can also be of use but in a different way. It is not a matter of their having clear and extensive knowledge of one and simply communicating it. Certainly a therapist, a spiritual director, a friend (even an enemy) can help one recognize things that otherwise would remain hidden—a habit or an emotional tone, for instance, that one has never recognized. But the knowledge gained by the subject will be different from that possessed by the onlooker. Although in any field no two people have exactly the same understanding of it, a far greater congruence is possible when people are studying some external object than when they are talking about themselves. There are things about oneself that can only be known with the help of others; there are things that only the person himself or herself can know. And there are aspects of any human being that remain mysterious.

What *can* be gained through systematic instruction are skills of introspection. Growth in self-understanding demands not only attention to the reactions of others, but also attention to one's own inner life. Self-knowledge is an ongoing awareness—of one's own feelings and thoughts, of the reactions of others to one's words and actions—more than an accumulation of facts.

Because self-knowledge is so different from most of what we call knowledge, humility—partly constituted by self-knowledge—should not be treated as if it were an intellectual accomplishment. The fact that self-knowledge is more like a skill than like information brings us back to Aristotle's notion of a virtue—the habitual doing of the right thing for the right reasons, supported by the right emotions. My definition of humility emphasizes this last aspect with the phrase "to be at ease with one's mistakes and flaws." Clearly ease cannot mean indifference. On the contrary, unless one feels something like sadness about one's limitations, one has not seen them for what they are, and the degree of sadness (and related emotions) should match the seriousness of the flaw. What is meant here by "being at ease" is not indifference but something subtler. It is an emotional condition that recognizes and responds to one's failings *in such a way that the self regains harmony and finds strength* and hence is less likely to fail in the same way in the future.

The ease spoken of here is not separate from recognition but part of what makes it possible. It might seem that we often recognize and hate our inadequacies, so that ease is not essential to self-knowledge. It should be obvious, however, that such hatred is likely to interfere with clear sight. Here as elsewhere pain and fear interfere with understanding. Patients who are told that they are terminally ill generally hear nothing else for a while: they may not even fully take in what they have been told. Students can freeze when called on or during exams. Most of us who write professionally have sometimes reacted to unfavorable reviews with a sort of blindness; a month later we can reread the comments and understand what was hidden by a haze of pain in the first reading.

The ordinary fact that pain blinds is often not recognized or taken seriously. Part of the reason, perhaps, is the truth in the proverb, "Once bitten, twice shy." Sometimes pain is instructive. We *do* learn quickly to avoid simple sources of severe pain. But most sources are not simple; the various causes of mistakes are not simple. Leape points out some of these causes; the cause might be lack of knowledge or a flawed system (too few doctors, too little sleep, too-similar labels on bottles). The problem might be the way the human mind works, setting up routines, responding to certain cues. Sometimes—and here I go beyond Leape—the cause is more personal: inattention to detail, an inner blind spot, a mistake in establishing priorities. When we ask, "Why didn't I recognize this pattern, or listen to this patient; why did I rely on a single test?" useful answers demand a lot of thought. Learning from the answers—changing one's behavior in the future—takes still more. While a burnt child can avoid the stove, the sources of mistakes are not so concrete. They cannot simply be avoided. Some of them, in fact, are unchangeable. So while clinicians' fear may make them want to avoid mistakes, it may also keep them from dealing with the mistakes they make.

In another sense, however, the proverbial stove is relevant after all. Most of us cannot put our hands on a hot burner; we cannot force ourselves into such pain. For someone without the humility described here, recognizing one's own faults may be as searing as a physical burn. Because there are degrees of pain, probably different in different domains, someone may be fully cognizant of some faults, perhaps be preoccupied and weighted down by them; that person may have other faults that he or she cannot afford even to acknowledge.

Clarity about oneself, then, demands not only skills of introspection but also a fundamental enabling attitude that might be called compassion toward oneself. Compassion is made up of an understanding that suffering is inevitable and of a simple sort of kindness. Because too much pain can interfere with self-knowledge, and compassion eases that pain, it follows that compassion *toward oneself* is an essential component of clear sight about oneself.

This treatment of compassion helps contrast the approach presented in this essay with Richards's approach. When he discusses compassion, it is as concern for the suffering of others; his only comment about concern for self is that it can be inordinate and block our recognition that others are worse off. As true as that is, it is superficial. It does not distinguish various ways in which one might be concerned about oneself, and various reasons for the self-absorption. Richards suggests that compassion is simply a matter of recognizing the proper proportion between one's own problems and those of others. In contrast, my point is that a sense of proportion is a consequence of more important things at the heart of humility, especially compassion toward oneself and skills of introspection. The self-absorption that Richards criticizes may be an overestimation of one's importance, as he suggests; paradoxically, however, it may also result from inadequate compassion toward oneself. It may be a fascination with what one cannot turn away from, because it is so unsettling.

My central claim—that a morally appropriate understanding of one's strengths and weaknesses depends upon certain attitudes toward oneself—is not unusual. Buddhists, psychotherapists, and many others take similar positions. For Buddhists, "loving-kindness" toward oneself (and others) is itself a skill, not just, as in my account, a condition for self-knowledge. For thousands of years Buddhists have practiced a guided meditation that fosters this attitude toward oneself, gradually expanding to include others. "The quality of *loving-kindness* is the fertile soil out of which an integrated spiritual life can grow. With a loving heart as the background, all that we attempt, all that we encounter, will open and flow more easily."[16] In contrast, the literature of psychotherapy treats self-love as an emotional configuration that results from either adequate parenting or good counseling. It speaks of redoing parenting, of modeling an attitude of acceptance that the client did not sufficiently encounter as a child and that, over time, he or she will internalize. Psychologist Cynthia Morgan reports that early in therapy clients may be unable to entertain the slightest suggestion of having done wrong; later, as they learn self-acceptance, such discussions become easier. In "The Fragility of the Moral Self: Self-Love and Morality," Laurence Thomas sums up the childhood experiences taken to be crucial: "the experience of others taking delight in [one's] accomplishments," learning that what one does matters, "that [one's] life has value independent of performances and physical appearances."[17] Note that the causal framework assumed—inadequate parenting—

is being vigorously debated.[18] We may eventually find that what forms us and what heals us are more diverse—that some causal factors, for instance, are cultural (think of the ways in which racism, sexism, constant competition, and an emphasis on beauty and youth make self-love difficult). We may learn that peers are more important than parents. We will probably find that genes are significant (but not straitjackets: genes usually make things more or less likely rather than inevitable). And we will probably recognize that emotional suffering, like physical suffering, can sometimes be healed by techniques whose theoretical grounding is misunderstood.

These are empirical issues, of course. They are mentioned as preparation for the argument that compassion toward oneself is a *moral* quality. Current controversies about child development are liberating. In suggesting different accounts of the self and its formation, they free us to take different stances toward the result.

COMPASSION TOWARD THE SELF
AS A MORAL ATTRIBUTE

In addition to being necessary for self-knowledge, compassion toward oneself is in itself a morally good quality; it helps make up humility, rather than simply being a means toward it. The argument presented here differs with one aspect of Laurence Thomas's paper on a similar subject. Because so much of what he says parallels my position here, our differences are particularly revealing.

Let me begin by outlining the points on which we agree. Thomas argues: "Persons with self-love value themselves appropriately; they are not disposed to undervalue themselves or their accomplishments, or to think more of themselves than the circumstances warrant."[19] Self-love makes a moral life possible; its absence explains certain kinds of immorality. According to Thomas, "Persons without a full measure of self-love will be much more easily threatened."[20] A moral life demands a clear sense of other people—their needs, their abilities, their trustworthiness, and so on. "Feelings of inadequacy can get in the way. A person with a very low opinion of himself will often be too consumed by his own inadequacies"[21] to see others clearly.

In spite of this general similarity, Thomas's position and mine diverge, sometimes in subtle, sometimes in fundamental ways. The most subtle difference is in terminology. Where he uses "self-love," I use "compassion for the self." *Love,* appropriate only towards what is good, emphasizes the intrinsic worth of the self. *Compassion* is a richer word—one that not only marks the worth of the self, but also calls to mind the suffering and limitations intrinsic to it. Compassion is more useful (and probably more feasible) as we gaze upon our flawed selves. Thomas and I may also differ about the moral status of how one treats oneself. He seems to share the blind spot found in much of contemporary moral theory.[22] At least he talks only about the importance of self-love for taking *others* seriously. He recognizes that one can fail to love oneself, but does not talk about the moral cost of not taking oneself seriously. Our most fundamental difference, however, is about the role of emotion in ethics. On this point Thomas is Kantian: "It is reason that tells each individual that she, herself, has intrinsic moral worth; and it is reason that informs her that all other persons likewise have intrinsic moral worth."[23] As a result, self-love can only be a *precursor* to morality, not a constituent of it. Self-love is a necessary condition for the right working of moral reasoning.

I think we will be better served by thinking of self-love—or rather, of compassion toward oneself—as a constituent of morality. One reason we shy away from granting the emotions moral status is that some of our understanding of morality confines it to that over which we have control—that is, our choices. But Bernard Williams and Thomas Nagel have pointed out inconsistencies within that tradition: there seems to be an irreducible element of luck in our moral standing.[24] In fact, the point of Thomas's article is to describe still another way in which our moral status is not directly within our own control. (His title, "The Fragility of the Moral Self," echoes Martha Nussbaum's *The Fragility of Goodness*, a work reminding us of what the Greeks understood about moral contingency.) I have argued elsewhere that the felt necessity to tie moral status solely to a person's choices derives in part from concepts of a just and judging God.[25] If we broaden our understanding of morality to that which is admirable and that which should be emulated—to the ideals that should guide our childrearing and policy making—it is easy to see that we want not just people who choose rightly but those whose selves are integrated with those choices (that is, people who need not struggle against their emotions and need not rethink each situation as it arises). As Justin Oakley has argued, emotions "help constitute or undermine such central human goods as understanding, strength of will, psychic harmony, love and friendship, and a sense of self-worth."[26] As I have described it here, compassion for oneself does just that.

Furthermore, as many have argued recently, our emotions are to some extent ways of knowing, and part of what it means to value something.[27] Compassion is a way of knowing and of valuing a self that is at once priceless and flawed. It is not just a precursor of morality; it is part of a fully moral self. It is part of many virtues; in particular, it is part of humility.

This analysis helps with some of the points philosophers have found puzzling. First, why should we call humility, defined as clarity about oneself, virtuous? Norvin Richards gives three reasons: a person who is clear about his or her own merits and demerits will be more ready to forgive others, will have better judgment about others, and will have reasonable expectations of him or herself.[28] Since these are good things, the trait that produces them, he reasons, is probably also good. Philosophers who deal with "modesty" rather than "humility" ground the former's goodness in a recognition of the equal moral worth of all human beings. Richards's explanation gives humility only an instrumental value. Philosophers of modesty rest their arguments on a debatable claim about necessary conditions for the trait. The position defended in this essay gives humility intrinsic moral value. It is the ability to look inward with clarity and ease. A virtue is an excellence, a perfection, and a strength: humility is all of these things.

I can now explain some intuitions presented earlier in this paper. First, humility is not so much a matter of accurately assessing one's comparative worth as something simpler and deeper; a person with humility is just not interested in these comparisons. Compassion and loving kindness toward oneself eliminate the need to seek rank through comparisons.[29] Second, I agree with the rabbinic tradition that humility adds savor to all human relationships. Humility as I have presented it here is an inner balance. Without it we will in various ways clutch and strike out at others. With it, we are free to see and value others as they are, neither desperate for their support nor distraught at the threat they may pose.

In summary, humility is a form of self-knowledge that essentially demands compassion toward oneself. Because self-knowledge is not primarily an intellectual activity but more like a skill, because it is part of a complex of attitudes that crucially includes self-love, and because it is a learned ability to look peacefully within and properly value what is seen—for all these reasons humility counts as a virtue. It is a disposition to recognize and respond readily to what is of value, just as courage is the disposition to recognize and respond when good things are in danger. Humility is a virtue that allows us not only to see our mistakes, but simultaneously to live with them and try to minimize them.

FOSTERING THE VIRTUE

Virtues are learned within a community. What sort of community best fosters humility? In answering that question, we will finally be able to unite the disparate approaches of David Hilfiker and Lucian Leape, the authors whose works were cited earlier in this essay. Both men want medicine to become a profession in which errors can be more easily acknowledged—Leape for the sake of patients (because errors will be fewer), Hilfiker for the sake of doctors (who need healthier and more honest ways to deal with their mistakes). Leape's critics worry about lessening a sense of personal responsibility. My analysis suggests that these three concerns—about errors, emotional health, and personal responsibility—are satisfied when a community encourages humility, a virtue that includes compassion toward oneself as part of candor about oneself. A community that fosters these attitudes is healthier and safer, as well as more moral.

What can be done to help promote such an environment? At Michigan State University, Tom Tomlinson has taken interesting steps in that direction. He has developed a course entitled "Ethics, Policy, and Law" for the College of Osteopathic Medicine, the final unit of which deals with error in medicine. Students read and hear three perspectives on the issue: First, a lawyer clarifies the so-called malpractice crisis, providing some balance to the exaggerated picture so common among clinicians. Then a risk manager provides a systems perspective on error. Each of these presentations is framed by relevant readings, including those of Leape. But the cornerstone of the unit, indeed of the course, is the week's final event—one that may be unique in medical education. During a two-hour panel, three or four physicians discuss mistakes they have made. Each describes an incident or two in detail, including his or her feelings about it; each talks about ways of dealing with mistakes once they are recognized. This year, for instance, one panelist said: "You have to go to confession. You may want to tell the family or patient, or you may not, but you must tell someone. It provides you with emotional release and with perspective. Sometimes you will discover that the outcome was unavoidable; on the other hand, you may find things are worse than you thought. But at least you will know. And you may be able to get help from your 'confessor' about how to avoid the same mistake in the future." The background reading for this session is Hilfiker's "Facing Our Mistakes."[30]

The panel is not always successful. Physicians are selected carefully, and even then there is no certainty about what will happen. Some physicians on the panel avoid the question, usually by describing a bad outcome that could not have been prevented, for example, an autopsy shows that the wrong diagnosis was made, but no one could have known the real facts while the patient was alive. Another avoidance strategy is talking about uncooperative patients or incompetent colleagues. This (unconscious) resistance is a sign of the strength of the barriers to openness within medicine. Experience indicates that it is helpful to choose a moderator who has been a panelist; he has the standing to prod the panelists who are avoiding the real subject. The sessions are moving, and are helpful to the presenters as well as to the audience.

The panel, of course, is only one small step toward an improved medical culture—toward a profession that encourages humility, as I have described it here. Hilfiker's self-disclosures, Leape's model systems, innovative education, further analyses of the virtues involved—all these and more will help bring the better climate that Hilfiker and Leape so eloquently, if so differently, urge us to create. Steps like these will help nurses, doctors, and therapists find the composure and the clarity to deal well with mistakes—to see them, minimize them, and yet live with them.

NOTES

1. L.L. Leape, "Error in Medicine," *Journal of the American Medical Association* 272 (21 December 1994): 1857. [Leape's article is reprinted as chapter 7 of this book—ED.]

2. D. Hilfiker, *Healing the Wounds* (New York: Penguin, 1987), 85.

3. I have heard such reactions from students and other audiences. C. Bosk takes issue with Leape along somewhat similar lines in his essay "Margin of Error: The Sociology of Ethics Consultation," printed as chapter 17 of this book.

4. D. Hume, *A Treatise of Human Nature* (Oxford, England: Clarendon Press, 1967), book 3, pt. 3, Sec. 2, p. 598.

5. N. Richards, *Humility* (Philadelphia: Temple University Press, 1992), xii.

6. A. Ben Ze'ev, "The Virtue of Modesty," *American Philosophical Quarterly* 30 (1993): 235-46; S. Hare, "The Paradox of Moral Humility," *American Philosophical Quarterly* 33 (1996): 235-40. Hare looks at the further paradox of knowing that one is morally superior to another (more honest, generous, just, or whatever). He resolves the paradox by arguing that although one may act more morally, one's intrinsic worth as deserving of moral treatment from others remains equal.

7. N. Richards, "Humility," *Encyclopedia of Ethics,* ed. L.C. Becker and C.B. Becker (New York: Garland, 1992).

8. Richards seems to be unaware of how close his own discussion is to contemporary Christian perspectives. Even 40 years ago the Catholic schools I attended laid little emphasis on medieval texts about worthlessness, and a great deal on what Richards now calls "accurate self-assessment."

9. R. Green, "Jewish Ethics and the Virtue of Humility," *Journal of Religious Ethics* 1 (1973): 54.

10. Ibid., 56.

11. Ibid.

12. Interestingly, when Green goes on to ask what might make this attribute morally good from a secular point of view, he turns to the same egalitarianism emphasized by the other philosophers mentioned here. Referring to Rawls's contractarianism, Green writes: "The whole enterprise of moral reasoning involves an abandonment of the knowledge of one's particular strengths and excellences in order to enter, *as one human being among others* [emphasis added], into the procedure of moral choice." Because of the constraints of Rawls's "original position," one would also "pay particular attention to the effect [of principles endorsed] on the poor and disadvantaged" (pp. 59, 61).

13. Others, of course, would argue that we cannot surpass the wisdom found in ordinary language, worked out as it has been over centuries and over millions of lives. That is a very strong claim. I believe instead only that we should pay the most serious attention to ordinary usage and to a word's history, but that we are not always and necessarily bound to accept the distinctions and values it encodes. The other objection that could be made is that philosophical attempts to redefine a word rarely work; language has a life of its own. As true as that is, some self-conscious attempts to reform language *have* worked: "woman" is now used symmetrically with "man," and "he" is rarely used today when "he or she" is meant. As noted earlier, Richards's reformative attempts are scholarly version of some 20th-century religious treatments of humility.

14. This is slightly paradoxical because the Greek and Hebrew traditions are in many ways quite different, and—since both are very important sources of contemporary Euro-American culture—contrasting them can be enlightening.

15. A classic source is L. Wittgenstein, *Lectures and Conversations on Aesthetics, Psychology and Religious Belief,* ed. C. Barrett (Berkeley: University of California Press, 1967).

16. J. Kornfield, *A Path with Heart: A Guide through the Perils of Promises of Spiritual Life* (New York: Bantam Books, 1993), 19-21.

17. L. Thomas, "The Fragility of the Moral Self: Self-Love and Morality," (working paper distributed by the Poynter Center, Indiana University, 1997).

18. M. Gladwell, "Do Parents Matter?" *New Yorker,* 17 August 1998, 54-64.

19. See note 17 above, p. 6.

20. Ibid., 4

21. Ibid., 6

22. See J. Andre, "The Equal Moral Weight of Self- and Other-Regarding Acts," *Canadian Journal of Philosophy* 17, no. 1 (March 1987): 155-65.

23. See note 17 above, p. 11.

24. T. Nagel, *Mortal Questions* (Cambridge, England: Cambridge University Press, 1979); B. Williams, *Moral Luck* (New York: Cambridge University Press, 1981).

25. The point is that a just God could not punish or reward us for things we could not help doing and being. See J. Andre, "Nagel, Williams, and Moral Luck," *Analysis* 43, no. 4 (October 1983): 202-7.

26. J. Oakley, *Morality and the Emotions* (New York: Routledge 1992), 78.

27. An excellent recent example is M. Stocker's "How Emotions Reveal Value," in *How Should One Live? Essays on the Virtues,* ed. R. Crisp (Oxford, England: Clarendon Press, 1996), 173-90.

28. See note 5 above, p. 18.

29. I owe this insight to an article on a trait similar to humility whose Italian name seems to defy translation: *la mitezza.* Although the author translates it as "meekness," "gentleness" seemed to me closer. N. Bobbio, "In Praise of La Mitezza," *Diogenes* (English edition) 44, no. 4 (Winter 1996): 3-38.

30. D. Hilfiker, "Facing Our Mistakes," *New England Journal of Medicine* 310, no. 2 (1984): 118-22. [Hilfiker's article is reprinted as chapter 6 of this book—ED.]

5

Mistakes in Context

John D. Lantos and Martha Montello

INTRODUCTION

Periodically, in our ethics consultation conferences, a question arises regarding mistakes and truth-telling. Should doctors tell patients every time they make a mistake? The cases are almost always interestingly ambiguous. The mistakes can be either minuscule but symbolically important, or catastrophic and irreversible. Often it is not clear who made the mistake or whether the mistake caused the bad outcome. The events create a sort of narrative angst. We do not like the story that is being told. There is tension but no resolution. Doctors are behaving badly, acting like there is a cover-up.

It is never clear, although always crucial, what the patient would want to hear or know. One view is that patients clearly want to be informed of all errors and have the right to be informed. The other view is that, at least for some errors, patients might be better off not knowing—just as airline passengers might be better off not knowing about a near miss that didn't hurt them, and about which there is nothing they can do.

The articulate, informed, and empowered sorts of people who tend to speak up at ethics consultation conferences all say, in the cozy comfort of the conference room, that they would certainly want to be told about mistakes if and as they happen. But it is unclear whether they really know what they are asking for. Researchers have found that, in the average intensive care unit (ICU), there are three or four mistakes per patient per shift.[1] Most of the mistakes are minor, some are serious, and some cause major consequences. All are identifiable as events where something was done wrong that could and should have been done better. So when we ask, "When you are in the ICU, do you really want to hear about every one of these mistakes?" people start thinking about other situations in life where we do not always get the whole truth. (Do we really want to know that the pilot has made a little error, flying at 31,000 when he should have been at 33,000? Do we really want to know that the chef forgot to put the bay leaf in the sauce?) Things start to get a little more complex. What is a mistake, anyway? What does disclosure really accomplish?

Medicine is a particularly complex area in which to define error because medicine is a particularly complex area in which to define perfection. It is hard to say, in a given situation, what "ideal" practice would have been, and so it may be hard to say how far from ideal any deviation might be. There may also be standards that incorporate complex social realities that we find uncomfortable but must grudgingly acknowledge; for example, a patient in a managed-care organization may be offered a different set of interventions than a patient with indemnity insurance. A patient in a small town may get different care than a patient in a big city. There are well-documented differences in the treatment of patients of different race, gender, age, or social class. We suspect that these differences reflect less-than-perfect treatment for one group or another, but we do not precisely define what constitutes an error, a mistake, or negligence.

All cultures make moral rules. Those rules define ideals and perfection on the one hand, and deviation or negligence on the other. We latch onto categories of right action and mistakes. The rules flow from our tendency to categorize. That tendency is not limited only to "cultures" in the anthropologic sense, but applies equally to subcultures, tribes, professions, religions, and moral and legal systems. Each social aggregate constructs its own specific normative hierarchy. Each has its own rules about who can or cannot, under certain circumstances, kill one another, have sex with one another, or exploit, be cruel to, or neglect one another.

We all live within a system of rules in which the dependency upon context becomes almost invisible. We lose the sense that our rules are simply our rules and that, more importantly, our rules are the grid, the background, the metric against which our judgments take place. With one part of our postmodern minds we know—as certainly as we know anything—that ours is but one culture, our rules but one set of rules; we are as tolerant of differences as any people could ever be. But with another part of our minds, we remain resolutely premodern, holding to certain moral certainties that we not only see as the bedrock of morality for ourselves but are willing to impose on others with all the evangelistic zeal of any religious missionary. As Americans, these bedrock values include respect for the individual as the indivisible locus of morality, which leads to derivative faith in things such as informed consent, democracy, and free markets. We are as blind to, as dependent upon, and as unquestioning of the culture-specific rules, boundaries, conventions, and taboos of our place and time as any Azande, Hopi, or Trobriand Islander.

THE CULTURAL RITUAL OF TORT LITIGATION

Medicine, too, is a moral and cultural system. It is embedded in the larger moral system of our political and economic culture in complex ways that include concepts of entitlement, human rights, professional obligations, contractual constraints, and negligence. In the United States, some of the ongoing work of keeping medicine firmly embedded in culture is accomplished through our system of tort litigation. This system incorporates a set of assumptions, presumptions, methodologies, and arcana that allow actions to be morally classified so that judgments can be rendered. By and through this system, we decide what should or should not count as an error or as a mistake. The judgments that are reached by the creaky machinery of the tort system are recognizably and almost proudly idiosyncratic. We know, for instance, that huge awards are made in many cases where impartial experts find no negligence and that, in most cases of known negligence, no awards are made.[2]

The system of tort litigation has about it the air of a mysterious lottery, ensconced at the center of a set of mechanisms and procedures that purport to be rational, accountable, and nonrandom. We pour money into the system for a set of activities that is loosely termed "discovery," and that is even more loosely conceptualized as a process of "fact finding." All of the players involved act as if the goal of the process is to discover the truth about what really happened, even though the procedures for discovering the truth are notoriously funky and arcane. That is part of the ritual, too. And, with the postmodern part of our minds, we recognize it as ritual, even though, when we are involved in it, it seems not just real but hyperreal. The end of the ritual can be to send a man to jail, to kill someone, or to impeach a president.

The ritual is real. It is just not real in the sense that the ritual actors must pretend to believe what they are saying. They do believe it, if only for that moment. When we observe, as outsiders, the rituals of other cultures, we are often surprised by the seeming gullibility of the "primitive" peoples. Do they really believe that when the witch doctor puts on a mask he becomes a god? And yet we believe that when a jury renders a verdict, it has acted with God-like authority. Or that when the doctor makes a mistake, the mistake caused the patient's death. And we are willing to punish people severely, even put people to death, based on the pronouncements of juries in these matters. We suspend disbelief at the same time that we bring our sophisticated skepticism to bear on the process, because we believe, as a culture, that there is such a thing as right and wrong, or that it is important to live as if there were.

One reading of such rituals is that they do not only "discover" the truth but that they also "construct" it. That view is too simple. Such rituals neither construct a truth out of whole cloth nor discover it somewhere out there in the universe, like a comet or a quark. Instead, they order and contextualize events into particular narrative truths. The function of the rituals is to take events that are frightening or disconcerting—for example, a patient who was doing well suddenly died—and to reshape them as part of a larger story that is less frightening or disconcerting. When these rituals work, both the event and the story make more sense than they did before. Put another way, they bring the conventional wisdom of the time to bear on the particular events that seem to disturb that conventional wisdom; and they create a culture-specific harmony between foreground and background, between event and context, between individuals and their culture.

A number of our institutional rituals for identifying, classifying, and responding to mistakes in medicine have this harmonizing function. The quality assurance approach seeks to compare healthcare by analogy to other sorts of activities or enterprises—the assembly-line production of cars or computers, or the routine maintenance of airplane engines—in which we have found ways to reduce errors. The analogy does not entirely work, for many interesting reasons and in many interesting ways. But it does work as ritual. We feel better, in certain ways, knowing that hospitals have committees to ensure that they will achieve continuous quality improvement and that, unless they do, the accreditors will notice and close them down.

The medical malpractice approach imagines an ideal world in which all care is perfect, or at least perfectible. That state of perfection is known as "the standard of care." It is thought that all doctors should achieve this standard. In the ritual, then, we identify cases in which care has fallen short of this standard, and we elaborately sacrifice the professionals who negligently allowed it to happen. The elaborate grandeur and formality of the ritual strengthens and preserves the illusion that these are rare and exceptional cases; that we spare no expense to find them; that we punish those responsible swiftly and severely; and that, as a result, whatever else happens in medical care is natural, normal, acceptable, and standard.

The foreground is defined by the background. The concept of mistake only makes sense against a context of nonmistake. In some cases, this dynamic is straightforward. If the surgeon meant to amputate the right leg but amputated the left instead, or if the internist meant to prescribe morphine but gave digoxin instead, there is little interpretation necessary. But these are the easy ones. The tougher ones, such as decisions about whether to tell the truth, or about whether whole classes of activities that are routine ought to be questioned, require a deeper analysis of the relationship between foreground events and background assumptions. This sort of analysis has been largely missing from the literature on mistakes in medicine.

How do we know, then, when the rituals for identifying and judging error are themselves in error? Because our sense of what constitutes a mistake is itself contingent upon the mores and rituals that define the larger cultural story, we can recognize and begin to evaluate mistakes only if we tell the smaller story and the larger story at the same time. This double action is precisely what most mechanisms for identifying and responding to errors cannot perform, because these mechanisms exist and make sense only in the context of the particular background cultural story of which they are a subplot.

TWO TYPES OF MORAL NARRATIVE

One area of inquiry that seeks a double-tracked appreciation of the complexity of judgments about right and wrong is literary fiction. Certain fictional narratives use the tension between the intracultural judgments of a specific time or place, on the one hand, and the implicit, presumably superior, judgments of the differently situated reader, on the other, to provide forward motion to the narrative and also to focus its moral message. These works appeal to us as readers in part for the way they imply that we are superior, in perception and discernment, to the characters about whom we are reading. But the works are also implicitly critical. Well-drawn characters more often than not resonate with readers. We are more like them than not; we could be them. There but for the grace of the author go we.

These narratives can play out in one of two ways. In one, the protagonist is a sympathetic character who defies the culture in which he lives. He is thus a renegade, but a renegade whose rebellion against the cultural norms of the time is made in terms that make it clear to the reader that he is right and his culture is wrong. In the other sort of narrative, the protagonist is an unsympathetic character who adheres to the cultural norms of the time and place. In his adherence, he represents for the differently situated reader an example of the dangers of conformist complacency. This form of narrative works when it forces us, as readers, to realize that the character is morally flawed, an example of what we should not be or become.

One of the best examples of the first sort of narrative is Mark Twain's novel, *The Adventures of Huckleberry Finn*.[3] Rendering one of the greatest fictional confrontations of misguided abstract principle with concrete lived experience, Twain portrays Huck's dilemma of whether to deliver Jim, an escaped slave, to freedom. In the context of pre–Civil War southern culture, his actions would clearly be wrong, and Huck knows it. Yet he is conflicted because the decision to help Jim feels intuitively right. Floating on their raft, heading down the Mississippi toward Cairo, Illinois, where the Mississippi joins with the Ohio River and where Jim will go ashore into free territory, Huck begins to agonize over whether he is doing the right thing.

Jim said it made him all over trembly and feverish to be so close to freedom. Well, I can tell you it made me all over trembly and feverish, too, to hear him, because I begun to get it through my head that he was most free and who was to blame for it? Why, me. I couldn't get that out of my conscience, no how nor no way. It got to troubling me so I couldn't rest; I couldn't stay still in one place. It hadn't ever come home to me before, what this thing was that I was doing. But now it did; and it stayed with me, and scorched me more and more. I tried to make out to myself that I warn't to blame, because I didn't run Jim off from his rightful owner; but it warn't no use, conscience up and says, every time, "But you knowed he was running for his freedom, and you could 'a' paddled ashore and told somebody." That was so I couldn't get around that no way. That was where it pinched.[4]

In one of the most widely known literary assaults on the norms dictated by allegiance to public morality—and particularly official Christianity—Huck comprehends that he is committing a grievous sin by helping Jim escape to freedom. His "good heart," as Twain calls it, does battle with his "conscience"—in reality the destructive moral system bred by a culture of slavery.

"The more I studied about this," thinks Huck, "the more my conscience went to grinding me, and the more wicked and low-down and onery I got to feeling. And at last, when it hit me all of a sudden that here was the plain hand of Providence slapping me in the face and letting me know my wickedness was being watched all the time from up there in heaven, whilst I was stealing a poor old woman's nigger that hadn't ever done me no harm, and now was showing me that there's One that's always on the lookout, and ain't agoing to allow no such miserable doings to go only just so fur and no further, I most dropped in my tracks. . . . Well, I tried the best I could to kinder soften it up somehow for myself, by saying I was brung up wicked, and so I wurn't so much to blame; but something inside of me kept saying, "There was the Sunday school, you could a gone to it; and if you'd a done it they'd a learnt you there, that people that acts as I'd been acting about that nigger goes to everlasting fire." It made me shiver. And I about made up my mind to pray; and see if I couldn't try to quit being the kind of boy I was, and be better. So I kneeled down. But the words wouldn't come. Why wouldn't they? It warn't no use to try and hide it from Him. Nor from *me* neither. I knowed very well why they wouldn't come. It was because my heart warn't right; it was because I warn't square; it was because I was playing double.[5]

Huck's complex set of moral considerations reflects the culture in which he has been raised, with its economic, moral, and religious systems and understandings about right and wrong. Having internalized those understandings, his "conscience" recognizes that turning Jim in is the right thing to do. But the scene's crucial choice reverses the traditional religious injunction to eschew his natural impulses and to rely on accepted moral rules, and yields instead the message that he has nothing but the truth of his inner feelings to guide him now. At the critical moment, a moral force he can scarcely articulate compels him to honor his friendship with Jim, with its own obligations that outweigh the moral dictates of his culture.

At last I struck the time I saved him and he was so grateful, and said I was the best friend old Jim ever had in the world, and the only one he's got now; and then I happened to look around, and see that paper [the letter offering to sell Jim]. It was a close place. I took it up, and held it in my hand. I was a trembling, because I'd got to decide, forever, betwixt two things. I studied a minute, sort of holding my breath, and then says to myself: "All right, then, I'll go to hell."[6]

For Huck, the experience of choosing to honor his allegiance to Jim, to reject the cultural norms that dictated that he should turn Jim in, has shifted his basis for making moral decisions. The reader has the clear sense that Huck will no longer struggle in the same way to decipher what constitutes a mistake. Cultural norms no longer hold the weight they did with him. He declares, "So, I reckoned I wouldn't bother no more about it, but after this always do whichever come handiest at the time."[7]

Wrapped in some of Twain's finest irony, Huck seems to believe that he's simply given up trying to figure out the whole right/wrong problem, commenting that he would feel bad with either decision he made and saying: "What's the use you learning to do right when it's troublesome to do right and ain't no trouble to do wrong, and the wages is just the same?"[8] But his understanding that the issue is now settled for him and his resolution henceforth "to do what is handiest at the time" tips his hand. The reader comprehends the importance of the word *handiest*—with its truest meaning located beyond mere "convenience" and closer to "close by," "close at hand"—the language mirroring the way he has come to his moral choice. By choosing his friendship with Jim—close at hand, tangible, and based in the commitments of personal relationship over time—as a greater good and a more compelling obligation than his duty to the abstract principles of social norms, he has established a basis for moral response that is consistent with his own character. A hands-on, practical morality that works for him.

As Antigone struggled with her decision to bury her dead brother over the prohibitions of her society and as Dimmesdale agonized before he knew he must repudiate his religious culture to acknowledge his commitment to Hester in *The Scarlet Letter,* Huck has discovered what it means to make a moral decision when the very culture he exists in is itself in error.

To a certain extent, the American gangster movie genre conveys this same theme. The heroes of *Bonnie and Clyde* and *Butch Cassidy and the Sundance Kid* are "wrong" to do what they do—rob banks, murder people, and so forth. But, implicitly, the banks are even more wrong. There is a larger injustice or error or transgression that exists embedded in the context, so that the smaller injustice seems to be the lesser of two evils. Don Corleone, in *The Godfather,* is the protector and benefactor of the helpless Italian-Americans, who cannot get justice from the corrupt system of American law. He is a deeply moral man—caring for his family and his community. And, as part of his morality, he must sometimes kill. But in this, the movie argues, he is no different from a government official, a congressman or senator, who also must sometimes make decisions to kill others, even innocents, in the service of a larger good. The romantic hagiography of the gangster boss draws us in. We identify with him and his struggles, even though, in general, we do not condone organized crime as moral force in society. He is, some basic way, a villainous, good man.

Modern literature is also replete with conventionally virtuous villains, fatally flawed by their unreflective adherence to immoral social norms or by their blindness to true but unconventional goodness. *Huckleberry Finn*'s Miss Watson, Jim's owner and a dutiful Christian, is the prototype in her determination to "live so as to go to the good place." This second form of narration, in which the protagonist is discovered by the reader to be fatally morally flawed but nevertheless demanding of our sympathies, finds its full expression in Kazuo Ishiguro's novel, *The Remains of the Day.*[9]

The narrative's protagonist, Stevens, is a butler working for a wealthy British family in the 1930s, on the eve of World War II. The scion of a long line of butlers, he takes his job seriously, aspiring to be the perfect butler, who discharges his duties with equanimity, with aplomb. He is not dispassionate, but his passions are all channeled into the icy facade of pure and unruffled competence that is the highest achievement of the butler's art. In a scene that perfectly portrays his character, the reader sees him working at a dinner party while his father is dying in an upstairs bedroom. He conquers his natural filial inclination to empathy, his nearly overwhelming desire to be with his father, and continues to perform his professional duties with precision. The novel's dramatic tension derives from the author's assumption that the reader will find the butler's heartless control while his father is dying to be morally problematic, even despicable. Few readers fail to perceive that the butler's idea of virtue is itself a repudiation of virtue.

Much later, after World War II has come and gone, after the estate has been sold to an American, after all notions of the excellent butler have virtually disappeared from the culture, the protagonist goes looking for some center of his life, seeking out a woman with whom he was once in love and to whom he almost once confessed of his love. His world is falling apart. There is no place for him or his kind. On the journey, he is confronted with the ugly truth about his former employer; he had been a sympathizer with the Nazis, had entertained several of them in his home, and had tried to facilitate an alliance between the British and Nazi governments.

In a climactic scene in the novel, the butler is working one evening when Herr Ribbentrop, the German Ambassador to England, is meeting with the Prime Minister. Stevens, the butler, is waiting on the dignitaries. A young cousin asks him whether he is concerned, embarrassed, or ashamed of his employer's actions in trying to broker an agreement with the Nazis. Stevens is not. That very same night, Miss Kenton, a maid for whom Stevens has shown some affection, tells him that she may be getting engaged and that, if she does, she will be leaving her current post. Stevens shows no emotion and, in his emotionlessness, drives Kenton to tears of anger and frustration. Taken together, these two events represent the breakdown of everything that Stevens believes in and holds dear—his professional life and his emotional life are about to crumble. He even senses it, for a moment, "At first, my mood was—I do not mind admitting it—somewhat downcast." But the mood passes. "I had, after all, just come through an extremely trying evening, throughout which I had managed to preserve a 'dignity in keeping with my position.' "[10] Stevens's emotional paralysis is shown to be the parallel of his political and intellectual paralysis. Our ease in condemning his emotional reserve helps us see how much more devastating his political apathy is.

Later, when asked about his own past, Stevens lies. He denies who he is and who he once worked for. In so doing, he implicitly acknowledges a vague awareness of the mistakes that he has made. But the reader recognizes that he has no real understanding of them. The reader comes to understand the insidious connection between a seemingly small complicity with evil and larger, universally recognized instance of monstrous evil. Providing a kind of moral dissonance, the tension between the butler's code of conduct and the presumed superior judgments of the differently situated reader renders an implicit critique of the prevailing culture.

NARRATIVE CONTEXT AND MEDICAL ERROR

What do these considerations have to do with a discussion of medical mistakes? In medicine, more than in most of life's arenas, we have a highly refined sense that we know what is right and what is wrong. Doctors encourage this sense, believing about themselves that they have practices, standards, and criteria for excellence that allow them to know that what they do is good. Interestingly, doctors have always had this sense, even when, as things turned out, what they were doing was wrong after all. And doctors have a way of dealing with that situation, also, in their tendency to see themselves as somehow more scientific, more perfect, than doctors of times past.

There is a hospital on the South Side of Chicago, where most of the patients are African-American. In the hospital's clinic for children with cystic fibrosis, there are a number of African-American patients. It used to be thought that cystic fibrosis did not occur in African-American patients. The story goes that the first case was discovered when a stupid medical student, who had not learned the demographics of the disease, ordered the diagnostic test for cystic fibrosis on an African-American patient with all the symptoms. If his attending physician had known, the student would have been condemned for the error. As it turned out, the student made the diagnosis, changed medical dogma, and saved a number of lives. We can only wonder how much of current dogma will go the same way.

At least since the early 19th century, there has been an implicit message of progress and perfectionism in medical discourse, a sense that we are getting better at knowing and understanding what works and what does not, why it works, how it works, and what constitutes a mistake. Most of this progress has been internal to medicine. That is, best practices and mistakes have both been defined by the profession and for the profession within the relatively rarefied context of professional discourse. There has been a sense that only doctors can judge other doctors—that decisions about what is right or wrong, good or bad, professional or inept are decisions about what a certain type of person with a particular type of training should do in a precisely defined context. The implicit assumptions of the training and the context often go unquestioned. Can a whole program of medical innovation be a mistake? Could we be wrong in thinking that curing certain diseases will make us healthier, happier, or better off? Can our emphasis on health as the supreme political good be a mistake?

The only way to approach such questions effectively is to recognize the version of the historical story that we tell—to see Huck or Stevens in context—and then to ask whether the story might be told a different way. We could then develop a critique of certain medical actions derived not from the sense that other doctors would have acted differently in similar circumstances but from a critique of the circumstances themselves. What might this critical exercise look like?

In his novel, *The House of God,* Samuel Shem imagines a topsy-turvy medical world in which the accepted dogma is all wrong, where nothing is what it seems, and where perfectly delivered medical care only has the effect of increasing the suffering of patients, while negligent care allows them to get better.[11] In Shem's novel, as in Twain's, everything that is supposed to be right turns out to be wrong. The climactic conversation occurs after one of Roy Basch's patients, Dr. Sanders, has just died of leukemia. Dr. Sanders' only wish was to die a painless death, but his death was horrible and deeply disturbing to Roy. Afterwards, Jo, the senior resident, wants Roy to get permission for a postmortem examination. She clearly views the death impersonally, as she does most of medical care—a dazzling scientific and technical achievement that has little to do with human interactions or human relationships. Roy refuses to seek permission for the examination, citing his loyalty to Sanders, loyalty that goes beyond the grave. When Jo questions him, Roy responds:

"I didn't want to see his body ripped to shreds in the morgue."

"That kind of talk has no place in modern medicine," Jo replies.

"So don't listen."

"The post-mortem is important. It is the flower of the science of medicine. . . . How do you think we're able to deliver such precise medical care to those entrusted to us? This ward—my ward—is looked up to in the House for being the most efficient and having the most successes with placement and handling the toughies with skill. My ward is a legend, dammit."

"Jo, go fuck yourself. . . . Do you want to know why it's become a legend? You don't want to hear."

"Of course I want to hear, even though I know already."

So I told her. I started by telling her about how Chuck and I had, after our original empirical test on Anna O, become fanatics at doing nothing and had lied to Jo about it, making up all forms of imaginary tests and buffing the charts. I told her how in modified form we'd done the same thing with the dying young, who went ahead and died, but died without the hassle, pain, and prolongation of suffering that their care might otherwise have produced.[12]

Drawing on the same dynamics that Twain used, Shem counts on the reader to negotiate the tension between Jo's view of medicine, which admires science, precision, and the pursuit of knowledge, and Roy's view, which calls for caring, compassion, and loyalty. On one level, we know that Roy and his mentor, the Fat Man, are wrong. They fail to follow the rules; refuse to order the correct diagnostic tests; and clearly do not follow practice guidelines, meet standards of care, or achieve the target goals of the continuous quality improvement monitors. They are distrusted by their superiors, as suggested by the following conversation between Roy and the chief of medicine:

"They have diseases and by God, we treat them: aggressively, objectively, completely, and we never give up."

"Well that's just it. . . . The more you do, the worse they get. When I tried it your way, they developed incredible complications. The best treatment for them is to do nothing."

"I don't understand. The Fat Man taught you that to deliver no medical care is the best thing you can do?"

"The Fat Man said that that was the delivery of medical care."

"To do nothing?"

"That's something."

"Ward 6-South is the best ward in the House. You mean to tell me it's from doing nothing?"

"That's doing something. We do as much nothing as we can without Jo finding out about it."

"But then why do doctors do anything at all?"
"The Fat Man says to produce complications."
"Why do doctors want to produce complications?"
"To make money."[13]

Parallels from compelling current dilemmas in medicine clarify the need for the double-tracked vision so well portrayed by authors such as Shem, Twain, and Ishiguro. One is the ongoing debate about euthanasia. Clearly, from one point of view, euthanasia is "wrong" today. That is to say, it is against the rules. However, some critics suggest that the rules themselves are wrong, and that doctors who refuse to provide euthanasia are as misguided by their obedience to immoral rules as any southern slaveholder. One could imagine a Huck Finn type of parable in which a clever but naïve doctor helps his patients to die, even though he knows it to be "wrong." Even more contentious and less obvious examples might include much of today's ICU care for extremely premature babies or for frail, elderly patients. Is such care a humanitarian ideal, or is it, as some authors have suggested, a bizarre form of torture? Is it altruistic or mercenary? Moral judgments about such matters, and thus about whether the doctors involved are making a mistake, cannot come from inside the profession or from examining particular cases; such judgements can come only from a view that examines both the case and the context, that critiques both our actions and our methods of criticizing our actions.

CONCLUSIONS AND DISCLAIMERS

One reading of this essay is that the authors are claiming that there is no such thing as right or wrong, that all moral norms and all medical events are so totally and inherently dependent upon context that judgment must be ever and always paralyzed. That would be an overreading. Instead, we are making the more modest claim that sometimes it is not enough to evaluate our actions and our moral beliefs within the frameworks that we have accepted. Often, when there is a true dilemma, it arises because the framework itself is weak. In those instances, a natural tendency is to shore up the framework, to emphasize its sturdiness and durability. Nothing is more dysphoric than watching a moral framework crumble. The moral narratives presented here suggest a different approach: sometimes, the only right thing to do is to question the framework; to help the slave escape; to subvert one's boss's meetings with a dangerous Nazi; or to lie to medical superiors, avoid providing standard medical care, and begin to ask soul-searching questions about what it means, really, to be a doctor.

NOTES

1. L.B. Andrews et al., "An Alternative Strategy for Studying Adverse Events in Medical Care," *Lancet* 349, no. 9048 (1 February 1997): 309-13.

2. T.A. Brennan, C.M. Sox, and H.R. Burstin, "Relation Between Negligent Adverse Events and the Outcomes of Medical-Malpractice Litigation," *New England Journal of Medicine* 335, no. 26 (1996): 1963-67.

3. M. Twain, *The Adventures of Huckleberry Finn* (New York: Modern Library, 1948).
4. Ibid., 181.
5. Ibid., 191.
6. Ibid., 223.
7. Ibid., 224.
8. Ibid.
9. K. Ishiguro, *The Remains of the Day* (New York: Vintage, 1988).
10. Ibid., 118.
11. S. Shem, *The House of God* (New York: Bantam Books, 1978).
12. Ibid., 164-5.
13. Ibid., 181-2.

Part 2

Error in Medical Practice

6

Facing Our Mistakes

David Hilfiker

Looking at the appointment book for July 12, 1978, I notice that Barb Daily will be in today for her first prenatal examination. "Wonderful," I think, remembering my joy as I helped her deliver her first child two years ago. Barb and her husband Russ are friends, and our relationship became much closer with the shared experience of that birth. With so much exposure to disease every day in my rural family practice, I look forward to today's appointment with Barb and to the continuing relationship over the next months.

Barb seems to be in good health with all the symptoms and signs of pregnancy, but her urine pregnancy test is negative. I reassure Barb and myself that she is fine and that the test just hasn't turned positive yet. Rescheduling another test for the following week, I congratulate her on her condition and promise to get all her test results to her promptly.

But the next urine test is negative, too, which leaves me troubled. Isn't Barb pregnant? Has she had a missed abortion? I could make sure right now, of course, by ordering an ultrasound, but the new examination is available only in Duluth, 110 miles away from our northern Minnesota village, and it is expensive. I am aware of the Dailys' modest income. Besides, by waiting a few weeks, I'll find out for sure without the ultrasound. I call Barb on the phone and tell her about the negative test, about the possible abortion, and about the necessity of a repeat appointment in a few weeks if her next menstrual period does not occur on schedule.

It is, as usual, a hectic summer, and I almost forget about Barb's situation until a month later when she returns. Still no menstrual period, no abortion. She is confused and upset, since, she says, "I feel so pregnant." I am bothered, too, especially because her uterus continues to be enlarged. Her urine test remains definitely negative.

I break the bad news to her. "I think you have a missed abortion. You were probably pregnant, but the baby appears to have died some weeks ago, before your first examination. Unfortunately, you didn't have the miscarriage to get rid of the dead tissue from the baby and the placenta. If a miscarriage does not occur within a few weeks, I'd recommend a reexamination, another pregnancy test, and if nothing shows up, a dilation and curettage to clean out the uterus."

Barb is disappointed and saddened: there are tears. Both she and Russ have sufficient background in science to understand the technical aspects of the situation, but that doesn't alleviate the sorrow. We talk in the office at some length and make an appointment for two weeks later.

When Barb returns, Russ is with her. Still no menstrual period, no miscarriage, and a negative pregnancy test. It is difficult, but it also feels right to be able to share in friends' sadness. Thoroughly reviewing the situation with both of them, I schedule the D and C for later in the week.

Friday morning, when Barb is wheeled into the operating room, we chat before she is put to sleep. The surgical nurses in our small hospital are all friends, too, so the atmosphere is warm and relaxed. After induction of anesthesia, I examine Barb's pelvis. To my hands, the uterus now seems bigger than it had two days previously, but since all the pregnancy tests were negative, the uterus couldn't have grown. I continue the operation.

But this morning there is considerably more blood than usual, and it is only with great difficulty that I am able to extract any tissue. The body parts I remove are much larger than I had expected, considering when the fetus died, and they are not the decomposing tissue I'd anticipated. These are body parts that were recently alive! I suppress the rising panic in my body and try to complete the procedure. I am unable to evacuate the uterus completely, however, and after much sweat and worry, I stop, hoping that the uterus will expel the rest within a few days.

Russ is waiting outside the operating room, so I sit with him for a few minutes, telling him that Barb is fine but that there were some problems with the procedure. Since I haven't completely thought through what has happened, I can't be very helpful in answering his questions. I leave hurriedly for the office, promising to return that afternoon to talk with them once Barb has recovered from the anesthesia.

In between seeing other patients in the office that morning, I make several rushed phone calls, trying to figure out what has happened. Despite reassurances from the pathologist that it is statistically "impossible" for four consecutive pregnancy tests to be negative during a viable pregnancy, the horrifying awareness is growing that I have probably aborted Barb's living child. I won't know for sure until several days later, when the pathology report is available. In a daze I walk over to the hospital and try to tell Russ and Barb as much as I know, without telling them all that I suspect. I tell them that there may be more tissue expelled and that I won't know for sure about the pregnancy until the next week.

I can't really face my own suspicions yet.

That weekend I receive a tearful call from Barb. She has just passed some recognizable body parts of the baby; what is she to do? The bleeding has stopped, and she feels physically well, so it is apparent that the abortion I began on Friday is now over. I schedule a time in midweek to meet with them and review the entire situation.

The pathology report confirms my worst fears: I have aborted a living fetus at about 13 weeks of age. No explanation can be found for the negative pregnancy tests. My consultation with Barb and Russ later in the week is one of the hardest things I have ever done. Fortunately, their scientific sophistication allows me to describe in some detail what I have done and what my rationale was. But nothing can obscure the hard reality: I have killed their baby.

Politely, almost meekly, Russ asks whether the ultrasound examination could not have helped us. It almost seems that he is trying to protect my feelings, trying to absolve me of some of the responsibility. "Yes," I answer, "if I had ordered the ultrasound, we would have known that the baby was alive." I cannot explain to him why I didn't recommend it.

Over the next days and weeks and months, my guilt and anger grow. I discuss the events with my partners, with our pathologist, and with obstetric specialists. Some of my mistakes are obvious: I relied too heavily on one particular test; I was not skillful in determining the size of the uterus by pelvic examination; I should have ordered the ultrasound before proceeding with the D and C. Other mistakes become apparent as we review my handling of the case. There is simply no way I can justify what I have done. To make matters worse, complications after the D and C have caused much discomfort, worry, and expense. Barb is unable to become pregnant again for two years.

As physicians our automatic response to reading about such a tragedy is to try to discover what went wrong, to analyze why the mistakes occurred, and to institute corrective measures so that such things do not happen again. This response is important, indeed necessary, and I spent hours in such a review. But it is inadequate if it does not address our own emotional and spiritual experience of the events.

Although I was as honest with the Dailys as I could be in those next months, although I told them everything they wanted to know and described to them as completely as I could what had happened, I never shared with them the agony that I underwent trying to deal with the reality of the events. I never did ask for their forgiveness. I felt somehow that they had enough sorrow without having to bear my burden as well. Somehow, I felt, it was my responsibility to deal with my guilt alone.

Everyone, of course, makes mistakes, and no one enjoys the consequences. But the potential consequences of our medical mistakes are so overwhelming that it is almost impossible for practicing physicians to deal with their errors in a psychologically healthy fashion. Most people—doctors and patients alike—harbor deep within themselves the expectation that the physician will be perfect. No one seems prepared to accept the simple fact of life that physicians, like anyone else, will make mistakes.

By the very nature of our work, we physicians daily make decisions of extreme gravity. Our work in the intensive-care unit, in the emergency room, in the surgery suite, or in the delivery room offers us hundreds of opportunities daily to miscalculate, often with drastic consequences.

And it is not only in these settings but also in the humdrum of routine daily care that a physician can blunder into tragedy. One evening, for instance, a local boy was brought to the emergency room after an apparently minor automobile accident. One leg and foot were injured, but he was otherwise fine. After examining him, I consulted by telephone with an orthopedic surgeon in Duluth, and we decided that I would try to correct what appeared on the x-ray film to be a dislocated foot. As usual, I offered the patient and his mother (who happened to be a nurse with whom I worked regularly) a choice: I could reduce the dislocation in our small hospital or they could travel to Duluth to see the specialist. I was somewhat offended when they decided they would go to Duluth. My feelings changed considerably when the surgeon called me the next morning to thank me for the referral. He reported that the patient had not had a dislocation at all but a severe posterior compartment syndrome, which had hyperflexed the foot, causing it to appear dislocated. The posterior compartment had required immediate surgery the previous night in order to save the muscles of the lower leg. I felt physically weak as I realized that this young man would have been permanently injured had his mother not decided on her own to take him to Duluth.

Although much less drastic than the threat of death or severe disability, perhaps the most frequent result of physician misjudgment is the wasting of money, often in large amounts. Every practicing physician spends thousands of dollars of patients' money every day in the costs for visits, laboratory examinations, medications, and hospitalizations. An unneeded examination, the needless admission of a patient to the hospital, even the unnecessary advice to stay home from work can waste large amounts of money—frequently, the money of people who have little to spare. One comes to feel that any decision may have important consequence.

The cumulative impact of such mistakes (and the ever-present potential for many others) has had a devastating effect on my own emotional health, as it does, I believe, for most physicians. For it is not only the obvious mistakes with obvious results that trouble us. Such mistakes as I made with Barb are fortunately rare occurrences for any physician, and an emotionally mature person may learn to cope with them. But there are also those frequent times when an obvious mistake may lead to less obvious consequences, when the physician errs in judgment, never to know how important the error was.

Some years ago, as I was rushing to an imminent delivery, a young woman stopped me in the hospital hall to tell me that her mother had been having chest pains all night. Should she be brought to the emergency room? I knew her mother well, had examined her the previous week, and knew of her recurring angina. "No," I responded, thinking primarily of my busy schedule and the fact that I was already an hour late because of the unexpected delivery. "Take her over to the office, and I'll see her there as soon as I'm done here." It would be a lot more convenient to see her in the office, I thought. About 20 minutes later, as I was finishing the delivery, our clinic nurse rushed into the delivery room, her face pale and frantic. "Come quick. Mrs. Martin just collapsed." I sprinted the 100 yards to the office to find Mrs. Martin in cardiac arrest. Like many physician offices at that time, ours was not equipped with the advanced life-support equipment necessary to handle the situation. Despite everything we could do Mrs. Martin died.

Would she have survived if I had initially agreed to see her in the emergency room where the requisite staff and equipment were available? No one will ever know for sure, but I have to live with the possibility that she might have lived if I had made a routine decision differently, a decision similar to many others I would make that day, yet one with such an overwhelming outcome.

There is also the common situation of the seriously ill, hospitalized patient who requires almost continuous decision making on the part of the physician. Although no "mistake" may be evident, there are always things that could have been done better: a little more of this medication, starting that treatment a little earlier, recognizing this complication a bit sooner, limiting the number of visitors, and so forth. If the patient dies, the physician is left wondering whether the care provided was adequate. There is no way to be certain, for no one can know what would have happened if things had been done differently. Usually, in fact, it is difficult to get an honest opinion from consultants and other physicians about what one could have done differently. (Judge not, that you not be judged?) In the end, the physician has to swallow the concern, suppress the guilt, and move on to the next patient. He or she may simply be unable to discover whether the mistakes were responsible for the patient's death.

Worst of all, the possibility of a serious mistake is present with each patient the physician sees. The inherent uncertainty of medical practice creates a situation in which errors are always possible. Was that baby I just sent home with a diagnosis of a mild viral fever actually in the early stages of a serious meningitis? Could that nine-year-old with stomach cramps whose mother I just lectured about psychosomatic illness come into the hospital tomorrow with a ruptured appendix? Indeed, the closest I have ever come to involvement in a courtroom malpractice case was the result of my treatment of an apparently minor wrist injury one week after it happened: I misread a straightforward x-ray film and sent the young boy home with a diagnosis of sprain. I next heard about it five years later, when after being summoned to a hearing, I discovered that the fracture I had missed had not healed, and the patient had required extensive treatment and difficult surgery years later.

As practicing primary-care physicians, then, we work in an impossible situation. Each of the myriad decisions to be made every day has the potential for drastic consequences if it is not determined properly. And it is highly likely that sooner or later we will make the mistake that kills or seriously injures another person. How can we live with that knowledge? And after a serious mistake has been made, how can we continue in daily practice and expose ourselves again? How can we who see ourselves as healers deal with such guilt?

Painfully, almost unbelievably, we physicians are even less prepared to deal with our mistakes than the average lay person is. The climate of medical school and residency training, for instance, makes it nearly impossible to confront the emotional consequences of mistakes; it is an environment in which precision seems to predominate. In the large centers where doctors are trained, teams of physicians discuss the smallest details of cases; teaching is usually conducted to make it seem "obvious" what decisions should have been made. And when a physician does make an important mistake, it is first whispered about in the halls, as if it were a sin. Much later, a case conference is called, in which experts who have had weeks to think about the situation discuss the way it should have been handled. The environment in which physicians are trained does not encourage them to talk about their mistakes or about their emotional responses to them.

Indeed, errors are rarely admitted or discussed once a physician is in private practice. I have some indication from consultants and colleagues that I am of at least average competence as a physician. The mistakes I have discussed here represent only a fraction of those of which I am aware. I assume that my colleagues at my own clinic and elsewhere are responsible for similar numbers of major and minor errors. Yet we rarely discuss them; I cannot remember a single instance in which another physician initiated a discussion of a mistake for the purpose of clarifying his or her own emotional response or deciding how to follow up. (I do not wish to imply that we don't discuss difficult cases or unfortunate results; yet these discussions are always handled so delicately in the presence of the "offending" physician that there is simply no space for confession or absolution.)

The medical profession simply seems to have no place for its mistakes. There is no permission given to talk about errors, no way of venting emotional responses. Indeed, one would almost think that mistakes are in the same category as sins: it is permissible to talk about them only when they happen to other people.

If the profession has no room for its mistakes, society seems to have even more rigid expectations of its physicians. The malpractice situation in our country is symptomatic of this attitude. In what other profession are practitioners regularly sued for hundreds of thousands of dollars because of a misjudgment? A lawyer informed me I could be sued for $50,000 for misreading the x-ray film that led to the young man's unhealed fracture. I am sure the Dailys could have successfully sued me for large amounts of money, had they chosen to do so. Experienced physicians who are honest with themselves can count many potential malpractice suits against them. Even the word "malpractice" carries the implication that one has done something more than make a natural mistake; it connotes guilt and sinfulness.

It is easy, of course, to understand why this situation has arisen. These mistakes are terrible; their consequences are drastic; and the victim or family should be compensated for medical bills, time lost from work, and suffering or death. But in our society, rather than establish a "patient compensation fund" (similar to worker's compensation) from which a deserving patient can be compensated for an injury that results from a legitimate mistake, we insist that the doctor be sued for "malpractice," judged guilty, and forced to compensate the patient personally. An atmosphere of denial is created: the "good physician" doesn't make mistakes.

The drastic consequences of our mistakes, the repeated opportunities to make them, the uncertainty about our own culpability when results are poor, and the medical and societal denial that mistakes must happen all result in an intolerable paradox for the physician. We see the horror of our own mistakes, yet we are given no permission to deal with their enormous emotional impact; instead, we are forced to continue the routine of repeatedly making decisions, any one of which could lead us back into the same pit.

Perhaps the only adequate avenue for dealing with this paradox is spiritual. Although mistakes are not usually sins, they engender similar feelings of guilt. How can I not feel guilty about the death of Barb's baby, the lack of adequate emergency care for Mrs. Martin, the fracture that didn't heal? Whether I "ought" to feel guilty is a moot point; most of us do feel guilty under such circumstances.

The only real answer for guilt is spiritual confession, restitution, and absolution. Yet within the structure of modern medicine there is simply no place for this spiritual healing. Although the emotionally mature physician may find it possible to give the patient or family a clinical description of what happened, the technical details are often so difficult for the lay person to understand that the nature of the mistake is hidden. Or if an error is clearly described, it is presented as "natural," "understandable," or "unavoidable" (which, indeed, it often is). But there is no place for real confession: "This is the mistake I made; I'm sorry." How can one say that to a grieving mother, to a family that has lost a member? It simply doesn't fit into the physician-patient relationship.

Even if one were bold enough to consider such a confession, strong voices would raise objections. When I finally heard about the unhealed fracture in my young patient, I was anxious that the incident not create antagonism between me and the family, since we live in a small town and see each other frequently. I was tempted to call the family and express my apologies and the hope that a satisfactory settlement could be worked out. I mentioned that possibility to a malpractice lawyer, but he was strongly opposed, urging me not to have any contact with the family until a settlement was reached. Even if a malpractice suit is not likely, the nature of the physician-patient relationship makes such a reversal of roles "unseemly." Can I further burden an already grieving family with the complexities of my feelings, my burden?

And if confession is difficult, what are we to say about restitution? The very nature of our work means that we are dealing with elements that cannot be restored in any meaningful way. What can I offer the Dailys in restitution?

I have not been successful in dealing with the paradox. Any patient encounter can dump me back into the situation of having caused more harm than good, yet my role is to be a healer. Since there has been no permission to address the paradox openly, I lapse into neurotic behavior to deal with my anxiety and guilt. Little wonder that physicians are accused of having a God complex; little wonder that we are defensive about our judgments; little wonder that we blame the patient or the previous physician when things go wrong, that we yell at the nurses for their mistakes, that we have such high rates of alcoholism, drug addiction, and suicide.

At some point we must bring our mistakes out of the closet. We need to give ourselves permission to recognize our errors and their consequences. We need to find healthy ways to deal with our emotional responses to those errors. Our profession is difficult enough without our having to wear the yoke of perfection.

ACKNOWLEDGMENT

This chapter originally was published as follows: D. Hilfiker, "Sounding Board: Facing Our Mistakes," *New England Journal of Medicine* 310, no. 2 (January 12, 1984): 118-22. ©1984, Massachusetts Medical Society. Used with permission; all rights reserved.

7

Error in Medicine

Lucian L. Leape

For years, medical and nursing students have been taught Florence Nightingale's dictum—first, do no harm.[1] Yet evidence from a number of sources, reported over several decades, indicates that a substantial number of patients suffer treatment-caused injuries while in the hospital.[2-6]

In 1964 Schimmel[2] reported that 20% of patients admitted to a university hospital medical service suffered iatrogenic injury and that 20% of those injuries were serious or fatal. Steel et al[3] found that 36% of patients admitted to a university medical service in a teaching hospital suffered an iatrogenic event, of which 25% were serious or life threatening. More than half of the injuries were related to use of medication.[3] In 1991 Bedell et al[4] reported the results of an analysis of cardiac arrests at a teaching hospital. They found that 64% were preventable. Again, inappropriate use of drugs was the leading cause of the cardiac arrests. Also in 1991, the Harvard Medical Practice Study reported the results of a population-based study of iatrogenic injury in patients hospitalized in New York State in 1984.[5,6] Nearly 4% of patients suffered an injury that prolonged their hospital stay or resulted in measurable disability. For New York State, this equaled 98,609 patients in 1984. Nearly 14% of these injuries were fatal. If these rates are typical of the United States, then 180,000 people die each year partly as a result of iatrogenic injury, the equivalent of three jumbo-jet crashes every 2 days.

When the causes are investigated, it is found that most iatrogenic injuries are due to errors and are, therefore, potentially preventable.[4,7,8] For example, in the Harvard Medical Practice Study, 69% of injuries were due to errors (the balance was unavoidable).[8] Error may be defined as an unintended act (either or omission or commission) or one that does not achieve its intended outcome. Indeed, injuries are but the "tip of the iceberg" of the problem of errors, since most errors do not result in patient injury. For example, medication errors occur in 2% to 14% of patients admitted to hospitals,[9-12] but most do not result in injury.[13]

Aside from studies of medication errors, the literature on medical error is sparse, in part because most studies of iatrogenesis have focused on injuries (eg, the Harvard Medical Study). When errors have been specifically looked for, however, the rates reported have been distressingly high. Autopsy studies have shown high rates (35% to 40%) of missed diagnoses causing death.[14-16] One study of errors in a medical intensive care unit revealed an average of 1.7 errors per day per patient, of which 29% had the potential for serious or fatal injury.[17] Operational errors (such as failure to treat promptly or to get a follow-up culture) were found in 52% of patients in a study of children with positive urine cultures.[18]

Given the complex nature of medical practice and the multitude of interventions that each patient receives, a high error rate is perhaps not surprising. The patients in the intensive care unit study, for example, were the recipients of an average of 178 "activities" per day. The 1.7 errors per day thus indicate that hospital personnel were functioning at a 99% level of proficiency. However, a 1% failure rate is substantially higher than is tolerated in industry, particularly in hazardous fields such as aviation and nuclear power. As W.E. Deming points out (written communication, November 1987), even 99.9% may not be good enough: "If we had to live with 99.9%, we would have: 2 unsafe plane landings per day at O'Hare, 16,000 pieces of lost mail every hour, 32,000 bank checks deducted from the wrong bank account every hour."

WHY IS THE ERROR RATE
IN THE PRACTICE OF MEDICINE SO HIGH?

Physicians, nurses, and pharmacists are trained to be careful and to function at a high level of proficiency. Indeed, they probably are among the most careful professionals in our society. It is curious, therefore, that high error rates have not stimulated more concern and efforts at error prevention. One reason may be a lack of awareness of the severity of the problem. Hospital-acquired injuries are not reported in the newspapers like jumbo-jet crashes, for the simple reason that they occur one at a time in 5,000 different locations across the country. Although error rates are substantial, serious injuries due to errors are not part of the everyday experience of physicians or nurses, but are perceived as isolated and unusual events—"outliers." Second, most errors do no harm. Either they are intercepted or the patient's defenses prevent injury. (Few children die from a single misdiagnosed or mistreated urinary infection, for example).

But the most important reason physicians and nurses have not developed more effective methods of error prevention is that they have a great deal of difficulty in dealing with human error when it does occur.[19-21] The reasons are to be found in the culture of medical practice.

Physicians are socialized in medical school and residency to strive for error-free practice.[19] There is a powerful emphasis on perfection, both in diagnosis and treatment. In everyday hospital practice, the message is equally clear: mistakes are unacceptable. Physicians are expected to function without error, an expectation that physicians translate into the need to be infallible. One result is that physicians, not unlike test pilots, come to view an error as a failure of character—you weren't careful enough, you didn't try hard enough. This kind of thinking lies behind a common reaction by physicians: "How can there be an error without negligence?"

Cultivating a norm of high standards is, of course, highly desirable. It is the counterpart of another fundamental goal of medical education: developing the physician's sense of responsibility for the patient. If you are responsible for everything that happens to the patient, it follows that you are responsible for any errors that occur. While the logic may be sound, the conclusion is absurd, because physicians do not have the power to control all aspects of patient care.[22] Nonetheless, the sense of duty to perform faultlessly is strongly internalized.

Role models in medical education reinforce the concept of infallibility. The young physician's teachers are largely specialists, experts in their fields, and authorities. Authorities are not supposed to err. It has been suggested that this need to be infallible creates a strong pressure to intellectual dishonesty, to cover up mistakes rather than to admit them.[23] The organization of medical practice, particularly in the hospital, perpetuates these norms. Errors are rarely admitted or discussed among physicians in private practice. Physicians typically feel, not without reason, that admission of error will lead to censure or increased surveillance or, worse, that their colleagues will regard them as incompetent or careless. Far better to conceal a mistake or, if that is impossible, to try to shift the blame to another, even the patient.

Yet physicians are emotionally devastated by serious mistakes that harm or kill patients.[19-21] Almost every physician who cares for patients has had that experience, usually more than once. The emotional impact is often profound, typically a mixture of fear, guilt, anger, embarrassment, and humiliation. However, as Christensen et al[20] note, physicians are typically isolated by their emotional responses; seldom is there a process to evaluate the circumstances of a mistake and to provide support and emotional healing for the fallible physician. Wu et al[21] found that only half of house officers discussed their most significant mistakes with attending physicians.

Thus, although the individual may learn from a mistake and change practice patterns accordingly, the adjustment often takes place in a vacuum. Lessons learned are shared privately, if at all, and external objective evaluation of what went wrong often does not occur. As Hilfiker[19] points out, "We see the horror of our own mistakes, yet we are given no permission to deal with their enormous emotional impact. . . . The medical profession simply has no place for its mistakes."

Finally, the realities of the malpractice threat provide strong incentives against disclosure or investigation of mistakes. Even a minor error can place the physician's entire career in jeopardy if it results in a serious bad outcome. It is hardly surprising that a physician might hesitate to reveal an error to either the patient or hospital authorities or to expose a colleague to similar devastation for a single mistake.

The paradox is that although the standard of medical practice is perfection—error-free patient care—all physicians recognize that mistakes are inevitable. Most would like to examine their mistakes and learn from them. From an emotional standpoint, they need the support and understanding of their colleagues and patients when they make mistakes. Yet, they are denied both insight and support by misguided concepts of infallibility and by fear: fear of embarrassment by colleagues, fear of patient reaction, and fear of litigation. Although the notion of infallibility fails the reality test, the fears are well grounded.

THE MEDICAL APPROACH TO ERROR PREVENTION

Efforts at error prevention in medicine have characteristically followed what might be called the perfectibility model: if physicians and nurses could be properly trained and motivated, then they would make no mistakes. The methods used to achieve this goal are training and punishment. Training is directed toward teaching people to do the right thing. In nursing, rigid adherence to protocols is emphasized. In medicine, the emphasis is less on rules and more on knowledge.

Punishment is through social opprobrium or peer disapproval. The professional cultures of medicine and nursing typically use blame to encourage proper performance. Errors are regarded as someone's fault, caused by a lack of sufficient attention or, worse, lack of caring enough to make sure you are correct. Punishment for egregious (negligent) errors is primarily (and capriciously) meted out through the malpractice tort litigation system.

Students of error and human performance reject this formulation. While the proximal error leading to an accident is, in fact, usually a "human error," the causes of that error are often well beyond the individual's control. All humans err frequently. Systems that rely on error-free performance are doomed to fail.

The medical approach to error prevention is also reactive. Errors are usually discovered only when there is an incident—an untoward effect or injury to the patient. Corrective measures are then directed toward preventing a recurrence of a similar error, often by attempting to prevent *that* individual from making a repeat error. Seldom are underlying causes explored.

For example, if a nurse gives a medication to the wrong patient, a typical response would be exhortation or training in double-checking the identity of both patient and drug before administration. Although it might be noted that the nurse was distracted because of an unusually large case load, it is unlikely that serious attention would be given to evaluating overall work assignments or to determining if large case loads have contributed to other kinds of errors.

It is even less likely that questions would be raised about the wisdom of a system for dispensing medications in which safety is contingent on inspection by an individual at the end point of use. Reliance on inspection as a mechanism of quality control was discredited long ago in industry.[24,25] A simple procedure, such as the use of bar coding like that used at supermarket checkout counters, would probably be more effective in this situation. More imaginative solutions could easily be found—if it were recognized that both systems and individuals contribute to the problem.

It seems clear, and it is the thesis of this article, that if physicians, nurses, pharmacists, and administrators are to succeed in reducing errors in hospital care, they will need to fundamentally change the way they think about errors and why they occur. Fortunately, a great deal has been learned about error prevention in other disciplines, information that is relevant to the hospital practice of medicine.

LESSONS FROM PSYCHOLOGICAL
AND HUMAN FACTORS RESEARCH

The subject of human error has long fascinated psychologists and others, but both the development of theory and the pace of empirical research accelerated in response to the dramatic technological advances that occurred during and after World War II.[26] These theory development and research activities followed two parallel and intersecting paths: human factors research and cognitive psychology.

Human factor specialists, mostly engineers, have been largely concerned with the design of the man-machine interface in complex environments such as airplane cockpits and nuclear power plant control rooms. Cognitive psychologists concentrated on developing models of human cognition that they subjected to empirical testing. Lessons from both spheres of observation have greatly deepened our understanding of mental functioning. We now have reasonably coherent theories of why humans err, and a great deal has been learned about how to design work environments to minimize the occurrence of errors and limit their consequences.

A THEORY OF COGNITION

Most errors result from aberrations in mental functioning. Thus, to understand why errors occur we must first understand normal cognition. Although many theories have been espoused, and experts disagree, a unitary framework has been proposed by Reason[26] that captures the main themes of cognitive theory and is consistent with empirical observation. It goes as follows.

Much of mental functioning is automatic, rapid, and effortless. A person can leave home, enter and start the car, drive to work, park, and enter the office without devoting much conscious thought to any of the hundreds of maneuvers and decisions that this complex set of actions requires. This automatic and unconscious processing is possible because we carry a vast array of mental models, "schemata" in psychological jargon, that are "expert" on some minute recurrent aspect of our world. These schemata operate briefly when required, processing information rapidly, in parallel, and without conscious effort. Schemata are activated by conscious thought or sensory inputs; function thereafter is automatic.

In addition to this automatic unconscious processing, called the "schematic control mode," cognitive activities can be unconscious and controlled. This "attentional control mode" or conscious thought is used for problem solving as well as to monitor automatic function. The attentional control mode is called into play when we confront a problem, either de novo or as a result of failures of the schematic control mode. In contrast to the rapid parallel processing of the schematic control mode, processing in the attentional control mode is slow, sequential, effortful, and difficult to sustain.

Rasmussen and Jensen[27] describe a model of performance based on this concept of cognition that is particularly well suited for error analysis. They classify human performance into three levels: (1) skill-based, which is patterns of thought and action that are governed by stored patterns of preprogrammed instructions (schemata) and largely unconscious; (2) rule-based, in which solutions to familiar problems are governed by stored rules of the "if X, then Y" variety; and (3) knowledge-based, or synthetic thought, which is used for novel situations requiring conscious analytic processing and stored knowledge.

Any departure from routine, ie, a problem, requires a rule-based or knowledge-based solution. Humans prefer pattern recognition to calculation, so they are strongly biased to search for a prepackaged solution, ie, a "rule," before resorting to more strenuous knowledge-based functioning.

Although all three levels may be used simultaneously, with increasing expertise the primary focus of control moves from knowledge-based toward skill-based functioning. Experts have a much larger repertoire of schemata and problem-solving rules than novices, and they are formulated at a more abstract level. In one sense, expertise means seldom having to resort to knowledge-based functioning (reasoning).

MECHANISMS OF COGNITIVE ERRORS

Errors have been classified by Reason and Rasmussen at each level of the skill-, rule-, and knowledge-based model.[26] Skill-based errors are called "slips." These are unconscious glitches in automatic activity. Slips are errors of action. Rule-based and knowledge-based errors, by contrast, are errors of conscious thought and are termed "mistakes." The mechanisms of error vary with the level.

SLIPS

Skill-based activity is automatic. A slip occurs when there is a break in the routine while attention is diverted. The actor possesses the requisite routines; errors occur because of a lack of a timely attentional check. In brief, slips are monitoring failures. They are unintended acts.

A common mechanism of a slip is *capture*, in which a more frequently used schema takes over from a similar but less familiar one. For example, if the usual action sequence is ABCDE, but on this occasion the planned sequence changes to ABCFG, then conscious attention must be in force after C or the more familiar pattern DE will be executed. An everyday example is departing on a trip in which the first part of the journey is the same as a familiar commuting path and driving to work instead of to the new location.

Another type of slip is a *description error*, in which the right action is performed on the wrong object, such as pouring cream on a pancake. *Associative activation errors* result from mental associations of ideas, such as answering the phone when the doorbell rings. *Loss of activation errors* are temporary memory losses, such as entering a room and no longer remembering why you wanted to go there. Loss of activation errors are frequently caused by interruptions.

A variety of factors can divert attentional control and make slips more likely. Physiological factors include fatigue, sleep loss, alcohol, drugs, and illness. Psychological factors include other activity ("busyness"), as well as emotional states such as boredom, frustration, fear, anxiety, or anger. All these factors lead to preoccupations that divert attention. Psychological factors, though considered "internal" or endogenous, may also be caused by a host of external factors, such as overwork, interpersonal relations, and many other forms of stress. Environmental factors, such as noise, heat, visual stimuli, motion, and other physical phenomena, also can cause distractions that divert attention and lead to slips.

MISTAKES

Rule-based errors usually occur during problem solving when a wrong rule is chosen—either because of a misperception of the situation and, thus, the application of a wrong rule or because of misapplication of a rule, usually one that is strong (frequently used), that seems to fit adequately. Errors result from misapplied expertise.

Knowledge-based errors are much more complex. The problem solver confronts a novel situation for which he or she possesses no preprogrammed solutions. Errors arise because of lack of knowledge or misinterpretation of the problem. Pattern matching is preferred to calculation, but sometimes we match the wrong patterns. Certain habits of thought have been identified that alter pattern matching or calculation and lead to mistakes. These processes are incompletely understood and are seldom recognized by the actor. One such process is *biased memory.* Decisions are based on what is in our memory, but memory is biased toward overgeneralization and overregularization of the commonplace.[28] Familiar patterns are assumed to have universal applicability because they usually work. We see what we know. Paradoxically, memory is also biased toward overemphasis on the discrepant. A contradictory experience may leave an exaggerated impression far outweighing its statistical importance (eg, the exceptional case or missed diagnosis).

Another mechanism is the *availability heuristic,*[29] the tendency to use the first information that comes to mind. Related are *confirmation bias,* the tendency to look for evidence that supports an early working hypothesis and to ignore data that contradict it, and *overconfidence,* the tendency to believe in the validity of the chosen course of action and to focus on evidence that favors it.[26]

Rule-based and knowledge-based functioning are affected by the same physiological, psychological, and environmental influences that produce slips. A great deal of research has been devoted to the effects of stress on performance. Although it is often difficult to establish causal links between stress and specific accidents, there is little question that errors (both slips and mistakes) are increased under stress. On the other hand, stress is not all bad. It has long been known that "a little anxiety improves performance." In 1908, Yerkes and Dodson[30] showed that performance is best at moderate levels of arousal. Poor performance occurs at both extremes: boredom and panic.[31] *Coning of attention* under stress is the tendency in an emergency to concentrate on one single source of information, the "first come, best preferred" solution. (A classic example is the phenomenon of passengers in a crashed aircraft struggling to open a door while ignoring a large hole in the fuselage a few feet away.) *Reversion under stress* is a phenomenon in which recently learned behavioral patterns are replaced by older, more familiar ones, even if they are inappropriate in the circumstances.[31]

The complex nature of cognition, the vagaries of the physical world, and the inevitable shortages of information and schemata ensure that normal humans make multiple errors every day. Slips are most common, since much of our mental functioning is automatic, but the rate of error in knowledge-based processes is higher.[26]

LATENT ERRORS

In 1979, the Three-Mile Island incident caused both psychologists and human factors engineers to reexamine their theories about human error. Although investigations revealed the expected operator errors, it was clear that prevention of many of these errors was beyond the capabilities of the human operators at the time. Many errors were caused by faulty interface design, others by complex interactions and breakdowns that were not discernible by the operators of their instruments. The importance of poor system design as a cause of failures in complex processes became more apparent.[32] Subsequent disasters, notably Bhopal and Chernobyl, made it even clearer that operator errors were only part of the explanation of failures in complex systems. Disasters of this magnitude resulted from major failures of design and organization that occurred long before the accident, failures that both caused operator errors and made them impossible to reverse.[26,32]

Reason[26] has called these *latent errors,* errors that have effects that are delayed, "accidents waiting to happen," in contrast to active errors, which have effects that are felt immediately. While an operator error may be the proximal "cause" of the accident, the root causes were often present within the system for a long time. The operator has, in a real sense, been "set up" to fail by poor design, faulty maintenance, or erroneous management decisions.

Faulty design at Three-Mile Island provided gauges that gave a low pressure reading both when pressure was low and when the gauge was not working and a control panel on which 100 warning lights flashed simultaneously. Faulty maintenance disabled a safety back-up system so the operator could not activate it when needed. Similarly, bad management decisions can result in unrealistic workloads, inadequate training, and demanding production schedules that lead workers to make errors.

Accidents rarely result from a single error, latent or active.[26,32] System defenses and the abilities of frontline operators to identify and correct errors before an accident occurs make single-error accidents highly unlikely. Rather, accidents typically result from a combination of latent and active errors and breach of defenses. The precipitating event can be a relatively trivial malfunction or an external circumstance, such as the weather (eg, the freezing of O-rings that caused the Challenger disaster).

The most important result of latent errors may be the production of psychological precursors, which are pathologic situations that create working conditions that predispose to a variety of errors.[26] Inappropriate work schedules, for example, can result in high workloads and undue time pressures that induce errors. Poor training can lead to inadequate recognition of hazards or inappropriate procedures that lead to accidents. Conversely, a precursor can be the product of more than one management or training failure. For example, excessive time pressure can result from poor scheduling, but it can also be the product of inadequate training or faulty division of responsibilities. Because they can affect all cognitive processes, these precursors can cause an immense variety of errors that result in unsafe acts.

The important point is that successful accident prevention efforts must focus on root causes—system errors in design and implementation. It is futile to concentrate on developing solutions to the unsafe acts themselves. Other errors, unpredictable and infinitely varied, will soon occur if the underlying cause is uncorrected. Although correcting root causes will not eliminate all errors—individuals still bring varying abilities and work habits to the workplace—it can significantly reduce the probability of errors occurring.

PREVENTION OF ACCIDENTS

The multiplicity of mechanisms and causes of errors (internal and external, individual and systematic) dictates that there cannot be a simple or universal means of reducing errors. Creating a safe process, whether it be flying an airplane, running a hospital, or performing cardiac surgery, requires attention to methods of error reduction at each stage of system development: design, construction, maintenance, allocation of resources, training, and development of operational procedures. This type of attention to error reduction requires responsible individuals at each stage to think through the consequences of their decisions and to reason back from discovered deficiencies to redesign and reorganize the process. Systemic changes are most likely to be successful because they reduce the likelihood of a variety of types of errors at the end-user stage.

The primary objective of system design for safety is to make it difficult for individuals to err. But it is also important to recognize that errors will inevitably occur and plan for their recovery.[26] Ideally, the system will automatically correct errors when they occur. If that is impossible, mechanisms should be in place to at least detect errors in time for corrective action. Therefore, in addition to designing the work environment to minimize psychological precursors, designers should provide feedback through instruments that provide monitoring functions and build in buffers and redundancy. Buffers are design features that automatically correct for human or mechanical errors. Redundancy is duplication (sometimes triplication or quadruplication) of critical mechanisms and instruments, so that a failure does not result in loss of the function.

Another important system design feature is designing tasks to minimize errors. Norman[28] has recommended a set of principles that have general applicability. Tasks should be *simplified* to minimize the load on the weakest aspects of cognition: short-term memory, planning, and problem solving. The power of *constraints* should be exploited. One way to do this is with "forcing functions," which make it impossible to act without meeting a precondition (such as the inability to release the parking gear of a car unless the brake pedal is depressed). *Standardization* of procedures, displays, and layouts reduces error by reinforcing the pattern recognition that humans do well. Finally, where possible, operations should be easily *reversible* or difficult to perform when they are not reversible.

Training must include, in addition to the usual emphasis on application of knowledge and following procedures, a consideration of safety issues. These issues include understanding the rationale for procedures as well as how errors can occur at various stages, their possible consequences, and instruction in methods for avoidance of errors. Finally, it must be acknowledged that injuries can result from behavioral problems that may be seen in impaired physicians or incompetent physicians despite well-designed systems; methods of identifying and correcting egregious behaviors are also needed.

THE AVIATION MODEL

The practice of hospital medicine has been compared, usually unfavorably, to the aviation industry, also a highly complicated and risky enterprise but one that seems far safer. Indeed, there seem to be many similarities. As Allnutt observed,

Both pilots and doctors are carefully selected, highly trained professionals who are usually determined to maintain high standards, both externally and internally imposed, whilst performing difficult tasks in life-threatening environments. Both use high technology equipment and function as key members of a team of specialists . . . both exercise high level cognitive skills in a most complex domain about which much is known, but where much remains to be discovered.[31]

While the comparison is apt, there are also important differences between aviation and medicine, not the least of which is a substantial measure of uncertainty due to the number and variety of disease states, as well as the unpredictability of the human organism. Nonetheless, there is much physicians and nurses could learn from aviation.

Aviation—airline travel, at least—is indeed generally safe: more than 10 million takeoffs and landings each year with an average of fewer than four crashes a year. But, it was not always so. The first powered flight was in 1903, the first fatality in 1908, and the first midair collision in 1910. By 1910, there were 2,000 pilots in the world and 32 had already died.[32] The US Air Mail Service was founded in 1918. As a result of efforts to meet delivery schedules in all kinds of weather, 31 of the first 40 Air Mail Service pilots were killed. This appalling toll lead to unionization of the pilots and their insistence that local field controllers could not order pilots to fly against their judgment unless the field controllers went up for a flight around the field themselves. In 1922, there were no Air Mail Service fatalities.[32] Since that time, a complex system of aircraft design, instrumentation, training, regulation, and air traffic control has developed that is highly effective at preventing fatalities.

There are strong incentives for making flying safe. Pilots, of course, are highly motivated. Unlike physicians, their lives are on the line as well as those of their passengers. But, airlines and airplane manufacturers also have strong incentives to provide safe flight. Business decreases after a large crash, and if a certain model of aircraft crashes repeatedly, the manufacturer will be discredited. The lawsuits that inevitably follow a crash can harm both reputation and profitability.

Designing for safety has led to a number of unique characteristics of aviation that could, with suitable modification, prove useful in improving hospital safety.

First, in terms of system design, aircraft designers assume that errors and failures are inevitable and design systems to "absorb" them, building in multiple buffers, automation, and redundancy. As even a glance in an airliner cockpit reveals, extensive feedback is provided by means of monitoring instruments, many in duplicate or triplicate. Indeed, the multiplicity of instruments and automation have generated their own challenges to system design: sensory overload and boredom. Nonetheless, these safeguards have served the cause of aviation safety well.

Second, procedures are standardized to the maximum extent possible. Specific protocols must be followed for trip planning, operations, and maintenance. Pilots go through a checklist before each takeoff. Required maintenance is specified in detail and must be performed on a regular (by flight hours) basis. Third, the training, examination, and certification process is highly developed and rigidly, as well as frequently, enforced. Airline pilots take proficiency examinations every 6 months. Much of the content of examinations is directly concerned with procedures to enhance safety.

Pilots function well within this rigorously controlled system, although not flawlessly. For example, one study of cockpit crews observed that human errors or instrument malfunctions occurred on the average of one every 4 minutes during an overseas flight.[32] Each event was promptly recognized and corrected with no untoward effects. Pilots also willingly submit to an external authority, the air traffic controller, when within the constrained air and ground space at a busy airport.

Finally, safety in aviation has been institutionalized. Two independent agencies have government-mandated responsibilities: the Federal Aviation Administration (FAA) regulates all aspects of flying and prescribes safety procedures, and the National Transportation Safety Board investigates every accident. The adherence of airlines and pilots to required safety standards is closely monitored. The FAA recognized long ago that pilots seldom reported an error if it led to disciplinary action. Accordingly, in 1975 the FAA established a confidential reporting system for safety infractions, the Air Safety Reporting System (ASRS). If pilots, controllers, or others promptly report a dangerous situation, such as a near-miss midair collision, they will not be penalized. This program dramatically increased reporting, so that unsafe conditions at airports, communication problems, and traffic control inadequacies are now promptly communicated. Analysis of these reports and subsequent investigations appear as a regular feature in several pilots' magazines. The ASRS receives more than 5,000 notifications each year.[32]

THE MEDICAL MODEL

By contrast, accident prevention has not been a primary focus of the practice of hospital medicine. It is not that errors are ignored. Mortality and morbidity conferences, incident reports, risk management activities, and quality assurance committees abound. But, as noted previously these activities focus on incidents and individuals. When errors are examined, a problem-solving approach is usually used: the cause of the error is identified and corrected. Root causes, the underlying systems failures, are rarely sought. System designers do not assume that errors and failures are inevitable and design systems to prevent or absorb them. There are, of course, exceptions. Implementation of unit dosing, for example, markedly reduced medication dosing errors by eliminating the need for the nurse to measure out each dose. Monitoring in intensive care units is sophisticated and extensive (although perhaps not sufficiently redundant). Nonetheless, the basic health care system approach is to rely on individuals not to make errors rather than to assume they will.

Second, standardization and task design vary widely. In the operating room, it has been refined to a high art. In patient care units, much more could be done, particularly to minimize reliance on short-term memory, one of the weakest aspects of cognition. On-time and correct delivery of medications, for example, is often contingent on a busy nurse remembering to do so, a nurse who is responsible for four or five patients at once and is repeatedly interrupted, a classic set up for a "loss-of-activation" error.

On the other hand, education and training in medicine and nursing far exceed that in aviation, both in breadth of content and in duration, and few professions compare with medicine in terms of the extent of continuing education. Although certification is essentially universal, including the recent introduction of periodic recertification, the idea of periodically testing *performance* has never been accepted. Thus, we place great emphasis on education and training, but shy away from demonstrating that it makes a difference.

Finally, unlike aviation, safety in medicine has never been institutionalized, in the sense of being a major focus of hospital medical activities. Investigation of accidents is often superficial, unless a malpractice action is likely; noninjurious error (a "near miss") is rarely examined at all. Incident reports are frequently perceived as punitive instruments. As a result, they are often not filed, and when they are, they almost invariably focus on the individual's misconduct.

One medical model is an exception and has proved quite successful in reducing accidents due to errors: anesthesia. Perhaps in part because the effects of serious anesthetic errors are potentially so dramatic—death or brain damage—and perhaps in part because the errors are frequently transparently clear and knowable to all, anesthesiologists have greatly emphasized safety. The success of these efforts has been dramatic. Whereas mortality from anesthesia was one in 10,000 to 20,000 just a decade or so ago, it is now estimated at less than one in 200,000.[33] Anesthesiologists have led the medical profession in recognizing system factors as causes of errors, in designing fail-safe systems, and in training to avoid errors.[34-36]

SYSTEMS CHANGES TO REDUCE HOSPITAL INJURIES

Can the lessons from cognitive psychology and human factors research that have been successful in accident prevention in aviation and other industries be applied to the practice of hospital medicine? There is every reason to think they could be. Hospitals, physicians, nurses, and pharmacists who wish to reduce errors could start by considering how cognition and error mechanisms apply to the practice of hospital medicine. Specifically, they can examine their care delivery systems in terms of the systems' ability to discover, prevent, and absorb errors and for the presence of psychological precursors.

DISCOVERY OF ERRORS

The first step in error prevention is to define the problem. Efficient, routine identification of errors needs to be part of hospital practice, as does routine investigation of all errors that cause injuries. The emphasis is on "routine." Only when errors are accepted as an inevitable, although manageable, part of everyday practice will it be possible for hospital personnel to shift from a punitive to a creative frame of mind that seeks out and identifies the underlying system failures.

Data collecting and investigatory activities are expensive, but so are the consequences of errors. Evidence from industry indicates that the savings from reduction of errors and accidents more than make up for the costs of data collection and investigation.[31] (While these calculations apply to "rework" and other operational inefficiencies resulting from errors, additional savings from reduced patient care costs and liability costs for hospitals and physicians could also be substantial).

PREVENTION OF ERRORS

Many health care delivery systems could be redesigned to significantly reduce the likelihood of error. Some obvious mechanisms that can be used are as follows:

Reduced reliance on memory.—Work should be designed to minimize the requirements for human functions that are known to be particularly fallible, such as short-term memory and vigilance (prolonged attention). Clearly, the components of work must be well delineated and understood before system redesign. Checklists, protocols, and computerized decision aids could be used more widely. For example, physicians should not have to rely on their memories to retrieve a laboratory test result, and nurses should not have to remember the time a medication dose is due. These are tasks that computers do much more reliably than humans.

Improved information access.—Creative ways need to be developed for making information more readily available: displaying it where it is needed, when it is needed, and in a form that permits easy access. Computerization of the medical record, for example, would greatly facilitate bedside display of patient information, including tests and medications.

Error proofing.—Where possible, critical tasks should be structured so that errors cannot be made. The use of "forcing functions" is helpful. For example, if a computerized system is used for medication orders, it can be designed so that a physician cannot enter an order for a lethal overdose of a drug or prescribe a medication to which a patient is known to be allergic.

Standardization.—One of the most effective means of reducing error is standardizing processes wherever possible. The advantages, in efficiency as well as in error reduction, of standardizing drug doses and times of administration are obvious. Is it really acceptable to ask nurses to follow six different "K-scales" (directions for how much potassium to give according to patient serum potassium levels) solely to satisfy different physician prescribing patterns? Other candidates for standardization include information displays, methods for common practices (such as surgical dressings), and the geographic location of equipment and supplies in a patient care unit. There is something bizarre, and really quite inexcusable, about "code" situations in hospitals where house staff and other personnel responding to a cardiac arrest waste precious seconds searching for resuscitation equipment simply because it is kept in a different location on each patient care unit.

Training.—Instruction of physicians, nurses, and pharmacists in procedures or problem solving should include greater emphasis on possible errors and how to prevent them. (Well-written surgical atlases do this.) For example, many interns need more rigorous instruction and supervision than is currently provided when they are learning new procedures. Young physicians need to be taught that safe practice is as important as effective practice. Both physicians and nurses need to learn to think of errors primarily as symptoms of systems failures.

ABSORPTION OF ERRORS

Because it is impossible to prevent all error, buffers should be built into each system so that errors are absorbed before they can cause harm to patients. At minimum, systems should be designed so that errors can be identified in time to be intercepted. The drug delivery systems in most hospitals do this to some degree already. Nurses and pharmacists often identify errors in physician drug orders and prevent improper administration to the patient. As hospitals move to computerized records and ordering systems, more of these types of interceptions can be incorporated into the computer programs. Critical systems (such as life-support equipment and monitors) should be provided in duplicate in those situations in which a mechanical failure could lead to patient injury.

PSYCHOLOGICAL PRECURSORS

Finally, explicit attention should be given to work schedules, division of responsibilities, task descriptions, and other details of working arrangements where improper managerial decisions can produce psychological precursors such as time pressures and fatigue that create an unsafe environment. While the influence of the stresses of everyday life on human behavior cannot be eliminated, stresses caused by a faulty work environment can be. Elimination of fear and the creation of a supportive working environment are other potent means of preventing errors.

INSTITUTIONALIZATION OF SAFETY

Although the idea of a national hospital safety board that would investigate every accident is neither practical nor necessary, at the hospital level such activities should occur. Existing hospital risk management activities could be broadened to include all potentially injurious errors and deepened to seek out underlying system failures. Providing immunity, as in the FAA ASRS system, might be a good first step. At the national level, the Joint Commission on Accreditation of Healthcare Organizations should be involved in discussions regarding the institutionalization of safety. Other specialty societies might well follow the lead of the anesthesiologists in developing safety standards and require their instruction to be part of residency training.

IMPLEMENTING SYSTEMS CHANGES

Many of the principles described herein fit well within the teachings of total quality management.[24] One of the basic tenants of total quality management, statistical quality control, requires data regarding variation in processes. In a generic sense, errors are but variations in processes. Total quality management also requires a culture in which errors and deviations are regarded not as human failures, but as opportunities to improve the system, "gems," as they are sometimes called. Finally, total quality management calls for grassroots participation to identify and develop system modifications to eliminate the underlying failures.

Like total quality management, systems changes to reduce errors require commitment of the organization's leadership. None of the aforementioned changes will be effective or, for that matter, even possible without support at the highest levels (hospital executives and departmental chiefs) for making safety a major goal of medical practice.

But it is apparent that the most fundamental change that will be needed if hospitals are to make meaningful progress in error reduction is a cultural one. Physicians and nurses need to accept the notion that error is an inevitable accompaniment of the human condition, even among conscientious professionals with high standards. Errors must be accepted as evidence of systems flaws not character flaws. Until and unless that happens, it is unlikely that any substantial progress will be made in reducing medical errors.

ACKNOWLEDGMENT

This chapter originally was published as follows: L.L. Leape, "Special Communication: Error in Medicine," *Journal of the American Medical Association* 272, no. 23 (21 December 1994): 1851-57. © 1994, American Medical Association. Used with permission; all rights reserved.

NOTES

1. Nightingale F. *Notes on Hospitals*. London, England: Longman, Green, Longman, Roberts, and Green; 1863.

2. Schimmel EM. The hazards of hospitalization. *Ann Intern Med.* 1964:60:100-110.

3. Steel K, Gertman PM, Crescenzi C, et al. Iatrogenic illness on a general medical service at a university hospital. *N Engl J Med.* 1981:304:638-642.

4. Bedell SE, Deitz DC, Leeman D, Delbanco TL. Incidence and characteristics of preventable iatrogenic cardiac arrests. *JAMA.* 1991:265:2815-2820.

5. Brennan TA, Leape LL, Laird N, et al. Incidence of adverse events and negligence in hospitalized patients: results of the Harvard Medical Practice Study I. *N Engl J Med.* 1991:324:370-376.

6. Leape LL, Brennan TA, Laird N, et al. The nature of adverse events in hospitalized patients: results of the Harvard Medical Practice Study II. *N Engl J Med.* 1991:324:377-384.

7. Dubois RW, Brook RH. Preventable deaths: who, how often, and why? *Ann Intern Med.* 1988:109:582-589.

8. Leape LL, Lawthers AG, Brennan TA, Johnson WG. Preventing medical injury. *Qual Rev Bull.* 1998:8:144-149.

9. Lesar TS, Briceland LL, Delcoure K, et al. Medication prescribing errors in a teaching hospital. *JAMA.* 1990:263:2329-2334.

10. Raju TN, Thornton JP, Kecakes S, et al. Medication errors in neonatal and paediatric intensive care unit. *Lancet.* 1989:2:374-379.

11. Classen DC, Pestonik SL, Evans RS, Burke JP. Computerized surveillance of adverse drug events in hospital patients. *JAMA.* 1991:266:2847-2851.

12. Folli HL, Poole RL, Benitz WE, Russo JC. Medication error prevention by clinical pharmacists in two childrens' hospitals. *Pediatrics.* 1987:79:718-722.

13. Bates DW, Boyle D, Vander Vliet M, et al. Relationship between medication errors and adverse drug events. *J Gen Intern Med.* In press.

14. Anderson RE, Hill RB, Key CR. The sensitivity and specificity of clinical diagnostics during five decades: toward an understanding of necessary fallibility. *JAMA.* 1989:261:1610-1611.

15. Goldman L, Sayson R, Robbins S, Conn LH, Bettman M, Weissberg M. The value of the autopsy in the three medical eras. *N Engl J Med.* 1983:308:1000-1005.

16. Cameron HM, McGoogan E. A prospective study of 1,152 hospital autopsies. I: inaccuracies in death certification. *J Pathol.* 1981:133:273-283.

17. Gopher D, Olin M, Donchin Y, et al. The nature and causes of human errors in a medical intensive care unit. Presented at the 33rd annual meeting of the Human Factors Society; October 18, 1989; Denver, Colo.

18. Palmer RH, Strain R, Rothrock JK, et al. Evaluation of operational failures in clinical decision making. *Med Decis Making.* 1983:3:299-310.

19. Hilfiker D. Facing our mistakes. *N Engl J Med.* 1984:310:118-122.

20. Christensen JF, Levinson W, Dunn PM. The heart of darkness: the impact of perceived mistakes on physicians. *J Gen Intern Med.* 1992:7:424-431.

21. Wu AW, Folkman S, McPhee SJ, et al. Do house officers learn from their mistakes? *JAMA.* 1991:265:2089-2094.

22. Berwick DM. E.A. Codman and the rhetoric of battle: a commentary. *Milbank Q.* 1989:67:262-267.

23. McIntyre N, Popper KB. The critical attitude in medicine: the need for a new ethics. *BMJ.* 1989:287:1919-1923.

24. Berwick DM. Continuous improvement as an ideal in health care. *N Engl J Med.* 1989:320:53-56.

25. Deming WE. *Quality, Productivity, and Competitive Position.* Cambridge: Massachusetts Institute of Technology; 1982.

26. Reason J. *Human Error.* Cambridge, Mass: Cambridge University Press; 1992.

27. Rasmussen J, Jensen A. Mental procedures in real-life tasks: a case study of electronic trouble-shooting. *Ergonomics.* 1974:17:293-307.

28. Norman DA. *To Err Is Human,* New York, NY: Basic Books Inc Publishers; 1984.

29. Tversky A, Kahneman D. The framing of decisions and the psychology of choice. *Science.* 1981:211:453-458.

30. Yerkes RM, Dodson JD. The relation of strength of stimuli to rapidity of habit formation. *J Comp Neurol Psychol.* 1908:18:459-482.

31. Allnutt MF. Human factors in accidents. *Br J Anaest.* 1987:59:856-864.

32. Perrow C. *Normal Accidents: Living With High-Risk Technologies.* New York, NY: Basic Books Inc Publishers; 1984.

33. Orkin FK. Patient monitoring during anesthesia as an exercise in technology assessment. In: Saidman LJ, Smith NT, eds. *Monitoring in Anesthesia.* 3rd ed. London, England: Butterworth Publishers Inc; 1993.

34. Gaba DM. Human errors in anesthetic mishaps. *Int Anesthesiol Clin.* 1989:27:137-147.

35. Cooper JB, Newbower RS, Kitz RJ. An analysis of major errors and equipment failures in anesthesia management: considerations for prevention and detection. *Anesthesiology.* 1984:60:34-42.

36. Cullen DJ, Nemeakal RA, Cooper JB, Zaslavsky A, Dwyer MJ. Effect of pulse oximetry, age, and ASA physical status on the frequency of patients admitted unexpectedly to a post operative care unit. *Anesth Analg.* 1992:74:181.

8

Mistakes in Medicine: Personal and Moral Responses

Joel E. Frader

TWO CASES

STEVEN

It was in the middle of my extended training in pediatrics.[1] It was early on a Saturday evening. I was on call on one of the general inpatient units of our hospital. It had not been a terribly busy day. I wandered into the pediatric intensive care unit (PICU) to check on a patient. Seven-year-old Steven Bertrum did not look terribly ill propped up in his bed. However, he had a serious disorder, one that could take his life or change it miserably. Until several days earlier he had been enjoying first grade and anticipating Thanksgiving. A few weeks earlier he had experienced what seemed to be an ordinary sore throat. It went away so quickly that his mother had not even taken him to see the doctor. A few days before his admission to the hospital, he began to feel weak and his urine turned dark. Then he developed swelling in his legs. At that point, he told his mother. Mrs. Bertrum telephoned Steven's pediatrician and arranged for an appointment the next day. However, the following morning, Steven felt too weak to get out of bed. When his mother answered his calls and entered Steven's bedroom, she immediately became dismayed. Steven appeared pale and shaken. Soon, Steven and Mrs. Bertrum were on their way to the emergency room of their local hospital where Steven's pediatrician had agreed to meet them. The doctor assessed the situation, noting the boy's high blood pressure, swelling, and poor circulation; he immediately arranged for our transport team to pick up Steven.

That Steven was in trouble was apparent even to medical novices. The story suggested acute renal failure. Most likely, Steven had inflamed kidney tissue as part of his body's reaction to a "strep throat." That is, his throat infection a few weeks previously had probably been caused by bacteria, group A streptococci, which can prompt the body's immune system to react against and damage parts of the kidneys. We thought Steven had post-streptococcal glomerulonephritis. In any event, his kidneys were not working adequately. His body was retaining fluid and waste products were not being eliminated properly. Among the things we learned in his first few hours with us was that he had a dangerous buildup of potassium in his blood. Largely for that reason, we started Steven on peritoneal dialysis. The therapy uses the lining of the abdominal cavity, the peritoneum, as a large surface across which one can draw out some of the elements of the blood the kidneys would normally remove. Through a tube inserted into the abdomen, one can run a solution designed to maintain the balance of many of the blood's minerals and chemicals. The system serves as a temporary, if somewhat crude, replacement for the kidneys in the hopes that the body will heal and normal kidney function will return.

Steven had been getting peritoneal dialysis and other treatment for many hours at the time I entered the PICU. We had removed some of the excess fluid from his body and improved his circulation. He felt better. I wanted to check on his electrolytes—some essential chemical elements of his blood. The most recent report from the laboratory was reassuring. The excess potassium was approaching normal. I called a more senior trainee to report the news. Together we called the faculty physician in charge of the child's care. We spent most of the time on the telephone discussing the things we needed to do in the next 12 to 24 hours, recognizing that the biochemical improvement told us nothing about whether Steven's kidney function would return on its own. Fortunately, most of the time it does in these situations. Among the topics we mentioned was the need to add potassium to the fluid running into the abdomen. We had to do that in order to maintain a chemical balance. If we put a normal (for the body) concentration of potassium in the dialysis fluid, then there would be no chemical "pressure" for potassium to continue to flow out of the blood. This was simple high school chemistry, not high-tech medicine.

A few hours later, I checked on the electrolytes again. By that time, Steven's blood potassium was normal. It was time to add potassium to the dialysis solution. Around midnight, I wrote an order to do just that. The order was, for me, just like hundreds of other orders I had written to add potassium to fluids going into patients. It was automatic. Only that was the problem. I should have written a different kind of order.

Doctors commonly add potassium to intravenous (IV) fluids when patients cannot or will not take in enough nutrients on their own. Under most circumstances, the precise amount of potassium we add to the IV solution does not matter all that much. The potassium simply supplements the larger amount already circulating in the patient's blood, and the kidneys remove any relatively small excess. So we generally add 20 to 40 milliequivalents (units) of potassium to every liter (1000 cc) of IV fluid. However, dialysis fluid should match the normal amount of potassium in the blood—a concentration only one-tenth that of IV fluids or 4 milliequivalents per liter. I ordered the potassium concentration for the dialysis fluid as if it were IV fluid. My order was mechanical—something I did all the time, without thinking.

I discussed the need to add potassium to the dialysate with Steven's nurse and ordered another set of blood chemistries for six hours later (I wanted to have the results for rounds the next morning). The nurse followed my written order precisely and also automatically.

Very early Sunday morning, I made a list of all my patients, their diagnoses, problems, and treatments and the things that needed to be attended to during the day. As per our routine, I "signed out" to Jeremy, the trainee on call that day. The two of us walked around to see each of the patients and to discuss what had been going on and what needed to be done. My work was done; I went home.

Shortly after I left the hospital, Jeremy got a call from the laboratory that Steven's potassium was very high again. The lab technician commented that the serum they had tested seemed dark and was probably hemolyzed, meaning the red blood cells had opened up and emptied their mineral-rich contents into specimen, raising the potassium level. That happens all the time in pediatrics, as the methods of drawing blood from children can damage the red cells. Thinking the lab finding was such an artifact, but mindful he was caring for a very sick patient, Jeremy arranged to send another set of chemistries immediately and went about doing other business. A little while later, before anyone knew the results of the repeat test, Steven's heart rhythm became wildly disturbed, a result of excess serum potassium. His heart stopped pumping effectively. Nothing the PICU nurses or doctors could do restored a normal beat. Steven died.

The staff was confused and upset about the unexpected disaster. Dialysis had been working. They set out to figure out what had happened. A review of the orders and notes in the chart quickly revealed the error. Jeremy picked up the telephone to call me. "Hello," I said. "You killed your patient," came the response.

Over the next several days, almost nothing else occupied my consciousness. Anyone could have made the same mistake, many people told me. We did not treat many patients with renal failure; we did not use peritoneal dialysis often. I had written an order for a familiar drug (potassium chloride) in a familiar way and the nurses had carried it out as written because it all seemed quite familiar and fine to them, as well. Others told me that Steven might not have recovered anyway, that he had a serious disease. The attending physician had decided to tell Steven's family that he had died of "complications." I was told I could not speak with the family to convey my condolences or my regrets. Clearly, those in charge worried I would reveal the error. For some that meant placing an additional burden on the family, that of guilt for having let *these* doctors treat their son. For others, it probably meant attempting to prevent a malpractice suit. For me it meant adding the guilt associated with deception to that stemming from my mistakes. In addition, I could not face Jeremy. In fact, I could not speak to him except out of absolute necessity for the rest of that year.

CINDY

Years later, I was working on a weekend afternoon in a "fast-track" clinic in a children's hospital. The children did not need true emergency care, but they had acute illnesses for which their parents or other caregivers sought medical attention. Cindy's family brought her because she had a high fever. The toddler had been sick for a little more than 48 hours. Two days earlier, just after the fever and irritability started, Cindy's pediatrician had examined her and diagnosed acute otitis media, or middle-ear infection. The physician had prescribed a usual oral antibiotic, which the child had taken since the afternoon of the visit with her doctor. Cindy had experienced many ear infections previously. In fact, she had experienced so many that she was scheduled for an operation, in a week or so, to place "tubes" through her eardrum to keep the middle ear aerated and cut down on the frequency of infections. On the day we saw Cindy, her mother and grandmother thought she was not getting any better. In fact, they thought she was worse. Perhaps her fever was higher and she was breathing "more heavily." Because her own doctor was not available that weekend, they brought Cindy to us, where her ear surgery was to happen.

One of the two doctors I was supervising that afternoon went in to see the patient. She took note of the family's concern. She learned some important information about Cindy's medical history. As an infant, Cindy had had a serious medical problem that required many weeks of inpatient treatment in several different hospitals, including ours. In addition to the main reason for her hospitalization as a newborn, she had developed a nosocomial infection—that is, she had become infected with a virus passed from another patient, probably through a member of the hospital staff. That infection had caused some respiratory difficulty; and although it had resolved completely, the family had been warned that children do not develop immunity to the particular offending virus, so she could have the infection again. In addition, babies who are infected with that virus have a somewhat higher chance of developing asthma. So, the family had been warned to watch out for "breathing problems." They were watching and they were worried.

The resident examined Cindy and came to discuss the case with me. She told me that the child looked quite sick. On examination, the ears appeared to be actively inflamed, with no evidence of the improvement that 48 hours of successful treatment might bring. She noted an abnormal breathing pattern, although she recognized that the youngster had considerable nasal congestion. The child was breathing through her mouth, and noisily. The family's worry had managed to infect the resident. She wanted to know if we should do blood tests and a chest x-ray. I said I wanted to examine the child to make my own assessment. We both entered the examining room. I sat down and held the child while the mother and grandmother went over their worries and some of the story. I then did a thorough examination, anxious not to miss anything, given the level of concern expressed by the family and the resident. The ears looked actively infected. The nasal passages were swollen and filled with thick mucous. No air was moving through the child's nose. But the lungs sounded perfectly clear. There was a normal amount of air moving in and out of the chest and no wheezing. There were no areas where the breath sounds were in any way abnormal. The rest of the examination was also normal. The child was alert and playful.

I told the family that the resident and I would step out and take a few minutes to discuss things, but we would be right back. In the conference area, I told the resident that I thought everything could be explained by the continued ear infection and nasal congestion. I did not think there was any pneumonia. I did not favor tests, as they would not be likely to lead to any change in what I we should do. Even if an x-ray showed some pneumonia, which I really doubted, the appropriate response would be to change to a different antibiotic, one designed to kill the bacteria that had developed resistance to first-line drugs. In our community, about 40 percent of the bacteria that infected ears had such resistance. The antibiotics that I would use now for this child would also work well for the common type of pneumonia that children develop outside of the hospital. So, tests would only delay things and not change my recommendations. The resident accepted this, though perhaps uncomfortably. We returned to the room with the family. I explained my findings and conclusion. The grandmother said she thought the child should be admitted to the hospital and we should "run tests." I went over my reasoning. After more conversation, I thought the family had accepted our perspective. We provided a prescription for a different antibiotic, instructions about the nasal congestion, and suggested they follow up with their pediatrician in 24 to 48 hours.

The next time I heard about that patient was the following afternoon. Someone, I do not remember who it was, came to tell me that the county coroner had requested the records from the previous day's visit. The emergency department doctors had pronounced the child dead at a community hospital that morning.

We had an urgent meeting of a committee to review such "adverse events." The hospital's medical director, the director of the emergency department, the risk manager, the hospital's chief malpractice defense lawyer, the resident, myself, and assorted others convened. We reviewed the record and the documentation of the visit. Fortunately, both the resident and I had written detailed, legible, and reasonably intelligent notes. We agreed that from the record and our recollection, nothing untoward had happened. We also agreed that we needed more information—in particular, the coroner's findings. I asked for and received permission to contact the family. I wanted to convey my condolences. I called many times, on two occasions leaving a message on an answering machine, but I never had a conversation with a family member.

Autopsy reports do not appear in the wink of an eye. No matter how anxious various persons might be to know some answers, the information almost always seems to take forever to materialize. This case was not exceptional. Only after many weeks—or perhaps it was months—we learned that the coroner had declared "bronchopneumonia" as the cause of death. Just a little while later, we received notification that the family had retained a lawyer, all our records were under subpoena, and we should expect filing of a malpractice action.

Another lethal mistake? This time I was not so ready to believe it. Even if the child had pneumonia, the little girl I saw the afternoon before was not anywhere near death from respiratory infection. The autopsy diagnosis made little sense. A few days later, when I first met with the attorney assigned to represent me, the hospital, and the resident, he agreed. Again, we needed more information. We needed a complete copy of the autopsy report and we needed an independent review of the autopsy findings.

Eventually we arranged for both. The autopsy report astounded me. There had been no cultures taken of blood or of the lungs. The description of the lungs and the weight of the lungs at autopsy were not consistent with pneumonia as a cause of death. It did not add up. And the pediatric pulmonary pathologist who finally had the opportunity to review the autopsy material agreed. In fact, he said, the slides from the autopsy did not show any evidence of pneumonia. It just was not there.

Well, the short form of the very long story is this. We went to trial. The plaintiffs had two experts who testified, via videotape, that we had practiced substandard medicine that led to the child's death. The first was the coroner, who by then had moved to another city. Interestingly, this coroner was an attorney as well as a pathologist. In his elected role as county coroner in our city, many felt he had a politically motivated grudge against our medical center. The other expert was a pediatric cardiologist from a large city. He was not just a heart specialist, but one who spent virtually all his time working in a cardiac catheterization laboratory. He testified that we had not met the standard of care for examining, testing, and treating a child with a respiratory illness in an ambulatory care facility. Our experts, who appeared in person, were a director of a pediatric emergency department in a hospital comparable to ours—someone who dealt daily with problems similar to the deceased patient's—and the pediatric pathologist who had reviewed the slides.

At the trial, I testified about what I had seen and done, about my reasons for my actions, and my belief that we had acted reasonably and responsibly. The pediatric emergency specialist testified that our medical behavior met the standard of care. The pathologist came with poster-sized blow-ups of the slides from the autopsy and exemplary slides of pneumonia from other patients. The visual evidence and the pathologist's clear, effective testimony seemed to be persuasive. After a relatively short period of deliberation, the jury rendered a verdict "for the defendants." Eleven of the 12 jurors felt there had been no malpractice. More than enough.

EXEGESIS

CATEGORIES

How can we make sense of what happened in these two situations? How would I know if I had made a mistake in the second case if we had not been sued? If we want to know the nature of the mistakes, we need a system for defining and categorizing mistakes. Dictionaries offer insight into how people use words, so perhaps starting there would help. The *American Heritage Dictionary* defines a mistake as an "error or fault."[2] In addition, I would say that in ordinary usage we can often hear an implication of blameworthiness, especially with respect to human action. People make mistakes and are at fault. Many people talk as if computers make errors, a statement, whether accurate or not, with a less moralistic quality.

Medical mistakes are very complicated when we try to sort them out. Sometimes we try to talk about mistakes as a matter of "bad outcomes." However, this does not always work. Outcomes can be less than desired without being a result of a faulty process. The patient may not respond to treatment even when everyone agrees the treatment has been appropriate. Alternatively, we may speak about a process approach to medical error. But this way of looking at things does not fully satisfy either. Inadequate processes do not always result in a bad outcome. Fortunately, we may discover mistakes in time to prevent harm, or the patient and those who make the mistakes may just get lucky—nothing bad happens and no one knows why.

Medical uncertainty makes it very difficult to decide if there has been a mistake. We often do not understand enough about all the factors in human physiology, pathology, psychology—not to mention their interaction—and the interventions we employ to ferret out cause and effect. Even when we have as much information as we might like in investigating a problem, we have trouble sorting out what went wrong and why. Medical reality is enormously complex. We face a host of patient-related circumstances—those just listed, as well as social and environmental factors and factors related to the care providers—that also have physiological, emotional, and social components. The complicated matrix and interplay confound us. We formally recognize this when we talk about "complications" of diseases and treatments. This term signifies a neutral (that is, nonblaming) way to say we do not control or understand everything about medical situations.

This complexity has several components. The first involves knowledge, especially scientific or clinical knowledge with inherent limitations. Some of the limits exist because the necessary scientific work, be it research in molecular biology or a controlled clinical trial, has not yet been done. Some of the limits exist because our techniques for measurement and statistical analysis of data only permit us to infer finite degrees of certitude, frequently less than we prefer. To provide a mundane example, picture a patient who appears in the emergency department with abdominal pain that began within the last few hours. The patient's story suggests possible appendicitis. The examination of the patient can add, to some degree, to the suspicion of a need for an operation, but cannot provide "proof." The patient's tolerance for pain, even the patient's particular anatomy, can make the diagnosis more or less difficult. Laboratory tests will not provide definitive information either, although they may add something. Ultimately, a surgeon will have to decide whether to take the patient for an operation, and only when the surgeon sees the intestinal appendage will he or she have the answer. In this setting, physicians formally acknowledge and expect uncertainty. In fact, a surgeon who only removes "hot" appendixes, as judged by pathologic examination, would risk criticism for operating on too few patients, for being too certain of his or her judgment.

Uncertainty operates at another level. We use the fact of uncertainty in different ways, depending upon our attitudes, values, and beliefs. For some, the inevitability of not knowing "for sure" becomes a warrant for taking considerable risks. For example, consider a previously healthy patient who is highly likely to die soon from an acute problem. One physician may use the lack of an established intervention as a justification for attempting a new treatment that might, in theory, save the patient—but might also produce a longer, more uncomfortable death. Other physicians, patients, or family members facing a similar situation might conclude that the use of a highly uncertain procedure would not be worth the chance of making things worse. Our interpretation, our acceptance or denial of medical uncertainty, can take us in different directions. Thus far, attempts to limit clinical uncertainty through health services research and the use of standardized patient care "pathways" or protocols based upon expert opinion or the development of consensus among clinicians have not had a large effect on variations in practice.

Given all this, we should not be surprised when we sometimes have a very hard time figuring out what happened when something appears to have gone wrong. Moreover, we rarely have the medical equivalent of aviation's "black box." Even when medical records are legible and helpful, different persons involved will have different perceptions of the same events. We will have an inevitable insufficiency of information most of the time, leading us to say we can not really tell if a mistake occurred. We may feel that someone has made a momentous error, but deem ourselves unable to prove it. Therefore, we hesitate to raise the issue with the person involved. Our desires to educate and prevent future harm, perhaps to punish, wane in the face of this uncertainty, aided, possibly, by our wish to avoid the unpleasantness associated with drawing attention to errors.

Although medicine has trouble defining, categorizing, and responding to error, the law claims to do better. The legal standard of negligence seems, in concept, quite clear.[3] One has committed malpractice if the plaintiff can (1) demonstrate that harm (damages) occurred (the damage may be physical or in the form of the more elusive "pain and suffering"); (2) show that the defendant had a particular duty (standard of care) under the circumstances; (3) prove that the defendant committed a breach of the duty (the mistake itself); and (4) establish that the breach caused the damages. Juries are charged as "fact finders" and must decide if all four of these elements are present, constituting professional negligence. Note that a mistake, pure and simple, does not alone make for malpractice. Note also that the apparent legal clarity only raises more questions. How does one clearly define the standard of care? In the law, different jurisdictions actually use different definitions. One could ask if trainees should be held to the same standard as faculty members and supervisors? Intuitively, we want to say "yes." However, on reflection, we see that the answer ought to vary with the specifics. Perhaps all residents should ask about drug allergies before starting a patient on penicillin. It is less clear that residents should know the nuances of possible adverse drug reactions used to treat hypertension in elderly patients with diseases involving multiple organ systems. Should the generalist have to uphold the same standard as the subspecialist? Again, it depends on such matters as how frequently one can expect each clinician to encounter similar problems, the availability of the relevant clinical information, and so on. Should the person practicing in a rural setting with fewer resources have to conform to the same standard as another in a large, resource-rich tertiary-care center? Similar responses apply. All these questions involve a certain degree of controversy with no universal normative, legal, or sociologic answer.

One can also look at errors in medicine from a different perspective. Sociologists have examined medical error. Bosk produced one of the most interesting and provocative examinations, based on his participant-observation on the surgical service of a large, urban teaching hospital.[4] He described three kinds of error: technical, judgmental, and normative. *Technical errors* involve instrumental issues having to do with knowledge and skill and mostly affect trainees (for example, the addition of the wrong concentration of potassium to dialysis fluid). *Judgmental errors* involve the inappropriate application of knowledge to the clinical situation (for example, drawing the wrong conclusion from available clinical and laboratory data). In Bosk's study, supervisory or attending surgeons typically make these judgmental errors, but much the same could be said of senior clinicians in any field. *Normative errors* involve the failure to acknowledge or "own up" to one's limitations; such errors elicit strong emotional reactions. A clinician commits a normative error when he or she does not seek the advice or intervention of a more experienced or skilled person under circumstances that call for greater knowledge or surgical proficiency. The surgeons in Bosk's study see normative errors as blameworthy; the other two kinds of errors, which are viewed as routine and expected, do not carry the same moral weight.

Now, one can readily imagine physicians and perhaps those outside of health-care asking: "Why should these distinctions matter?" Perhaps an example from the mass media can help. In *Heartsounds*, Martha Weinman Lear's story of her physician-husband's struggle with heart disease, we have the following account. Dr. Lear had a serious myocardial infarction (MI). After considerable hand wringing, he underwent coronary artery bypass grafting. He did not recover well after surgery: his cardiac function did not improve as expected, and he had considerable problems with memory and other neurologic symptoms. Mrs. Lear pressured her husband's cardiologist to find an answer to what had happened. The physician conducted a careful review of all Dr. Lear's records and inferred that during the bypass surgery the patient probably suffered an additional heart attack that was not recognized at the time. The cardiologist and Mrs. Lear discussed the situation and decided not to provide this new interpretation to Dr. Lear. Later, the patient discovered the cover-up and became infuriated. However, his anger focused on the deception, not the fact of the intraoperative MI or even that his physicians failed to recognize what had happened. To Dr. Lear, the real moral harm—the betrayal—involved his doctor's and his wife's conspiracy of silence.[5] This demonstrates the personal and ethical significance of normative error, rather than technical or judgmental error.

This discussion invites a related question. Are there "innocent" mistakes? Perhaps technical and judgmental errors fall into such a category from some perspective, although not necessarily from others, such as that of legal liability. However, an important point here is that raising the question of innocence suggests that we assume the validity of blameworthiness. We seek a responsible agent. We want to extract retribution and compensation. When we acquiesce in this view, we miss a great deal. What seems better is consideration of error in medicine with appreciation of the context and inevitability of error. We want a system to humanize patients, families, and professionals, rather than one that objectifies everyone in an adversarial manner.[6] In addition, we need to help patients and the public to have realistic expectations of medicine and the people who provide care.

Of course, healthcare providers need to take some responsibility for creating the host of misperceptions that feed the mistrust and fuel the public relations and malpractice nightmares that haunt professionals and healthcare institutions. Media hype, whether in the form of sensationalistic journalism or advertising, leads naïve individuals to believe that medicine may just be able to cure anything. In one city, a hospital advertises its technically advanced surgical procedures in a way that allows prospective patients to believe that the doctors will not really have to "cut" them, open them up, or hurt them. This new surgery seems a little like Erica Jong's "zipless" sex act, requiring nothing messy or invasive. In another city, a series of advertisements for an academic medical center states that what goes on there is "amazing," implying perhaps that nothing could go wrong in such an environment. Our zeal for a competitive edge may bring us rather too close to bald commercialism for everyone's good.

REALITY

Just how big a problem do we have? It is hard to know for sure. Lesar and colleagues found 3.1 medication errors for every 1,000 orders written on the inpatient service of a teaching hospital.[7] They rated 58 percent of those to have "significant" potential for adverse effects. In a subsequent paper, the same lead author reported a trend toward an increasing frequency of errors over the nine-year period of 1987 to 1995.[8] In the last year of the study they found 4.14 "clinically significant" errors per 1,000 orders written. Using death certificate data to "capture" medication-related deaths for patients in and out of the hospital, Phillips and colleagues found that 7,391 people in the United States died from medication errors in 1993 and that the number of deaths per year increased by more than two and a half times between 1983 and 1993.[9] In a 1994 article, Leape estimated approximately 180,000 deaths per year in the United States from preventable, unintended healthcare-related acts—an alarming figure by almost any standard.[10] Andrews and colleagues conducted a prospective observational study that suggests the incidence of error may be yet higher than that estimated by others.[11]

Leape's work has brought great insight to the problem of medical error. He helps us understand that the general culture and social organization of medicine have impeded efforts to take constructive steps to prevent mistakes or reduce their seriousness. According to Leape, medicine insists on seeing errors as isolated incidents, rather than recognizing underlying patterns that arise from the nature and structure of our medical care system. This tendency to miss the forest (or avoid painful truths) is reinforced by the fact that, although mistakes are quite common, most errors do no not result in harm. Moreover, physicians especially are socialized to strive for perfection or infallibility. Therefore, errors come to be seen as a failure of character for the person responsible. This, in turn, creates a psychological incentive to cover up mistakes. The fear of reprisal also has another consequence. When an individual has to hide what happens, it blocks opportunities to "share" the emotional impact (sense of guilt, sorrow, and so forth) with others. Leape also reminds us that the malpractice system in the United States adds an element of terror that discourages open communication about and rational responses to errors. Wu and colleagues discuss the barriers to disclosure of mistakes more comprehensively, noting the potential harms (negative patient reaction; psychological stress on the physician; and the loss of referrals, privileges, or other status) that may result.[12]

Leape helps us to understand that "human error" often is beyond the control of the individual(s) involved. That medicine has failed to recognize the insights that industry has learned from cognitive sciences and other disciplines only adds to the tragedy of the preventable deaths, disability, and suffering caused by mistakes. In particular, Leape focuses on two concepts contributed by modern psychology—slips and mistakes. Slips result from "glitches" in automatic mental processes. Mistakes involve errors of conscious thought. The two notions involve different external conditions and different mechanisms.

Slips happen when, during routine actions, an individual experiences a diversion of his or her attention or failure in the usual internal monitoring processes. As a result, a surgeon may take the right action (perform the indicated operation) but do it on the wrong object (right instead of left arm). Or a nurse may fail to notice that the package that just arrived for her patient from the blood bank does not match the patient's red cell type and start to infuse the mismatched blood anyway. These kinds of errors increase when the individuals involved suffer from sleep deprivation or fatigue from other causes; when persons have used substances that alter mental states; when boredom, anger, fear, anxiety, or other strong emotional states are active; or when environmental factors such as poor lighting or loud noises interfere with concentration. Of course, sleep deprivation, terror in confronting critical illness or death, and suboptimal work conditions pervade medical settings.

The *mistakes* that Leape discusses come in two subcategories: rule-based and knowledge-based. Rule-based errors involve misapplication of expertise, more or less analogous to Bosk's judgmental error. Knowledge-based errors happen very commonly in medicine. They often involve a "first-time" situation where the individual has no routine approach. These errors may entail a lack of relevant information or misinterpretation of the situation. We make these because of the way our minds work. Our memories rely on bias: the brain knows that certain events, diseases, and so forth, occur commonly. Hence, we perceive what we know to be frequent, even if some of the information points in another direction. One can easily order the wrong dose of potassium for the dialysis fluid. We also have a tendency to fixate on what comes to our minds first. We reinforce this by seeking data that confirm our early impression and because we want to believe in the validity of our choices. A well-known example in pediatrics involves the diagnosis of pain in a young child's lower abdomen on the right side. We tend to think first of appendicitis and forget about another important diagnosis—intussusception, where the bowel telescopes on itself and chokes off its own blood supply. Pediatricians must remind themselves to think about what to consider, rather than simply jumping to the conclusion that right-lower quadrant pain amounts to appendicitis. The conditions that favor slips also increase the likelihood of mistakes. Stress predisposes healthcare workers to all these errors.

According to Leape, we can create systems to reduce the incidence of error. We can increase safety by building error-detection mechanisms in complex processes. A good example is the use of computerized medication-ordering programs that (1) require clinicians to give the patient's weight or body surface area and (2) check the dose ordered against standardized doses per pound, per kilo, or per square meter. If the ordered dose falls outside the usual range, the system challenges or refuses the order. In the case of Steven presented above, if I had been required to type "dialysis fluid" and specify a potassium concentration, a good system would have caught the dosing error. We can also improve the presentation of information on dials, video screens, or other kinds of display. We can reduce the precursors to error, for example, by using "night-float" systems so that residents who care for patients during the day do not have to stay up most or all of the night and continue their work through the following afternoon or evening. We can increase standardization or simplify components of care, for example, by providing drugs in easy-to-use and well-labeled containers. We can increase the extent to which we monitor for errors and nonpunitively provide feedback. We can also increase the explicit attention to and training for safety and error reduction. We will still have to remember, however, that no matter what we do, as long as we have humans involved in action, people will make mistakes. The dream of a completely understood, error-free system will remain just that—a reductionist ideal that we cannot achieve.

Nevertheless, we can do better. Many components of our society have a head start on medicine with regard to minimizing mistakes. Leape leans heavily on the model of aviation. He notes that the aviation industry appropriately assumes that human errors will occur. In response, the industry uses buffers and redundancy, and takes advantage of automation to balance human operators. Much of what aviators do involves standardized activity with strict protocols and checklists. Training too is very standardized and pays a great deal of explicit attention to safety. Perhaps most importantly, those in aviation accept a high level of external control and institutionalized mechanisms organized around safety. Physicians, by contrast, insist on the preservation—indeed, the essential value—of minimal regulation and maximal individualism.

Medicine could do much of what industry has done. Routine error investigation—even when there has been no damage—could lead to the discovery of systemic faults. Correction of these faults could save money (as a result of fewer complications, shorter hospital stays, less expended in the malpractice system, and so forth), not to mention improve outcomes and satisfaction. As noted, we could rationalize work schedules, ensure safer physical environments for workers and patients, and provide a more supportive psychosocial environment (to reduce stress). We could begin to see mistakes as "treasures," opportunities to learn, rather than occasions for punishment.[13] We need to change our attitudes toward the meaning and reality of error. I have to admit, I have a hard time seeing my experience with Steven as any kind of good fortune. Even so, I learned to be much more circumspect when in uncharted clinical waters, and I hope I learned how to approach others who make mistakes in a more constructive way than the one used by my superiors and colleagues.

The matter of attitude deserves more attention. My own experience of committing error, or worrying that I did, makes me very aware of the personal, painful burden of error. One feels tremendous regret, remorse, and diminished self-worth when harm has come about, even when it is unclear who or what caused the harm. We will not, cannot, and perhaps should not eliminate these responses. However, the environment ought not to reinforce the misery. We want to do what we remind parents and teachers to do: separate the behavior from the person. We must not imply that those who make mistakes—even serious ones—are necessarily bad or evil persons.[14]

We must also realize that errors will evoke strong reactions from those around the person identified as making the mistake. Predictably, attending physicians get angry when residents or fellows err, normatively or technically. Trainees often express the view that any such negative response is hurtful and their supervisors should "swallow" their distress. However, common sense tells us that anger under the circumstances is itself understandable, and psychology teaches us that striving too forcefully to repress anger may have dire consequences. The more pragmatic concern involves the manner in which one expresses wrath and the degree of distress communicated. When supervisors and educators become upset—when they "lose it," as we have all seen happen—with subordinates who have erred, there is a need for restraint. The anger is best expressed in private. Public humiliation invites retaliation and defensiveness and inhibits self-reflection. Passionate utterances should be brief. When such orations become excessive, they warrant an apology. It is important to go beyond fury or exasperation. The subordinate—be it a medical student, resident, or junior colleague—needs the person in authority to extend sympathy, to provide nurturance, to encourage learning from what happened, and to promote healing. While none of my supervisors yelled at me in the case of Steven, neither did they provide a path for learning or healing. I do not know if this resulted from their own discomfort with what had happened or if it had to do with a style of education that simply avoided dealing with feelings. I hope I have done better when the roles have been reversed, but I have found it difficult to make accurate assessments of my own behavior in those circumstances.

RECOGNITION

We need to know about errors to learn from them, to create schemes for reducing their recurrence, to understand the factors that make them more or less likely. Nevertheless, we need to do more. We must, as Hilfiker says, face our mistakes. "As physicians our automatic response . . . is to try to discover what went wrong. . . . This response is important. . . . But it is inadequate if it does not address our own emotional and spiritual experience of the events. . . . We must bring our mistakes out of the closet. . . . Our profession is difficult enough without having to wear the yoke of perfection."[15]

Without responding to the powerful, nonrational aspects of our reactions to our errors, we compound the problem. Clinical mistakes— especially those that result in harm such as disability, suffering, or death—have devastating effects on those involved. We are crippled ourselves; we not only mourn, we feel the weight of responsibility for causing the grief. We question our professional and personal worthiness. Most of us cannot simply point to contributing and collateral factors and distance ourselves through repression and denial. In addition, as with dealing with other types of grief, it often helps to talk about it.

Even that, of course, does not lead to absolution, to complete catharsis. Paget, a sociologist, expressed this well. "The sorrow of this work is not only that mistakes are inevitable but also that they will go on happening in the tomorrows of medical work. Physicians must act in the face of this great looming presence of mistakes. They must also dwell, it seems, in a strange linguistic silence of this realm of being mistaken, for no adequate language captures their work or their conduct going awry with an even hand."[16]

We have an understandable tendency to hide our mistakes. In the case of Steven, I was told that revealing the error that led to his death would "not right the wrong, not bring him back." We would only add to the parents' misery. "Successfully" covering up mistakes can keep patients and family members from seeking compensation or retribution through the malpractice system. Many in medicine feel that the litigation process involves excessive costs, monetary and psychological, and works unjustly, depending more on the verbal skills of the advocates than on discovering facts. Others, recognizing the structural and cultural defects in our healthcare system, say that, until the system takes a corrective, rather than a punative approach, the risks to career and reputation exceed the value of openness.

We have similar rationales for keeping the knowledge or suspicions of others' mistakes under wraps. In addition to the arguments just given, we have to face the issue of group solidarity—the guild mentality, by no means unique to medicine, in which we hold that no outsider could possibly understand or judge the situation fairly. If we "rat" on others, we also risk injury to our own reputations, with the possible loss of referrals (and hence, income) and even a fear of litigation for libel. For some, openness about error in medicine will undermine trust in the profession. Other people point to the fact that, under many circumstances, we have no legal duty to report or reveal the errors others may have committed.

But powerful reasons counterbalance these notions. From the point of view of medical ethics, there is the issue of truthfulness. Even if one rejects a rule-based notion that one should not lie, one has to consider the consequentialist view that knowing the truth may enhance and empower the patient's or family member's position in seeking compensation or satisfaction—whether monetary or otherwise. If we withhold information, we undermine the autonomy of the patient or family members and narrow their options. Besides, we do want to take responsibility for and police our own. Only by taking self-criticism and self-regulation seriously can we attempt to engender public trust in the profession. In addition, as noted, acknowledging errors can be the first step toward learning, personal and systemic, and toward corrective and preventive measures.

In addition, unanticipated outcomes might never happen unless the truth emerges. I learned that lesson from my malpractice trial in the case of Cindy. I still do not know why that child died; I never will. There was no pneumonia, and pneumonia could not have been the cause of her death. Even knowing the stakes—that is, the outcome of a malpractice action—many smart people who reviewed Cindy's chart and the autopsy findings could not overcome the terrible uncertainty. Perhaps someone smarter or cleverer could have seen what was coming on that afternoon in our urgent care clinic and intervened in a way that might have prevented the tragic loss.

Knowing I had not made the specific mistake I was charged with in the malpractice suit—failure to diagnosis and appropriately treat pneumonia—did not completely expunge my sense of guilt or self-doubt. This is one of the legacies of clinical uncertainty. Convincing the jury that we were not "bad doctors" helped some. And there was an interesting effect of the trial I could not have foreseen. One of my colleagues spoke with the child's mother after the trial. She had sat through all the proceedings, as had I. It seemed she felt a kind of relief, too. Instead of being angry over injustice, over losing, she had heard what our experts had said and had some of the same response as the jury. The trial had brought about a kind of inner cleansing for her, as well. She did not have to berate herself for having trusted our hospital and its doctors, for having brought her sick child to us. Having the truth come out brought about a kind of renewal for her, one nobody expected.

CONCLUSION

Mistakes in medicine can have serious consequences for patients, their loved ones, and those providers of medical care who have more or less responsibility for the acts or omissions we call mistakes. In the case of Steven, I made a terrible, fatal error. Note, however, that I was not alone. The other trainee and the attending physician, knowing the relative lack of experience we had with such a situation, could and perhaps should have done more to be certain I knew and understood how to order the potassium for the dialysis fluid. The nurses did not question the order. Perhaps they should have looked up how to constitute dialysis fluid, given how infrequently they had to prepare it. Jeremy might have paid more attention to the laboratory's report of elevated serum potassium. He probably fell into the same trap that I did, responding on "autopilot." Most likely, Jeremy assumed that what he usually experienced, elevated potassium due to artifact, explained the situation he confronted with the lab report of Steven's electrolytes. He might have stepped back and considered the context, Steven's renal disease, and taken the findings more seriously. Note that Jeremy, as far as I know, never bore any of the responsibility for what happened—in his own mind, in the minds of our attending physicians, or in my mind. The incident, it seems, probably was a multifactorial system error of the sort Leape wants us to notice and prevent. But no one responded that way.

Unfortunately, we compounded the medication error when we failed to provide the facts about Steven's death to his family. I believe that the attending staff felt that informing the parents would only produce psychological harm. There may have been other factors involved—administrative or legal advice, for example—but I did not know of any. As a group, we transformed technical error into normative error. We made a mistake into a moral wrong. I could have changed that; I could have contacted the family against the wishes of my superiors. I wanted them to know the truth, for its own sake; I wanted for them to be able to determine how to react, knowing all that happened, for them not to have to bear whatever sense of responsibility they may have felt for what happened. I did not tell the family on my own. I lacked the courage to do so, knowing that such deviance would likely have severe consequences for my career, at least in academic medicine. As a result, not only did we deceive the family, we did nothing to prevent another trainee from making the same mistake in that institution in the future. I had no organized help working through the experience. It took many, many years for me to come to terms with those events.

In Cindy's case, I do not believe we made a medical error; at least I am convinced we did not commit malpractice (that is, provide substandard care). We did not do what we were accused of doing: failing to diagnosis or treat appropriately the alleged cause of death. In fact, it appeared that the coroner made a serious mistake—one that led unjustly to years of anguish for the child's family, a resident physician, and myself, and resulted in needless, substantial expenditure in the costs associated with litigation. Whether we might have missed something that could have prevented Cindy's death, I cannot know. I think about it, uncomfortably, from time to time.

What have I learned from these experiences and from reading the literature on medical error? Mistakes often have a larger set of causes than the technical or moral failings of the individual most readily identifiable as responsible; yet powerful forces prevent us from dealing with the wider, more complex systemic problems. Covering up results in further harm, usually for most of the involved parties. Dealing openly, even if it has to happen within the context of adversarial conflict in a flawed legal system, can help provide a measure of healing. Finally, uncertainty looms large. We need to confront uncertainty in medicine more. We need to acknowledge its role in clinical situations much more explicitly than we do. We need to educate the public generally and our patients and families specifically about what we do and do not know, what we can and cannot know. Acceptance of indeterminacy may make the practice of medicine more tolerable for caregivers and recipients alike. Reducing fear may reduce the stress on everyone. That, in turn, may help reduce error.

NOTES

1. The two stories closely parallel my experience. The first case is actually a composite drawn from various times in my career—times when I had very different roles in how the drama played out. I have changed the content and other information that might identify specific persons for two reasons. In part, I wish to protect the privacy of some of those involved, although the latter case is a matter of public record. More importantly, some individuals still could be hurt, in various ways, from accounts of the "real" cases. The reader should understand that so many similar stories—with precise, accurate portrayals—could be told that the details simply do not matter.

2. *The American Heritage Dictionary,* 3rd ed. (New York: Delta Trade Paperbacks, 1992), 534.

3. G.J. Annas, *The Rights of Patients: The Basic ACLU Guide to Patient Rights,* 2nd ed. (Carbondale, Ill.: Southern Illinois University Press, 1989), 240.

4. C.L. Bosk, *Forgive and Remember: Managing Medical Failure* (Chicago: University of Chicago Press, 1979).

5. M.W. Lear, *Heartsounds* (New York: Pocketbooks, 1980).

6. W.M. Tierney, "Laughter and Balance: A Letter to a Junior Resident," *Journal of General Internal Medicine* 13, no. 4 (1998): 271-2.

7. T.S. Lesar et al., "Medication Prescribing Errors in a Teaching Hospital," *Journal of the American Medical Association* 263, no. 14 (1990): 2329-34.

8. T.S. Lesar, B.M. Lomaestro, and H. Pohl, "Medication-Prescribing Errors in a Teaching Hospital: A 9-Year Experience," *Archives of Internal Medicine* 157 (1997): 1569-76.

9. D.P. Phillips, N. Christenfeld, and L.M. Glynn, "Increase in U.S. Medication-Error Deaths Between 1983 and 1993," *Lancet* 351 (1998): 643-4.

10. L.L. Leape, "Error in Medicine," *Journal of the American Medical Association* 272, no. 23 (1994): 1851-7. [Leape's article is reprinted as chapter 7 of this book—ED.]

11. L.B. Andrews et al., "An Alternative Strategy for Studying Adverse Events in Medical Care," *Lancet* 349 (1997): 309-13.

12. A.W. Wu et al., "To Tell the Truth: Ethical and Practical Issues in Disclosing Medical Mistakes to Patients," *Journal of General Internal Medicine* 12 (1997): 770-5.

13. D. Blumenthal, "Making Medical Errors Into 'Medical Treasures,' " *Journal of the American Medical Association* 272, no. 23 (1994): 1867-8.

14. C.P. Lape, "Disclosing Medical Mistakes," *Journal of General Internal Medicine* 13, no. 4 (1998): 283-4.

15. D. Hilfiker, "Facing Our Mistakes," *New England Journal of Medicine* 310, no. 2 (1984): 118-22. [Hilfiker's article is reprinted as chapter 6 of this book—ED.]

16. M.A. Paget, *The Unity of Mistakes: A Phenomenological Interpretation of Medical Work* (Philadelphia: Temple University Press, 1988), 139.

9

Learning to Keep a Cautious Tongue: The Reporting of Mistakes in Neurosurgery, 1890 to 1930

Rosa Lynn Pinkus

INTRODUCTION

Accomplished neurosurgeons understand that a prerequisite to good practice is the acquisition of good clinical judgment. They also candidly admit that one of the best routes to good judgment is the exercise of bad judgment. At first, this turnabout seems to be a rehearsal of the old adage, "We can learn from our mistakes." In a clinical practice such as neurosurgery, however, where mistakes can maim a patient or cause death, the adage assumes new meaning. How surgeons tolerate the harm that can come from their mistakes, how they categorize and forgive them, and what steps they take to prevent neophytes from making them has been the topic of one book-length study.[1]

This essay examines these questions historically, using case reports in neurosurgical practice and law during the 40 years from 1890 to 1930, the period during which neurosurgery attained full status as a surgical subspecialty.[2] During the last decades of the 19th century and the first decades of the 20th, surgeons published case reports that included the admission of errors that caused death or morbidity to patients. Proceedings from national meetings also documented debates in which neurosurgeons publicly questioned the honesty of their colleagues' statistical claims of success. This was a time when the boundaries for what counted as acceptable practice were being set, and the overt and explicit admission of error served to educate others who were learning the new specialty. Discerning truth from error was, in fact, a central part of Harvey Cushing's campaign to create the special field of neurological surgery.[3] These years, therefore, provide an opportunity to examine how a profession defines mistakes and then attempts to prevent them.

By 1930, the open and frank discussion of clinical misjudgment and technical error, along with the particularized case report, had all but disappeared from scholarly journals. Instead, journal articles included a tacit admission of errors that was couched in rhetoric of improved method. To the generalist, these reports provided evidence of the improvements in care that pioneers in neurosurgery had promised.[4] To the knowledgeable practitioner, such articles served as a constant reminder that harm could occur even in the hands of new surgical specialists, but the details were missing. This essay examines how the integration of the scientific method into the standardization of residency education and the changes in law contributed to the disappearance of the explicit publishing of mistakes.[5]

A SURGEON'S MISTAKES ARE UNIQUE

Of all physicians, the surgeon's interventions are most visible and his therapeutic expectations are most specific.   —Charles Bosk

In his oft-quoted book, *Forgive and Remember: Managing Medical Failure,* Bosk reported the results of 18 months of his participation at and observation of a major academic teaching surgical service. The phrase "forgive and remember" refers to a "shorthand for the complex moral code developed by surgeons to keep track of mistakes made during the residency years and to gauge which are routine and which are not, which are forgiven and which others cause irreparable damage to the surgeon's career. It also specifies the social control mechanisms used by the group to insure that the tacit knowledge is learned by those wishing to become surgeons."[6]

Bosk conducted an ethnographic study on two different surgical services in "Pacific Hospital." He observed how "failure," especially on the part of surgical residents, was tolerated. Bosk found that these surgical services distinguish, at least implicitly, between different sorts of error or mistaken action. *Technical error* is one in which the professional discharges role responsibilities conscientiously, but his or her technical skills or information fall short of what the task requires; every surgeon can be expected to make this sort of mistake occasionally. *Judgmental error* is one in which a conscientious professional develops and follows an incorrect strategy; these errors can also be expected. The third type of error, *normative error,* violates standards of conduct, particularly by a failure to discharge obligations conscientiously. Bosk concluded that technical and judgmental errors were subordinated in importance to normative errors; normative errors are especially serious, because a pattern indicates a defect of moral character, where moral character is understood in terms of good faith or conscientiousness.[7]

This overview of Bosk's work is included in the third and fourth editions of Beauchamp and Childress's influential text, *Principles of Biomedical Ethics.*[8] The first two editions, published in 1979 and 1983, emphasized theoretical and principled approaches to medical ethics and explained their value as action guides articulating the "moral minimum" expected of professionals. Beauchamp and Childress use Bosk's work as an example of the role that assessment of "virtue and character" plays in justifying moral decisions and in deciding when actions are praiseworthy or when persons should be blamed for wrongdoing. Rather than creating the morality that guides professional decisions and actions, ethical theory supplements and offers a reflective stance by which those decisions and actions may be analyzed and justified.[9]

Beauchamp and Childress cite Bosk's findings in order to clarify how surgery's tacit moral codes contribute to an understanding of the role that virtues play in medical practice. While Beauchamp and Childress point to the importance of character traits in the profession of surgery, they do not examine why or if this emphasis on virtues is unique to surgeons. They also neglect to define two other types of errors Bosk identified—quasi-normative and exogenous errors.[10] These two errors are important in understanding the particularities of surgery. A *quasi-normative error* occurs when a resident does not follow the attending physician's technique but uses a variation learned from another attending physician. This attests to the influence that the mentor is to have on training residents. An *exogenous error* is one caused by personnel in nursing or anesthesia and implies that there are boundaries in defining "the group." Thus, Bosk understood the particularities of surgical practice. Beauchamp and Childress sought to identify what was common in surgical practice and virtue theory and, in so doing, they overlooked some central aspects of surgical practice.

It is precisely the nature of the surgical craft and the surgeon's beliefs about it (that is, the particularities), however, that combine to create the tacit knowledge of the group. Bosk observes:

The specific nature of surgical treatment links the action of the physician and the response of the patient more intimately than in other areas of medicine. In many branches of internal medicine the physician's interventions are relatively nonspecific. This fact allows internists to attribute failure to the inevitable pathophysiology of the disease process rather than to the nature of treatment itself. . . . Of all physicians, the surgeon's interventions are most visible and his therapeutic expectations are most specific. These features intimately link the surgeon's action to the patient's condition.[11]

This link between the surgeon's actions and the patient's response has several consequences. First, it clarifies that the only acceptable reason to subject a patient to the risk and trauma of surgery is the expectation that the operation will cure or palliate the patient's condition. The expectation of success legitimates surgical action. Such an expectation, asserts Bosk, does not govern action to the same degree in other specialties. Second, it makes the surgeon more accountable than other physicians.[12] Hence the focus on categorizing errors that Beauchamp and Childress identified. The fact that technical errors and judgmental errors were subordinated to moral ones is the final consequence of the intimate link between patient and surgeon. Bosk identified one of the few tacit assumptions to surgical practice as full and honest disclosure—that is, truthfulness. According to Bosk, this principle or maxim "both protects attendings and at the same time frees them for other activities."[13] The implicit context in which this principle is so important is one that is characterized by a group effort. Truthfulness engenders trust, and trust is the virtue that cements relationships. The line that distinguishes a moral error from a technical or judgmental one is an individual's failure to meet the tacit requirement that good-faith behavior imposes. According to Bosk: "Moral errors disqualify one from civil treatment by the group. This fierce response is to effectively extinguish the behavior which evoked it. When the behavior is not extinguished in the individual, the individual is extinguished in the group."[14]

DEFINING MISTAKES: VALUES IN CONTEXT

Knowing what scientists value we may hope to understand what problems they will undertake and what choices they will make in particular circumstances.   —Thomas Kuhn

Neurosurgery is a professional discipline whose modern historical roots coincide with the emergence of the elite moral vision of academic medicine that Bosk found 75 years later on the surgical service at "Pacific Hospital." An examination of the development of this particular surgical subspecialty, in fact, should add depth and perspective to Bosk's conclusions. Bosk's framework provides a baseline to define what is actually meant by an error or mistake. What were the underlying values of the pioneering surgeons who sought to create the profession of neurosurgery during the years from 1890 to 1930? How did these values contribute to the current definition and reporting of mistakes or errors? Clarifying the historical context within which errors were first defined and reported is the major theme of this essay.

Case reports written between 1890 and 1930, in both neurosurgical practice and the law, provide a focus for this examination. These were the years when neurosurgery gained formal status as a surgical subspecialty. It was a time also when the first wave of malpractice cases, which actually began as early as 1840, gained momentum and appeared to "haunt" surgeons and physicians.[15] The two trends are not unrelated. Surgeons who wanted to create subspecialties were typically trained in Germany where they were taught the latest scientific underpinnings to practice. They disdained practitioners in the United States who represented a therapeutically impoverished and divided medical profession. The infighting, back stabbing, and competition among competing sects for dominance resulted in a general societal mistrust of doctors. Surgeons trained abroad in the scientific method joined the ranks of medical reformers to establish new standards for medical education. In effect, practitioners who were unable to attain the specified training were ousted. A first attempt to unite the divided profession focused on writing codes of ethics and the internal enforcing of moral codes.[16] By the second decade of the 20th century, these extralegal attempts gave way to the creation of state licensure and other regulatory mechanisms, including the law, to redress patients' grievances.

Harvey Cushing was the leader of the elitist surgeons of this era, holding professorships sequentially at Johns Hopkins, Harvard, and Yale. It is against a backdrop of medical reform on the one hand, and the vigilance of lawyers on the other, that his efforts to create a specialty called neurological surgery took place. Cushing was well aware of the political nature of this goal. He understood that a campaign to create a new surgical subspecialty was complex. Not only would he have to expose the blatant incompetence of medical practitioners who—within traditional bounds of practice—legitimately used their license to operate, but also he would have to criticize general surgeons who were technically competent but harmed patients by their ignorance of the delicate neuronal structures and of complex anatomic and neurological diagnostic skills. These criticisms, in turn, would have to be supported by evidence to justify training one subgroup of specialists to focus on surgical intervention in the brain.

Given the mistrust of the public toward a dueling medical profession and the distrust of generalists toward specialty surgeons, Cushing planned to articulate technical and moral standards for the new profession. In keeping with other surgeons who sought to reform their profession, he opted to create a postgraduate educational program wherein the new standards could be taught.[17] A new moral climate, in sum, was necessary for a beneficial application of the new techniques. In 1905, Cushing contributed an article entitled "The New Field of Neurological Surgery" to the *Journal of Surgery, Obstetrics and Gynecology*, which was soon to become the official journal of the American College of Surgeons.[18] The journal itself marked the beginning of a professional collaboration of ideas.

Cushing's colleague Frank Martin, one of the founders of the American College of Surgeons, stated the objectives for the publication: "to advance specialist knowledge, to give practitioners a review of the literature in their fields, and to bring together in an outstanding journal the divisions of surgery included in the title."[19] The journal was an immediate success. It gave Martin and other leaders of elite surgical subspecialties a vital line of communication with the ordinary practicing surgeon. Cushing's article on brain tumors, for example, offered the practitioner a text on surgery. Five years later, the first Clinical College of Surgeons was held in Chicago. This was a "hands-on" practicum, where any surgeon could observe an expert perform the new technical procedures that were described in the journal. By 1913, the forum's organizers disparaged its success, for it forced them to confront a basic educational dilemma: "Should the primary focus of surgical education be on upgrading the lowest common denominator to a standard of comparative safety; or should it be to create a relatively small, recognizable group of quality?"[20]

In 1913 the American College of Surgeons was established, and its founders identified the standardized teaching of residents in hospitals as one of its aims. The debate over whether to train an elite group of students in standardized techniques or upgrade the lowest common denominator already in practice was answered. Over the next 25 years, the American College of Surgeons successfully carved out the form and structure of internship and residency amidst a complex political landscape comprised of the American Medical Association, private foundations, medical schools, and hospital administrations—a network that was the forerunner of the present-day Joint Commission on Accreditation of Healthcare Organizations (JCAHO).

The model for the reforms was the system of residency at Johns Hopkins, which began in 1898 and existed, essentially unchanged, until 1941.[21] Under this system, a medical graduate wanting to become a neurosurgeon undertook eight years of training. The student spent the first year as a surgical intern; the second as a fellow in experimental surgery; the third and fourth learning surgical pathology, fractures, trauma, and plastic surgery. Then, the surgeon-to-be spent two years in neurosurgery, one as an assistant resident and the other as a resident. In the seventh year, the trainee earned the position of first assistant in general surgery. Finally, he or she was rewarded with the coveted position of chief resident in general surgery. Thus, neurosurgery remained a branch of general surgery—but a special branch, indeed. By 1939, the American College of Surgeons reported that it had accredited a total of 35 medical schools to offer surgical training programs. Of these 35, only 12 had residency programs in neurosurgery and, of these, the available slots varied from one to three. A total of 24 new positions for neurosurgical residency were available in 1939.[22]

The upgrading of medical education created a cadre of professionals who not only were elitist by distinction of training, but also had generally come from wealthy families. Only the wealthy could delay wage earning for eight years. A balance had to be struck, however, between keeping surgery elitist and ensuring that the long years of internship and residency training would be respected. Creating the form and structure needed to teach a surgical subspecialty, therefore, was clearly an accomplishment. It did little, however, to prepare mentors like Cushing for the problems and the responsibilities associated with young men in training living in the hospital. Nor did it attend to trainees' prevalent practice of leaving the residency and setting up practice before completing the course.[23]

GENIUS WITH A SCALPEL

It is easier to evolve the truth from error than from uncertain
confusion.   —Harvey Cushing

A review of Harvey Cushing's published articles and speeches provide insight into the strategy he used to meet his challenges. Cushing combined the technical lessons he had personally learned from his experiences performing surgery on Halsted's service with the moral tenets central to defining a "good physician" taught to him by the legendary Sir William Osler and other role models. This two-pronged approach informed the professional maxims or rules he specifically designed to guide new practitioners. For example, after describing in exquisite technical detail the dangers of operating on patients who had "inaccessible" brain tumors, Cushing reasoned: "In affording a measure of relief to these distressing cases, one may fulfill the chief of his duties as a physician . . . to prolong life and at the same time alleviate suffering." But, he was quick to add, "the mere lengthening of a patient's months or years without rendering them more livable, is . . . no justification whatsoever of an operative procedure."[24]

Quoting Sir Francis Bacon, Cushing emphasized, "It is easier to evolve truth from error than from uncertain confusion."[25] This maxim provided him with an ethical justification for reporting mistakes. It also gave him a rationale for constructing "definitive rules" for surgical intervention in specific cases. Aiming criticism again at the general surgeon, Cushing cited a range of harmful mistakes that occurred in patients who had been "needlessly subjected to laminectomy (a method of fusing the spine, usually to treat back pain)." In the hopes of "ordering the confusion" surrounding decisions to operate on patients with spinal cord lesions, he divided all spinal injuries into three categories and provided not only technical criteria for operating on each, but moral justification as well. For example, "In a fracture-dislocation where evidence of a complete transverse lesion [of the spinal cord] is found on clinical exam," he stated, "[an] operation can do no harm, but it is an unjustifiable ordeal for both patient and operator."[26]

The pairing of technical description and moral prescription characterized all of Cushing's early writings. They conveyed his recognition that advancement and promotion of a new subspecialty carried with it a double responsibility. Learning the technique and science of neurosurgery was not enough. Cultivating judgment based on ethical principles regarding the proper use of the technique was equally important. Cushing's experience had taught him that a neurosurgeon with proper training could, for example, diagnose a tumor at an early stage and intervene surgically to prevent severe and irreversible morbidity. This early diagnosis and intervention, in fact, provided one prime justification for the new profession. "Allowing a patient to become blind from the pressure of a tumor which does not directly implicate the optic paths" wrote Cushing in 1910, "is comparable to procrastination in appendicular disease until the onset of general peritonitis."[27] He also knew from his own mistakes that "the operation, in the hands of the inexperienced, must usually end with the first protrusion of the naked brain through an open dura, and when abandoned in this way, paralysis, a separated wound, an infected fungus, meningitis and each are, alas, too common."[28]

Cushing acquired his judgment, in part, by making mistakes. He knew that some mistakes were to be expected. As a pioneer in the field, he had to separate the gross and unforgivable errors made by incompetent generalists from the ones made by trainees under the watchful eye of a mentor. The message he kept repeating was that only specialists trained beyond medical school in the Hopkins' residency model could acquire the skills and judgment needed to become competent in neurosurgery. "[The] transformation of surgery from practices based almost wholly on an anatomical knowledge of the surface and extremities of the body, to ones based on the physiological activity of the viscera, has come rapidly," recalled Cushing. He attributed physicians' "reluctance or hesitation to accept surgery as an oft-needed form of therapy . . . for many . . . intracranial conditions . . . to the fear of surgical foolhardiness and its consequences."[29] He asked medical practitioners who were in a position to refer patients for surgery to look to the accomplishments of mechanical and surgical therapeutics. "The patients' risks," he concluded, "were about equal between the physician who knows nothing of surgery and the surgeon who possesses no alternative but the knife."[30]

As part of his campaign to set high, yet attainable, standards of excellence in neurosurgery, Cushing published detailed case reports of both his successes and his failures. His biographer J.F. Denzel reports that when Cushing began operating in 1900, "there were no established methods, no basic procedures. He had to improvise every technique, invent every instrument as he went along, solving each problem as it came up before he could go on to the next."[31] Cushing was a conscientious and disciplined pioneer. His routine involved dictating his case reports as soon as the operation was completed: "Without removing his gown or even his gloves he immediately wrote up the entire procedure, from start to finish, while it was fresh in his mind, complete with sketches, diagrams and directions."[32]

In 1902, for example, he reported a series of his cases in order to convince the reader of the unforgiving nature of brain disease and the narrow margin within which errors can be reversed.[33] He also spoke to the importance of moral and technical accountability. Akin to what Bosk labeled the "horror story," a true-life morality play that carried with it dire warnings of failed judgment, one case in particular identified an error in judgment that ultimately led to a patient's death. "Frank W., colored, aged forty years, entered Dr. Halsted's service at 8 a.m. on November 23, 1902. On the evening of November 21st he was supposed to have fallen from a bicycle; was found in the street in a semi-conscious condition, and was taken to the station-house as an inebriate."[34]

In the hospital, the man's stupor increased, his blood pressure became elevated, and he began to exhibit signs of respiratory distress. Cushing, familiar with these symptoms, attempted to relieve the intracranial tension and, if possible, to evacuate the clot. These were both successfully accomplished during surgery.

Two strips of rubber protective, to serve as drains, were passed into the cavity of the clot through the track which had been made. The bone flap was loosely replaced, no sutures whatever being taken in the skin. Strips of gauze were placed between the edges of the scalp and a loose gauze dressing over all. It was hoped in this way to allow for an elevation of the flap in safety-valve-like fashion, should there be once more a considerable increase in intracranial tension. On the day following surgery, the patient's condition had generally improved.

Owing to the great amelioration in the gravity of symptoms, it was thought probable that recovery would ensue, and at an ill-advised moment late in the afternoon of this date the dressing was removed, the drains withdrawn, the bone flap replaced, and the scalp sutured in place. A slight bulging of the brain was found at this time, and some compression was necessitated in readjusting the osteoplastic flap in position. . . . *This misjudged procedure evidently turned the balance against the patient* [emphasis added]. His former stuporous condition . . . again reappeared. Nourishment could no longer be taken and respiratory difficulty again became evident. When seen on the following morning, the error of the previous day was apparent, and although the bone flap was once more elevated . . . his condition gradually became worse . . . and at midnight, three and a half days after the operation, death occurred.[35]

Bosk concluded that such stories are told because, like confession, the admission of mistakes somehow absolves a surgeon of blame. Perhaps this was also true for Cushing. It is equally possible that he was acting the role model of one who admits mistakes so that, in Bosk's words, the audience would both "forgive and remember."

The appearance of this case suggests that the danger described was not generally known by a readership who needed to recognize it and that it was the ethical responsibility of the perpetrator to prevent the error from occurring anywhere again. Learning from one's mistakes was one useful way to attain both the judgment and the skill to discern when unilateral decision making was justified. Cushing's own experience taught him that, when a mistake occurred, it was preferable to publish the error and warn others how to avoid it. The admission of mistakes and the truthful reporting of results among peers, therefore, was important for the development of the profession.

In 1905 Cushing reported a series of six cases, each involving newborn infants.[36] One child had been diagnosed three days after her uneventful birth as having a cephalhematoma (blood under the scalp, usually an innocuous complication of birth) of the left parietal region. The swelling increased rapidly, and by the fifth day the infants' right pupil was enlarged, her pulse became slow, and she had difficulty taking nourishment. Fearing an intracranial hemorrhage, Cushing prepared the child for operation: "The clot overlying the skull was removed. There was no indication of any connection between it and the intracranial contents. After the evacuation of this clot and exposure of the parietal bone, the latter was turned back almost in its entirety as in the preceding cases. As was expected, a tense, plum-colored dura was brought into view. The dura was opened and a large clot about a centimeter in thickness, which seemed to cover the entire hemisphere, was disclosed. Much of this clot escaped as soon as the opening was made, and other large pieces of it were lifted off from the surface with a blunt instrument and removed."[37]

Having described the technical aspects of the procedure, Cushing then shifted his attention to a retrospective review of his judgment to continue operating at this point: "Possibly, I should have been satisfied with the relief which this partial operation would have afforded. It doubtless would have been wise to have postponed further interference to another and later occasion, but the child's condition seemed to justify an effort to more thoroughly remove the clotted blood which was within easy access over the anterior and posterior poles of the hemisphere. While [we were] irrigating away some of the blood, the child suddenly stopped breathing. Under artificial respiration, the heart beat continued for some minutes, but all efforts to restore spontaneous breathing were unavailing."[38]

Cushing extended this quest for veracity by reporting his experiences performing surgery to his residents and new graduates. A time when the boundaries for what counted as acceptable practice for the profession were being set, these years provided Cushing with a unique opportunity to influence what these practices were. This information, intended for his colleagues, was also public knowledge. In 1905, the *Baltimore Sun,* riding on the public interest in the new surgical procedures, began publishing Cushing's failures. They printed the name of each patient and the distance he or she had come to undergo the operation. Then, a few days later, they ran a follow-up story announcing that the patient had died.[39] By 1908, however, adverse public reaction to the new specialty began to wane. In that year, in fact, Cushing's successful removal of a tumor from the esteemed General Wood made headline news and "Cushing became known as the greatest brain surgeon in the country."[40]

The publication in 1912 of Cushing's "epoch-making" book on pituitary tumors, which contained the results of 47 cases, symbolized the progress he and his fellow reformers had made in setting new standards for practice. His route of access to tumors set the standard for the next 15 years, reduced mortality from about 30 percent to 5 percent, and "offered patients a reasonable chance of prolonged or even permanent improvement from a state of seriously impaired vision."[41] Recognition in 1915 by legal experts of these standards reconfirmed that they were widely publicized. In that year, the Supreme Court of North Dakota heard *Van Woert v. Modern Woodmen of America*, an insurance appeal by the widow of a man who had died of a "tumor of the brain."[42] Van Woert's widow appealed Modern Woodmen of America's refusal to pay $3,000 of her husband's insurance benefits. In applying for these benefits, Mr. Van Woert had to answer 35 questions, two concerning what we now refer to as a "preexisting condition." Although he had been treated for vision problems, he answered "No" to a query regarding whether he had been treated by or consulted a physician in the past seven years concerning a personal ailment. He also specifically answered that he did not have a tumor and failed to supply the names of physicians and dates of treatment. The widow claimed her late husband had misunderstood the cause of his vision problems and did not intend to deceive the insurance company.[43]

Testimony at trial included detailed evidence from three physicians who diagnosed and treated Van Woert from 1907 until his death in 1911: Dr. Carr, a generalist; Dr. C.E. Riggs, "a specialist in the line of neuro diagnosis," and Harvey Cushing, of the Department of Neural Surgery at Harvard Medical School (by this time, he had left Johns Hopkins University). Because the insurer probably would not have issued the policy had it known about the man's condition, the court held that the withholding of information—even if unintentional—was material and vitiated the policy. (Van Woert believed his condition originated from a kick in the head by a horse). Thus, Mrs. Van Woert never received her $3,000.[44]

This case attests to the influence Cushing had in setting a standard of practice for the field. The court relied on the combined and unanimous testimony of Van Woert's three physicians, specifically, the detailed medical expertise of Harvey Cushing, who was "in charge of the department of neural surgery of Harvard Medical College, and formerly was in charge of the same department in Johns Hopkins University. He [wrote] a book upon disorders of the pituitary body and is one of the recognized authorities in the United States upon the subject. He testified that in his opinion Van Woert had been suffering from the disorder, to wit, tumor of the pituitary body, for many years, and that the same was in existence as early as 1907."[45]

Cushing's testimony, and that of the others, demonstrated a shared knowledge of the details of the pituitary tumor. They documented the onset of symptoms: atrophy of the optic nerve, projectile vomiting, gradual loss of vision, vertigo, severe headaches, loss of memory, and trouble distinguishing well-defined odors and tastes. They also testified about the standard treatment: operation for the "tumor of the pituitary body, one of the ductless glands located at the base of the brain about 1 or 2 inches back of the eye."

The year this trial took place provided an ominous foreshadowing for Cushing—indeed, for the country as a whole. In the spring, Harvey Cushing was a personal observer on the Western Front of the war that was raging in Europe. He served with a Harvard unit in the American Ambulance at Neuilly, France. When he returned to the United States, he was instrumental in organizing and then directing one of the two base hospital units that would be sent to France in May 1917. Cushing served as a surgeon for Base Hospital No. 5 until June 1918, when he was transferred to Medical Headquarters of the American European Front as senior consultant in neurosurgery. He remained there until the war's end in December.[46]

In January 1919, Cushing was ordered to England to oversee the reconstruction of base hospitals. There, he witnessed the

tragic aftermath of the war for the returning "heroes." First, most found someone younger and more vigorous than themselves holding down their former jobs. Many disillusioned veterans were seen literally begging for work. Not the least disillusioned were middle-aged medical officers entitled to wear four blue chevrons on their sleeves, perhaps even a wound stripe or two and some pieces of ribbon on their breast. Home again, but broken in spirit after their four wasted years, they must start in once more at the bottom, replace their out-of-date office equipment and try to recapture some of their lost practice if it ever could be captured. It was a depressing time.[47]

On February 20, 1919, Cushing embarked on his trip home. When he returned, he too was to find that much had changed in the four years that he had been away.

THE DOUBLE-EDGED SWORD:
SETTING STANDARDS VERSUS GETTING SUED

Malpractice is virtually impossible to demonstrate in the absence of practice; no one can be convicted of doing established procedures poorly if no procedures have been established.   —James C. Mohr

Cushing's vast operative experience in World War I reinforced the validity of his previous mandate: to standardize procedures so as to train a competent cadre of neurosurgeons. One of his most visible means of doing this was to launch harsh criticism of Walter Dandy, MD, his gifted and creative student. Dandy tended to report the success of innovative procedures and tests without cautiously warning others of their inherent danger. Cushing's attacks on Dandy have been attributed to a feud, but more than personal animosity was at the root of the criticism. In keeping with his consistent teachings of "learning from mistakes," Cushing's campaign more than likely was aimed at discouraging others, who were not as gifted as Dandy, from practicing his inherently dangerous procedures on an unwary public.[48]

Cushing's reaction to Dandy's promotion of ventriculography is one such case. This technique involved the injection of air into the ventricles before taking an x-ray of the brain. The technique proved to be quite valuable in the identification of the position and size of an intracranial mass. While Cushing was manning the front in Europe during the war, Dandy remained at Hopkins, finally becoming Halsted's chief resident in 1918. In 1917, he devised this innovative procedure. He perfected the technique and optimistically reported his findings at the 1922 American Association of Neurological Surgeons meeting. Cushing publicly challenged him and demanded that he profile a full statistical account of his mortality and morbidity rates. Dandy was "stung" by Cushing's questioning of his "veracity," and he felt his character had been undermined.[49] Indeed, he believed he was reporting what had been called the most important neurosurgical technique of the century.

One year later, Dandy published his results, which spoke to the specifics Cushing had demanded. Referring to ventriculography, he reported: "It is very dangerous. There has been a tremendous mortality from its use. However, if judiciously used and only by one thoroughly skilled in intracranial surgery, the danger is minimal. I had three deaths at the beginning of the series. Since then, I have had none. . . . Certainly the danger in proper hands is small compared to the danger attending cranial operations based on guesswork."[50]

The published discussion that followed Dandy's report was focused on critically examining his statistics to decide whether cerebral pneumography (another name for ventriculography) does or does not help in the localization of brain tumors. "We have to balance" wrote a commentator, "its value against its faults."[51] Critics found that Dandy's published statistics were contradictory. Again, his honesty was questioned (this time in print), and the eminent surgeon was placed in the defensive posture of explaining the discrepancies.

Dandy's critics regarded his skill as a superior neurosurgeon as a dangerous yardstick against which to gauge other surgeons. Although Dandy could practice ventriculography without mortality, his critics found that "in hands other than Dandy's, the death rate was 3%." More to the point, they warned that if this was the mortality rate in the hands of the average neurological surgeon, the rate would be higher among general surgeons. "We must not allow cerebral pneumography to suggest to the uninitiated a rule of thumb and simple way of locating brain tumors. We must warn of the mortality and the need of experience in making as well as interpreting cerebral pneumogram."[52]

Cushing and Dandy both agreed that guesswork was not a basis for surgical intervention. Cushing had, for his professional lifetime, tried to discredit the blind exploration of the brain, insisting instead that a thorough understanding of neurology should be a prerequisite for neurosurgical training. He feared that incompetent surgeons would rely upon the risky innovation of ventriculography as a shortcut to diagnosis and that the rigorous educational criteria he had outlined would be bypassed. There was, in fact, no way to prevent practitioners from using this high-risk technique. The more conventional route of conducting a careful neurological examination was, in Cushing's estimation, the less harmful route. Not everyone all had the patience for Cushing's conservative approach. "The neurological surgeons have been too much to the right politically speaking!" wrote a critic examining Dandy's statistical inconsistencies. "They have not had enough of the radical about them. Dr. Dandy is on the extreme left! That is a good thing. It is courageous conduct which will make neurological surgery a living thing."[53]

Given that political battle lines were being drawn within the profession, Cushing remained consistent in articulating his new conventional standards. He accused Dandy of acting in an irresponsible manner when he reported his preliminary results for a new operation, the complete removal of a tumor of the eighth cranial nerve (acoustic neuroma) at the base of the skull.[54] Attempting a difficult and risky suboccipital exposure, Dandy described complete success based on a single case report. Cushing wrote a scathing letter to the editor of the *Bulletin of the Johns Hopkins Hospital* claiming that both Dandy and the editor acted irresponsibly in publishing this case without reference to the larger series complete with mortality figures and end results. In a personal letter to Dandy, he stated: "After all it is as important for you as it is for me that you stand in a high plane of professional ethics."[55] Dandy was shocked. He defended his report as merely staking claim to the procedure, clearly a major issue for him. Either he was unaware that others might use his description and operate on unsuspecting patients, or he simply did not accept responsibility for the actions of others. Cushing's critical attacks of 1922 and 1923 foreshadowed the vicious campaign he would conduct regarding tic douloureux.

Tic douloureux is a relatively rare disease. Although the etiology is still disputed, the symptoms are unmistakable: lancinating facial pain occurring with excruciating ferocity. Since ancient days, the disease had been treated with varying degrees of success by a litany of medical procedures. The fact that spontaneous remissions occurred complicated assessing the efficacy of treatment. Yet, from 1894 to 1901, some effective surgical techniques had been developed. One in particular, the Spiller-Frazier procedure, had gained the confidence of surgeons.[56] However, its complications included possible disturbance to the eye, loss of the motor branch to the nerve, loss of sensation in the face, occasional facial paralysis, and hemiplegia. Technically perfected and easily replicated, it fell within Cushing's range of acceptable therapies.

In 1925, Walter Dandy developed and published a new approach.[57] Using the same risky incision he pioneered operating on acoustic tumors, he sectioned the trigeminal nerve at the brainstem and reportedly achieved good results. If the surgeon used specialized tools and technique, he reported, none of the complications associated with the Spiller-Frazier procedure occurred. Complications from surgery at the brainstem still include death and neurologic devastation. Cushing's published disapproval of this technique was so thorough that it was not until the 1960s, with the introduction of the microsurgical technique, that Dandy's procedure entered the mainstream of neurosurgical procedures. The political loyalty of Cushing's followers not only affected how they practiced their craft, but shaped how later generations would as well.[58]

LEARNING TO KEEP A CAUTIOUS TONGUE

*As to your conduct on the stand in a case against you: you will be
honest, of course, but for goodness sake be honest briefly.*
                                    —Frederick J. Cotton

Reformers like Cushing sought to curb abuse of their profession by creating state licensing boards, backing the reforms of the American College of Surgeons, and crafting standard residency programs. These restrictive means, however, would take decades to have the desired effect. In 1932, physician Harold Foss wrote: "Unsupervised operations performed . . . without justifying indications were never as prevalent as at the present time. Lack of surgical judgement and technical skill are accounting for an enormous amount of unnecessary hospitalization, invalidism, and, all too frequently, fatal terminations. Unless this condition is corrected, some day the public will find it out, when it will in all probability offer its own solution."[59]

Patients caught in the cross fire of mutual mistrust and fear between generalists and specialists did pursue their own avenues to gain compensation for the harms that were inflicted on them. They availed themselves of legal counsel. The general acceptance by jurists of contingency fee agreements during the first decade of the 20th century was another development that encouraged redress against malpractice. Contingency fees had the practical advantage of enabling patients to bring malpractice claims against physicians without any real financial risk on their own part. By 1915, this arrangement was legitimized.[60] Physicians witnessed the "first wave of malpractice," which had begun slowly in 1850.[61] Foss's comments document that this trend was widespread by 1930.[62]

In 1844, the *Boston Medical and Surgical Journal* warned: "Western New York is becoming a dangerous ground for the surgeon, according to court dockets." Nine years later, the same journal included an editorial note titled "Liability of Physicians and Surgeons," that discussed the trend of "a few gentlemen" to refuse to perform certain services without written agreement to protect them against prosecutions.[63] The journal even claimed that "the lawyers pretend that they have us at their mercy," and "[their] pleasure would be to ruin [a physician] if money could be obtained thereby."[64] To conclude, it advised readers that malpractice suits require expert witnesses. "Yet who," it asked, "would dare say, absolutely and without qualification, that death might have been prevented?"[65]

In 1878, Eugene Sanger, a physician from Maine, published a scathing exposé of malpractice law.[66] From experience, Sanger told his readers: "During the last few months, I have wasted one whole month of my time in the Court House, and been put to more than $2,000 expense, to defend two of the simplest acts of surgery, for which I received ninety cents pay."[67] Sanger also offered anecdotal accounts of numerous other physicians who were forced to spend significant sums of money to defend against malpractice, even when they settled their cases without trial. He felt the collected cases "illustrate[d] the dangers from jealous rivals, tricky lawyers, impecunious and ignorant patients, of family conspiracies and of the unholy alliance of the sachel [sic] and scalpel."[68] He even remarked that his reporting of suits in Maine alone would startle other physicians and make them vow to abandon medical practice. Sanger warned that it was not safe to practice under the existing laws; he referred to the increasing trend of contingent fee arrangements when he noted that it costs a poor man almost nothing to bring a claim that could both raise public sympathy and earn him an award. He emphasized that it was a false idea to think that anyone could escape suit by using extra care. Sanger even claimed that some surgeons were being blackmailed into settling. Concluding his arguments, he offered two resolutions to the Maine Medical Association: (1) "that, with the existing State laws on civil malpractice, it is unsafe to practice surgery among the poor";[69] and (2) that a five-person committee should present the subject to the legislature. The association adopted both resolutions.[70]

Sanger was not alone in his accounts of the legal climate for medical practitioners. In 1879, the Medical and Surgical Society of Baltimore pledged its members mutual defense in court.[71] By 1911, George W. Gay warned the public, lest they be complacent about winning claims, that physicians were united against malpractice suits and would defend one another in court.[72] Gay wrote about the great expense in time and energy that a physician suffered after being dragged through the courts for three to four years to defend a malpractice suit.[73] The *New England Journal of Medicine* also continued to report the perils of malpractice suits and in 1929 published an article whose author blamed greed, not the pursuit of justice, for a marked increase in malpractice cases.[74] In 1934, the journal reported that approximately 20,000 suits had been brought against physicians during the past five years.[75]

Articles documented that self-exalting remarks of physicians, who inadvertently condemn other physicians, were a major cause of suits.[76]

Not surprisingly, the message of keeping a cautious tongue was repeated frequently in the literature of the time.[77] For example, articles discouraged physicians from bolstering their own reputation by remarking on the errors or poor techniques of other practitioners or by answering patients' hypothetical questions; such practices, physicians were warned, could lead to malpractice cases.[78] Stetson and Moran concluded that between 65 and 80 percent of malpractice cases were due to the remarks of other physicians; further, they reported that in 45 percent of those cases, the remarks were not intended to be malicious but led patients to believe that they had been wronged.[79] The following rules are a summary of the wise advise offered by Stetson, Moran, and Gay to safeguard against a malpractice suit:

1. Keep a cautious tongue.
2. Follow proper procedures for use of the x-ray.
3. Maintain accurate and complete records,[80] especially surgical notes.[81]
4. Adhere to the code of medical ethics and application of the golden rule in care of patients who have been previously attended by another physician.
5. Be knowledgeable of the accepted forms of treatment.[82]
6. Secure consent before performing surgery. If there is reason to believe that the parties are not of good character, require written consent.[83]

If sued, physicians were urged to stay close-mouthed and not to talk to anyone, especially the plaintiff, about the case.[84] In 1932, the *New England Journal of Medicine* included a thorough review of malpractice law and provided specific advice to physicians who were being sued: instructing them on what to say, how to behave, and what to expect of court procedure.[85]

CONCLUSION: A MISTAKE BY ANY OTHER NAME

The moment the physician departs from the usual and accepted mode of treatment of a case, he renders himself liable to action should the termination be unsatisfactory.   —George Gay

Cushing's truthfulness in reporting mistakes did not falter during his career. Yet, by 1928, the success of the Board of Surgery in its creation of standardized residency programs, the integral use of the scientific method in medical education, and the threat of malpractice worked together to prompt a different style of journal reporting. The sheer numbers of cases reported obviated an individualized story of each operation. The now familiar style of case presentation, commonplace by 1928, is demonstrated in Exhibit 9-1.

The care that Cushing exercised in his operating room is particularly notable when one considers that until the 1940s, appendectomy had a 20 percent mortality rate.[86]

Instead of discussing particularities of patient characteristics and the detailed context in which procedures were performed, surgeons and surgical departments began to use standardized tables and charts to summarize information about series of cases. Remnants of an earlier "nonscientific" style existed. In describing the removal of tumors, authors reverted to using such terms as "egg-shaped," or "the sized of a 'walnut' or a 'hazelnut.' "[87] Generally, however, a more standard scientific style of communication was emerging.

Within this more standard, scientific style of communication, the admission of mistakes was buried within lessons for improved technique. R.E. Semmes,

Exhibit 9-1
Case Presentation

Diagnosis	Number of Patients	Mortality Rate During Surgery(%)
Glioma	609	17.8
Adenoma	271	5.3
Meningioma	188	10.3
Neurinoma	131	11.5
Congenital tumors	90	11.7

From J. Eisenhardt, "Recent Advances in Neurological Surgery," *Archives of Surgery* 18 (1927-1935): 1929.

for example, reviewed the frequency of various sinus infections, meningitis, and brain abscesses, and assessed whether the current state of knowledge offered useful surgical intervention for these maladies. He discussed the surgical techniques employed by Sachs and Dandy and warned of a rare complication: thrombosis of the cavernous sinus. After describing how to diagnose the infrequent complication, he gave the general advice that any corrective surgical intervention that had been attempted would only hasten death (in other words, once the complication is diagnosed the prognosis is practically hopeless).[88] How many deaths, one might ask, taught Semmes this lesson?

Likewise, Howard Nafzinger, a physician who completed his residency under Cushing, wrote this list of instructional directives for neurosurgeons operating in the posterior fossa:

If the operator is careful to test bone thickness by percussion he will avoid possible accidents when dealing with the paper thin areas occasionally met. Prior to opening of the dura the reduction of intracranial pressure is often necessary to prevent sudden herniation and brain contusion. For dural closure, as for closure of the deep scalp and skin, trials of many materials and many types of sutures have caused a return to the fine silk suture. Closely spaced sutures in the deep layer of the scalp best control bleeding. . . . In the presence of intracranial pressure the bleeding is lessened during the operative performance by an early reduction of pressure. The full crossbow incision divides the entire occipital nerve supply, leaving the most prominent portion of the occiput anesthetic. The risk of decubitus, if the weight of the head is allowed to rest indefinitely in this area, is obvious.[89]

Artful lessons are given without the admittance of the specific errors that taught them.

Some mistakes were still described in journal articles, but these tended to be, in Bosk's term, "exogenous." In 1928, Dandy—a surgeon not known for admitting his mistakes—reported the death of a patient caused by a silver clip slipping from the middle cerebral artery. He advised that his "recent use of flat clips" afforded him a feeling of greater security. Particular detailed case reports also can be found, but these were reserved for reporting deaths or complications arising from unusual occurrences. In this context, Dandy implied that the error could not have been avoided.[90]

By the 1930s, mistakes were largely delegated to courtroom hearings, surgery reports, or mortality and morbidity conferences. In 1933, for example, the Superior Court of Pennsylvania heard an insurance appeal, *Ellis v. Jones & Laughlin Steel Co.*, in which the petitioner sought compensation after her husband died from a head injury.[91] The man was working on a locomotive at the steel plant, when he fell eight feet and struck his head. Prior to the accident, he was known to have a "nickel-sized" sarcoma, but after the fall the tumor swelled to the size of a "small hen's egg." The legal question was whether the fall and the treatment he received from the company doctor, a local surgeon, and finally a resident in Walter Dandy's clinic, "so aggravated and accelerated the growth of the sarcoma from which [decedent] was then suffering as to be the predisposing cause of his death."[92] The court affirmed the decision of the Commonwealth court, which awarded insurance compensation to Ellis's widow, but the company appealed the decision.

The case remained on the docket for a variety of reasons and was not heard again until nine years later, setting a precedent for allowing medical testimony from experts not present at the original trial. The "original players" in the court drama were Charles H. Gano, the defendant's "company" physician; H.E. McGuire, chief surgeon for the defendant at the South Side Hospital; and Deryl Hart, assistant resident surgeon at Johns Hopkins Hospital, where the patient was finally transferred several days after the accident. An excerpt from McGuire's original testimony sets the stage:

There was a swelling there about half the size of an egg, which had a small incision in it. The man gave me a history of having this lump a couple of years, and I thought probably it was a cyst which became larger. On cutting through the scalp I came right into brain tissue, with a terrific hemorrhage. I did not proceed any farther: I passed some deep sutures through the skull, closing the wound, which stopped the hemorrhage. Then we took x-rays which disclosed he had a tumor of the brain which ate its way through the skull on account of the pressure. I told the family about operating on the man, and that I refused to do it because I thought the man would die.[93]

The growth increased in size and was twice as large when Ellis left as it was when he entered the hospital. Hart testified, in substance, that when Ellis entered Johns Hopkins Hospital the patient was hardly able to walk and was suffering with intracranial pressure from osteosarcoma of the skull and was vomiting. Because the physicians believed that the patient could not survive more than a few days unless the sarcoma could be removed, they attempted to perform an operation; however, they found that the ravages of the tumor were so extensive that a successful operation was impossible.

McGuire expressed the opinion that the sarcoma was not "due" to the injuries received while working on the locomotive. His cross-examination, however, on this matter reads:

Q. You say that the blow could not have had any effect on the sarcoma?
A. I did not say that. If he had this blow, it increased in size due to the condition of the tumor and the scalp.
Q. But you are not in position to state to what extent the blow could increase it?
A. No, I didn't see it before.[94]

New testimony in 1932 by neurosurgeons L.H. Landon, Lester Hollender, and Walter Dandy led the court to reach the following conclusion:

We find from all the evidence that the blow to the back of decedent's head on December 16, 1924, while in the course of his employment, caused a swelling of the pre-existing sarcoma as the result of a hemorrhage occasioned by the blow. We further find that the incision made into the sarcoma by Dr. Charles H. Gano on the same day aggravated the growth of this sarcoma, and that the operation of Dr. H.E. McGuire in cutting into the sarcoma, the scalp, and the brain tissue, although with reasonable cause, precipitated a terrific hemorrhage and greatly accelerated the growth of the sarcoma, and that the accidental injury and surgical interference were the instant and accelerating cause of the growth of the sarcoma as to be the predisposing and superinducing cause of the death of the decedent some two months and nine days following the accident.[95]

The testimonies of the neurosurgical experts resulted in an award of $4,142.28.

These testimonies also helped document several trends that had developed: (1) standard treatment for brain tumors, in this case, was defined; (2) neurosurgical residency programs at select universities (Johns Hopkins, Yale, University of Pennsylvania) set the standard treatment; (3) general surgeons were no longer qualified, vis-à-vis new specialized knowledge, to treat neurosurgical disorders; (4) company physicians, in particular, could be found negligent in their casual treatment of accidents.[96] These broad trends have been well documented and applauded for the advancements they represented. That they also encouraged neurosurgeons to "keep a cautious tongue" when they wrote about complications and errors has been overlooked.

The cautious tongue, however, has not stopped surgeons from discussing their errors with one another. "There is one place," wrote Atul Gawande in 1999, "where doctors can talk candidly about their mistakes. . . . It is called the Morbidity and Mortality Conference—or, more simply, 'M&M.' "[97] Attesting to the long-term influence of Cushing and his peers, this conference usually "takes place once a week, at nearly every academic hospital in the country."[98] Bosk describes the mandatory attendance at these conferences of all medical students, interns, residents, and surgeons, as well as department chairs. He points to the central part the conference plays in transforming "private troubles" into public issues. The conference is a mechanism of social control that enables the surgeon to learn to "take responsibility for his failures."[99] This institution survives because, despite frequent challenges, laws protect the M&M proceedings from legal discovery.[100]

Even within the protected walls of the M&M conference, the circumspect lessons taught by lawyers linger. Reports of complications "involve a certain elision of detail and a lot of passive verbs. No one screws up a [laminectomy]" writes Gawande. Instead, "a [laminectomy] was attempted without success."[101] Unlike a courtroom, however, where the rule is to be truthful but brief, the M&M is a cultural ritual that poses a "correct" view of a mistake. It conveys the message voiced by Cushing almost a century ago: avoiding error is largely a matter of experience and surgical judgment. Staying informed, being alert to the ways things can go wrong, attempting to head off each potential problem before it happens is a virtue.[102] On the other hand, the lesson passed on in the tacit acceptance of "keeping a cautious tongue" and by the weekly scheduling of the M&M conference is to affirm that mistakes are also an inevitable part of neurosurgical practice. While the legal, medical, and social context has changed since 1930, the realities of being a surgeon have not.

ACKNOWLEDGMENTS

My heartfelt appreciation goes to Nathan Kottkamp, a JD/MA student in the University of Pittsburgh Health Law Bioethics and Program, for the legal background references and the preparation of earlier drafts of that material; Ellen Conser, graduate student in Medical Humanities at Michigan State University, for reviewing and summarizing resources, both general and historical; and Elizabeth "Betsy" Stow for her patient and excellent technical assistance in formatting, deciphering complex endnotes, and editorial comments.

Portions of an article by the author, "Politics, Paternalism, and the Rise of the Neurosurgeon: The Evolution of Moral Reasoning," *Medical Humanities Review* 10, no. 2 (Fall 1996): 20-44, have been reprinted in this chapter with the gracious permission of *Medical Humanities Review;* ©1996, all rights reserved.

NOTES

The epigraphs that begin several of the sections above are from the following works: Charles Bosk, *Forgive and Remember: Managing Medical Failure* (Chicago: University of Chicago Press, 1979; Thomas Kuhn, "The Historical Structure of Scientific Discovery," in *The Essential Tension: Selected Studies in Scientific Tradition and Change* (Chicago: University of Chicago Press, 1977), 165-77; Harvey Cushing, "The Special Field of Neurological Surgery," *Bulletin of the Johns Hopkins Hospital* 16, no. 168 (March 1905): 83; James C. Mohr, from the case *Van Woert v. Modern Woodmen of America,* 151 N.W., p. 225; Frederick J. Cotton, "Medicine, Ethics and Law," *New England Journal of Medicine* (13 March 1032): 590; George W. Gay, "Suits for Alleged Malpractice," *Boston Medical and Surgical Journal* 165, no. 10 (1911): 411.

1. C. Bosk, *Forgive and Remember: Managing Medical Failure* (Chicago: University of Chicago Press, 1979).

2. R.L. Pinkus, "Innovation in Neurosurgery: Walter Dandy in His Day," *Neurosurgery* 14, no. 5 (1984): 625.

3. H. Cushing, "The Special Field of Neurological Surgery: Five Years Later," *Bulletin of the Johns Hopkins Hospital* 21, no. 236 (November 1910): 325-39.

4. Ibid.

5. R. Brown, *Rockefeller Medicine Men: Medicine and Capitalism in America* (Berkeley: University of California Press, 1979), 60-133; P. Starr, *The Social Transformation of American Medicine* (New York: Basic Books, 1982); R. Stevens, *American Medicine and the Public Interest* (New Haven, Conn.: Yale University Press, 1971).

6. Bosk, *Forgive and Remember,* see note 1 above, 39.

7. Ibid., 37-67.

8. T.L. Beauchamp and J.F. Childress, *Principles of Biomedical Ethics,* 3rd and 4th ed. (New York: Oxford University Press, 1989, 1994).

9. Ibid., 366-94.

10. See note 1 above, pp. 67-70.

11. Ibid., 29.

12. Ibid.

13. Ibid.

14. Ibid., 61.

15. J.C. Mohr, *Doctors and the Law* (New York: Oxford University Press, 1993), 76-101. The second wave is said to have started in 1960.

16. T.L. Beauchamp and R.R. Faden, *A History and Theory of Informed Consent* (New York: Oxford University Press, 1986), 76-101.

17. R.A. Kessel, "Higher Education and the Nation's Health: A Review of the Carnegie Commission Report on Medical Education," *Journal of Law and Economics* 15, no. 1 (1972): 115-27; I.R. Brown, *Rockefeller Medicine Men,* see note 5 above; K.M. Ludmerer, *Learning to Heal: The Development of American Medical Education* (New York: Basic Books, 1985).

18. H. Cushing, "The New Field of Neurological Surgery," *Journal of Surgery, Obstetrics, and Gynecology* 1, no. 1 (1905).

19. R. Stevens, *American Medicine,* see note 5 above, p. 79.

20. Ibid.

21. W.L. Fox, *Dandy of Johns Hopkins* (Baltimore, Md.: Williams & Wilkins, 1984), 20.

22. B.C. Pevehouse, "Residency Training in Neurological Surgery, 1934-1984: Evolution over 50 Years of Trial and Tribulation," *Journal of Neurosurgery* 61 (1984): 999-1004.

23. H.L. Foss, "A Plan for the Systematic Instruction and Supervision of Interns and Resident Physicians," *Journal of American College of Surgeons* 6 (1931): 29-31.

24. Cushing, "The Special Field of Neurological Surgery," see note 1 above.

25. Ibid.

26. See note 3 above, p. 331.

27. Ibid., 326.

28. Ibid., 327.

29. Ibid.

30. Ibid.

31. J.F. Denzel, *Genius with a Scalpel: Harvey Cushing* (New York: Messner, 1971), 79.

32. Ibid.

33. H. Cushing, "The Blood Pressure Reaction of Acute Cerebral Compression, Illustrated as Cases of Intracranial Hemorrhage," *American Journal of Medical Science* 125, no. 16 (June 1903): 1038-44.

34. Ibid., 1040.

35. Ibid., 1041.

36. H. Cushing, "Concerning Surgical Interventions for the Intracranial Hemorrhages of the New-Born," *American Journal of Medical Sciences* (October 1905): 563-81.

37. Ibid., 578.

38. Ibid., 579.

39. See note 31 above, p. 79.

40. Ibid.

41. G. Horrax, *Neurosurgery: An Historical Sketch* (Springfield, Ill.: Thomas, 1952): 84-5.

42. *Van Woert v. Modern Woodmen of America,* 151 N.W., p. 225.

43. Ibid.

44. Ibid., 228.

45. Ibid., 226.

46. Ibid., 79.

47. H. Cushing, *From a Surgeon's Journal* (New York: Little, Brown in association with *Atlantic Monthly,* 1936).

48. R.L. Pinkus, "Politics, Paternalism, and the Rise of the Neurosurgeon: The Evolution of Moral Reasoning," *Medical Humanities Review* 10, no. 2 (1996): 20-44.

49. See note 21 above, pp. 162-3.

50. W.E. Dandy, "Localization of Brain Tumors by Cerebral Pneumography," *American Journal Roentgenology Radium Therapy* 10, no. 8 (1923): 611-1.

51. Ibid., 613. Following Dandy's journal article there were "comments"; the author of the comments is not identified.

52. Ibid., 614.

53. Ibid.

54. W.E. Dandy, "An Operation for the Total Extirpation of Tumors in the Cerebello-Pontine Angle: A Preliminary Report," *Bulletin of the Johns Hopkins Hospital* 33 (1922): 344-5.

55. See note 49 above.

56. See note 2 above, pp. 623-31.

57. W.E. Dandy, "Section of the Sensory Root of the Trigeminal Nerve at the Pons: Preliminary Report of the Operative Procedure," *Bulletin of the Johns Hopkins Hospital* 36 (1925): 105-6.

58. See note 2 above, pp. 623-31.

59. H.L. Foss, "A Plan for the Systematic Instruction and Supervision of Interns and Resident Physicians," *Journal of American College of Surgeons* 6 (1931): 29-31.

60. P. Karsten, "Enabling the Poor to Have Their Day in Court: The Sanctioning of Contingency Fee Contracts, A History to 1940," *DePaul Law Review* 47, no. 231 (1998): 1-25.

61. A.A. Sandor, "The History of Professional Liability Suits in the United States," *Journal of the American Medical Association* 163, no. 6 (9 February 1957): 459-66.

62. See note 16 above, pp. 109-289.

63. Editorial, "Liability of Physicians and Surgeons," *Boston Medical and Surgical Journal* 48 (1853): 506.

64. Ibid., 507.

65. Ibid.

66. E.F. Sanger, "Malpractice," *Transactions of the Maine Medical Association* 6 (1878): 360-82.

67. Ibid., 361.

68. Ibid., 365.

69. Ibid., 382.

70. Ibid.

71. J.C. Mohr, *Doctors and the Law* (New York: Oxford University Press, 1993), 119 and 289, n. 50.

72. G.W. Gay, "Suits for Alleged Malpractice," *Boston Medical and Surgical Journal* 165, no. 10 (1911): 411.

73. Ibid., 354.

74. "Why Are Malpractice Suits [sic]?" (editorial), *New England Journal of Medicine* 200, no. 2 (1929): 93-4. (Note: *New England Journal of Medicine* was the successor to the *Boston Medical and Surgical Journal*.)

75. H.G. Stetson and J.E. Moran, "Malpractice Suits, Their Cause and Prevention," *New England Journal of Medicine* 210, no. 26 (1934): 1381.

76. See note 72 above, pp. 353-411; and see note 74 above, p. 93.

77. See notes 72, 74, and 75 above.

78. See note 72 above, p. 354; see note 75 above, p. 1382.

79. See note 75 above, pp. 1382-4.

80. Ibid., 1385.

81. See note 72 above, p. 409.

82. See note 75 above, p. 1385.

83. Ibid., 1383.

84. See note 72 above, p. 410.

85. F.J. Cotton, "Medicine, Ethics and Law," *New England Journal of Medicine* 208, no. 11 (16 March 1932): 590-2.

86. R. Porter, *The greatest benefit to mankind: a medical history of humanity from antiquity to the present* (London: HarperCollins, 1997), 597-627.

87. See note 16 above, p. 78; *Ellis v. Jones & Laughlin Steel Co.*, 169 A, p. 264.

88. R.E. Semmes, "A Review of the Intracranial Complications of Ear, Nose, and Throat Infection from the Neuro-Surgical Standpoint," *Transactions of the American Lanryng., Rhin., and Oton. Society* 35 (1927): 518.

89. H. Nafzinger, "Brain Surgery: With Special Reference to Exposure of the Brain Stem and Posterior Fossa; The Principle of Intracranial Decompression, and the Relief of Impactions of the Posterior Fossa," *Clinical Surgery* 246 (February 1928): 244-7.

90. W. Dandy, "Removal of Right Cerebral Hemisphere for Certain Tumors with Hemiplegia: Preliminary Report," *Journal of the American Medical Association* 90, no. 11 (1928): 824.

91. *Ellis v. Jones & Laughlin Steel Co.*, 169 A. 264. The *Ellis* case set an important precedent in insurance law because it allowed testimony of medical experts who had never seen the deceased.

92. Ibid., 264.

93. Ibid., 263.

94. Ibid., 266.

95. Ibid., 268.

96. P. Starr, *The Social Transformation of American Medicine* (New York: Basic Books, 1982).

97. A. Gawande, "When Doctors Make Mistakes," *New Yorker*, 1 February 1999, 48.

98. Ibid.

99. See note 1 above, pp. 114, 121-2.

100. See note 97 above, p. 49.

101. Ibid.

102. See note 48 above, p. 31.

10

Rush from Judgment

James Lindemann Nelson

INTRODUCTION

Readers of the Sunday *New York Times Magazine* consumed coffee and croissants over a rather apocalyptic paragraph on 19 April 1998: "Three jumbo jets crashing every two days. If the airlines killed that many people annually, public outrage would close them overnight. Hospitals kill that many patients every year because of missed diagnoses, medication mishaps and other preventable errors."[1]

But readers of the *Times* are a hearty lot, and it takes more than a few downed jumbo jets to shake them. So Michael Weinstein, author of the article in question, continues:

Medical errors account for up to a quarter of the deaths from heart attack, stroke and pneumonia. Perhaps half of the nation's diabetics are treated improperly. Up to 85 percent of prescribed treatments lack scientific validation. An intensive-care unit committed nearly two errors per patient each day, a third of which were potentially serious. Surgeons in some parts of the country perform mastectomies rather than lumpectomies on Medicare patients 35 times more often than those in other regions, and for no apparent medical reason. Rates of heart surgery vary by a factor of three. One study found that nearly 20 percent of coronary angiographies lacked medical justification. A quarter of the surgeries to implant tubes in children's ears are inappropriate and a third are questionable.[2]

Having concluded this epic catalogue, Weinstein is ready to sketch out a solution. His leading theme is consumer choice—let people make informed choices about which physicians, hospitals, health plans, and clinics they want to attend, and the ValuJets of the medical world will be grounded. But for consumer choice to be effective, physicians and their health organizations have to be accurately graded; for accurate grading, there must be reliable data informing standards of good practice.

Both consumers and clinicians need better ways of determining what works and what doesn't, as well as mechanisms that will reliably instill improved practice techniques in healthcare providers. The man for this job, as Weinstein sees it, is Dr. Robert H. Brook, of Rand and the University of California at Los Angeles. According to Weinstein, Brook

has developed criteria for determining when medical procedures—like coronary bypass surgery, mastectomies and hysterectomies—are appropriate and when they are ineffective or needlessly risky. Brook's work is the source of many of the statistics given at the beginning of this article, and it could tell physicians and health plans how best to practice medicine if they would listen. But few do. The doctors who perform unwarranted treatments are rarely incompetent, let alone villainous. Their decisions are more often based on habit and presumption. In a sensible system, decisions would be solidly rooted in Brook's clinical evidence.[3]

Albeit couched in more sober prose, calls for increased medical accountability, backed by similar concerns about poor practice on the part of physicians and other health professionals, are common in the literature. Practices designed to elicit greater conformity to the "clinical evidence" as elicited by Brook and fellow workers in this particular vineyard are increasingly in place, especially in managed-care contexts. The path-breaking work by J.E. Wennberg and colleagues on apparently unmotivated "small-area variations" in hospitalization rates and the use of various procedures has seemingly underscored the role of irrational elements in physicians' decision making. It has contributed significantly to the "outcomes movement," the effort to discipline the practice of medicine by the use of practice guidelines based on outcomes studies—statistical analyses of extensive databases.

Because such studies and the resultant guidelines are thought to be potential money savers, as well as mortality and morbidity savers, managed-care organizations have been highly interested in incorporating them into medical practice and review. Even Congress—at least for a moment—was swept along in the wake of this enthusiasm. In 1989 it founded the Agency for Health Care Policy and Research, which for a brief, busy time had the charge to conduct outcomes research and to frame and disseminate the ensuing practice guidelines.

The movement to base clinical practice more firmly on clinical evidence would seem to be squarely on the side of the angels. Who wouldn't be in favor of avoiding error, rooting out irrationality, improving outcomes, and decreasing costs—especially if all that stands in the way is "habit and presumption"? However, although it may seem curious, there is something of a countermovement too. The countermovement tends to focus around the idea of "clinical judgment"—a much-invoked but analytically elusive idea that is taken to refer to some special faculty informing knowing and acting that physicians (in particular) develop as a result of their exacting training and experience.

Defenses of clinical judgment seem suspicious—in part because of its elusiveness, in part because of the perception that judgment-guided clinical practice is rife with serious error, and in part because it seems decidedly a property of individuals in a time when systematic and structural change seems the most popular way to reduce problems. The whole notion has the aspect of a hidebound holdover from prescientific medicine. Still, it is this apparently perverse direction of thought that is explored in this chapter, which supports a nondismissive, though also nondogmatic approach to clinical judgment. The considerations presented here are drawn largely from recent work in *naturalized epistemology* described and discussed below; they not only provide reason to continue to take clinical judgment seriously, but also hint at ways judgment might be improved.

To finish off the stage setting, it is necessary to do a bit of splitting and lumping. First, a distinction. One might divide medical errors into accidents and mistakes. While ordinary usage is not always precise in how it employs these terms, it is handy for present purposes to have some way of distinguishing one kind of error—such as giving a patient what everyone would allow to be an incorrect drug or dosage, or subjecting a patient to a procedure clearly not indicated by her health status—from another kind, such as the common practice of prescribing grommets (ear tubes) for otitis media when outcomes studies indicate that no benefit ensues. Grabbing the wrong syringe exemplifies the first kind of error, which is referred to here as an *accident*. But should it indeed be the case that grommets are pretty much valueless for otitis media, then their use exemplifies the second sort of error, which is referred to here as a *mistake*. It is the presence of systematic mistakes that is targeted by enthusiastic proponents of outcomes studies and practice guidelines.

No one, obviously, has a good word to say for accidents. The mistake category is a bit trickier, however. This is not because anyone is more prone to cheer for laxity about mistakes than about accidents, but because whether the outcomes movement truly has a good grasp on what will reduce mistakes, or reduce them optimally, is still an open question.

Second, a consolidation. The discussion that follows refers rather loosely to clinical evidence, outcomes studies, evidence-based medicine, and clinical pathways and guidelines. It is fairly insouciant about distinguishing between the perspectives of various possible users of the information and directions contained therein; physicians, patients *qua* patients and patients *qua* consumers, administrators, and policy makers are all among the various constituencies. For many purposes, carefully marking these differences would be crucial. But the focus here is on assumptions about the character of ourselves as knowers and about the world as an object of knowledge, which seem to run through much of the diagnosis of the problem of medical mistakes and the suggestions for its cure.

AMBIGUITIES OF EVIDENCE, COMPLEXITIES OF RESISTANCE

To get a better handle on medical mistakes, and what kinds of techniques will reduce them, it is reasonable to start out with an account of physicians as epistemic agents—what is the nature of the knowledge they claim to have and employ? Work by clinical epistemologists such as Sandra Tannenbaum, Marx Wartofsky, and Hilde Lindemann Nelson suggests the following picture: much of the knowledge physicians have and employ rests on their grasp of biological models that provide them with a picture of how human physiology is altered by disease processes.[4] In using these models to make sense of the data with which patients present them, and to fashion strategic recommendations for responding to those interpreted data, physicians exercise clinical judgment. This clinical judgment is an epistemic faculty not exhaustively reducible to the application of rules;[5] it is nourished by a broad mass of experience—much of it clinical, but also much of a general cultural character.[6] These models, and the skills of judgment, are produced, imparted, honed, and practiced in communities and sub-communities of knowledge and interpretation.[7]

This framework within which physicians match general biological models to specific human idiosyncrasies is referred to here as the *clinical-judgment model*. It has not been a direct focus of much attention by people interested in understanding and reducing medical mistakes. But there seems no reason in principle why it could not itself become an object of investigation and systematic improvement. One considerable advantage of doing so is as much ethical as epistemic. Consider the much discussed difficulties many physicians are alleged to have with fitting a patient's disease into the broader context of a patient's life—difficulties often alleged to have a great deal to do with the focus on science in healthcare education and practice. But the general epistemic framework described here is hospitable to the process of understanding the narrative of the patient's life. Moving back and forth between the general biophysical models provided by basic science, and the peculiarities of a particular patient presenting before a given physician, is also a complex task of understanding and constructing a certain kind of meaning. If physicians tend to need further encouragement to take whole persons seriously, at least the enterprise of doing so may not be so radical a departure from the interpretive skills they already draw upon, as is often thought.[8]

These matters are ordered differently in the world of evidence-based medicine. There, the crucial information is not based on models, but on statistics; the focus is not on *how* something—whether it be a disease or a treatment—works, but on *whether* it works. There seems to be a no-nonsense, cut-to-the-chase appeal in basing one's clinical decisions on the outcomes of large studies. Medicine, after all, is an applied practice, not a contemplative one, and knowing how things work is beside the point unless it helps us understand how to act usefully.

One way to understand the clinical-evidence movement is that it aims to provide practitioners with more pertinent data to enrich the basis of knowledge that informs their judgment. But there is reason to think that clinical evidence, outcomes data, and practice guidelines will not simply supplement, but supplant clinical judgment. Apart from fiscal pressure toward this end that might be exerted by managed care, there are more directly substantial reasons to call the clinical-judgment model into question. Consider the magnitude of the mistakes problem, as outlined by Weinberg. Consider that physicians' reluctance to comply with guidelines is seen as a function of a kind of intellectual indolence, rather than a principled defense of an alternative method of clinical reasoning and decision making. And there is yet another powerful consideration on which skeptics about physicians' judgment might rely—the evidence that clinicians are conspicuously poor at the kind of reasoning involved in interpreting the significance of several interacting, probabilistic considerations that bear on diagnosis and decision making. Influential work by Paul Meehl done in the 1950s purports to show that the diagnostic predictions of clinicians are much less accurate than diagnoses generated by simple statistical models.[9] Subsequent work on human inference, lead by Amos Tversky and Daniel Kahnemann, has done nothing to restore confidence.[10]

Here, then, is the difficulty. Overreliance on the rote clinical application of clinical evidence might well coarsen the more context-sensitive, interpretive approach to understanding what is happening with a particular patient, with the consequent possibility of lowering, rather than raising, the accuracy of diagnosis and treatment. Further, it seems not unreasonable to fear that such overreliance might also blunt what tendencies there might be within a physicians's own epistemic disposition to be sensitive to the full range of significant individuating features of patients. Yet the image of those medical jumbo jets being continually crashed by habit-encrusted physician-pilots with shaky holds on the canons of inductive inference seems too powerful to be effectively rebutted by seemingly speculative epistemic and ethical concerns. To vindicate the model of clinical judgment as an appropriate area for study as part of an overall effort to improve clinical decision making requires interrogating each figure in this image.

HOW MANY OF US ARE GOING DOWN IN FLAMES?

There is some room to cavil here. Some doubt exists as to whether the problem of small-area variations, which seems a paradigm of medical irrationality and unreliability, is really so dire as scholars like Wennberg and popularizers like Weinstein have made it seem. A body of responsible opinion suggests that the extent of small-area variations in particular has been exaggerated by artifacts of sampling and analytic techniques. For instance, Michael Schwartz and colleagues found that the magnitude of variation correlated with how many years of data are used, as well as how the data are analyzed.[11] When variation is explored using a technique known as "systematic component of variation" (or SCV—currently the most widely used measure), and the data considered are drawn from one year, dramatic and distressing results can ensue. However, using statistical analytic techniques based on Bayes's theorem, and considering data drawn from three years of practice, Schwartz and colleagues found much smaller rates of variation:

Analyses using 1 year of data produced higher estimates of systematic variation than multi-year analyses. Empirical Bayes [EB] techniques, which account better for the greater unreliability of observations from areas with small populations than the SCV approach, found less variation than did the SCV statistic. Relative to EB estimates using 3 years of data (the approach that best validated), the SCV statistic with 1 year of data overestimated the median amount of systematic variation by over 70 percent. With 3 years of data, it over-estimated systematic variation by 55 percent.[12]

In the light of alternative analytic possibilities, one has to wonder whether the picture Weinstein paints is based on brute facts or on contestable statistical inference.

IS UNREFLECTIVE CONSERVATISM ON THE PART OF PHYSICIANS THE CULPRIT?

It is perhaps worth noting here that doctors' resistance to complying with practice guidelines is a widespread phenomenon; according to a study by Roberto Grilli and Jonathan Lomas, who examined 143 recommendations published in clinical literature in the English language between 1980 and 1991, the mean compliance rate was 54.5 percent.[13] But it is not altogether clear that "habit and presumption" are the leading causes of physicians' reluctance to reduce medical mayhem by practicing in accord with clinical evidence. A more careful assessment of what is behind the reluctance of many doctors to jump aboard the clinical evidence bandwagon may tell a more interesting story.

Consider, for example, Donald J. Murphy's catalogue of reasons that physicians resist adopting practice guidelines based on outcomes data. "Many factors influence physicians' compliance with guidelines. These include their attitudes about utilization review, government regulations, physician profiling, uncertainty, private industry, clinical autonomy, sponsors of the guidelines, necessity and appropriateness of care, opinion leaders, conflict in guidelines, . . . the value of guidelines in general, . . . patients' expectations."[14]

I do not mean to suggest that there is anything sacrosanct about these attitudes; they may themselves, of course, be more or less open to criticism. But the picture painted here of how to account for physicians' recalcitrance is at least far more complex than is suggested in the *New York Times;* that, at least, is worth bearing in mind in thinking about effective ways of improving how doctors make decisions. And there may be a yet deeper moral: some part of doctors' dubiousness about practice guidelines and their sources may be traceable, not just to dislike of various encroachments on their autonomy, but to real problems in the guidelines.

Murphy, for example, brings to light complexities in the very notion of measurement, on which much of the whole structure of evidence-based medicine, outcomes research, and clinical guidelines must rest. He argues that professional judgment cannot be eliminated by reliance on clinical evidence, since judgment is itself required for determining *what* should be measured, *who* should be taking the measurements, and *how* the measurements are conveyed to patients.

In the absence of good judgment with respect to these considerations, the goal of better clinical evidence may lead us in search of precision that is specious. Consider, for example, a patient reflecting on her therapeutic options after a myocardial infarction (MI). Guidelines based on general outcomes studies recommend that she undergo a battery of further tests to stratify her risk for a subsequent MI to the limits of currently available precision. But if those limits represent only a small gain over what information is currently in hand, and if the extra information would seem very unlikely to alter the patient's choice, pursuing it in the name of compliance with guidelines of good practice seems unjustified.

Further, outcomes studies may yield data that are inaccurate. For example, measures of patients' preference are often regarded as pertinent to assessing outcomes. However, those preferences are often taken by survey instruments administered by "unbiased" research assistants rather than by physicians who have a working relationship, perhaps of years standing, with the subjects. But studies so conducted have yielded results that experienced clinicians find very counterintuitive. Murphy's example concerns patients' preferences for cardiopulmonary resuscitation (CPR):

The literature is replete with studies suggesting that a fair percentage of seniors (10 to 30) would opt for CPR in the event of an advanced chronic disease such as Alzheimer's. A study involving my patients at a geriatrics clinic indicates that only 5 percent of seniors would want CPR under the conditions of chronic illness where the life expectancy was less than one year. All of these studies—even the one involving my patients—overestimates the percentage of seniors opting for CPR. Why? Because physicians have approached this complex question as researchers, not as clinicians having trusting relationships with patients. As a clinician, I believe the percentage of seniors who would want CPR in the setting of advanced dementia is less than 1 percent. I have talked with hundreds of seniors about CPR, and I know of only one who would want CPR regardless of her condition and prognosis.[15]

Is this just another indictment of the insufficiently scientific clinician? Or does it suggest that human subjects may respond differently—and not necessarily "more accurately"—to strangers than to people they have reason to trust?

But perhaps all that these considerations amount to is reassurance that maybe not quite so many planes are falling out of the sky as we were given to think, and that physicians' scruples about changing the epistemic basis of their practice is not solely a matter of intellectual indolence. Such reassurance may not seem fully comforting. After all, even if the scenario depicted in the *Times* were inflated by several orders of magnitude, we still would be left with a problem of serious proportions.

Nor is all the resistance on the part of physicians to evidence-based medicine based on well-founded skepticism about its accuracy, pertinence, or applicability. In a recent Hastings Center study, investigators found that among the sources of physicians' resistance to outcomes studies and clinical guidelines were "profit," "ego," and "ignorance." For example:

Economic motivation was at times explicitly or implicitly a source of resistance. Some physicians claimed that the outcomes data carry normative conclusions that prefer cost-cutting to quality of care. . . . More commonly reported, at the opposite end of the spectrum, was motivation based on economic gain as a formidable source of resistance to implementing outcomes data. In several cases, most notably those that required extensive physician-patient interaction, such as smoking cessation counseling, physicians were more likely not to adhere to the recommendations because it was not in their financial interests to provide lengthy, costly, time-consuming counseling. In other cases, such as the placement of ear tubes for otitis media, it was in the financial interests of the ENT [ear, nose, and throat specialist] we interviewed to provide more costly procedures and to avoid recommendations about watchful waiting. Even though for some general practitioners there was no direct financial compensation for not following the recommendations, they received indirect benefit through referrals and professional reciprocity.[16]

So we have here a complex picture. Outcomes research and practice guidelines seem to have serious epistemic limits, and they apparently are not very user-friendly, from a physician's point of view. But concerns about the limitations of outcomes research and practice guidelines do not in themselves show us that medical practice is not rife with serious error. And even if the picture of unmotivated and irrational practice variations we inherit from Wennberg and consequent work is overstated, it would still be a serious matter if very much of that sort of thing were going on at all. There is reason to believe that mistakes and accidents are far from negligible features of life in contemporary medicine. There is further reason to believe that resistance to changing the present situation is robust, complex, and varied. Reasonable worries about whether outcomes data and practice guidelines are really promising ways of reducing error and enhancing the quality of care jostle with indifference and self-interest. Finally, and perhaps most fundamentally, the sort of Meehl-inspired skepticism about the reliability of physicians' reasoning abilities dovetails with considerations of the sort provided by Murphy to make the matter even murkier: if good judgment is required to obtain and apply outcomes data and practice guidelines, and it is just the reliance on the judgment of professionals that has got us into this fix, do we really have any reliable way of escape?

NATURALIZED EPISTEMOLOGY MEETS MEDICINE

The concerns inspired by Meehl, then, are perhaps the most serious reasons to wonder whether medical mistakes can be substantially reduced by a serious study of clinical judgment or by greater reliance on outcomes studies and clinical guidelines. While Meehl's classic work impugns the inferential skills of physicians, subsequent work in the same area suggests that there is nothing particularly problematic about doctors in this respect. To gain an inkling of the way the problem extends beyond the clinic to human judgment as such, consider this classic experiment from the literature on human statistical inference:

Let us suppose that you wish to buy a new car and have decided that on grounds of economy and longevity you want to purchase one of those solid, stalwart, middle-class Swedish cars—either a Volvo or a Saab. As a prudent and sensible buyer you go to *Consumer Reports,* which informs you that the consensus of their experts is that the Volvo is mechanically superior, and that the consensus of the readership is that the Volvo has the better repair record. Armed with this information, you decide to go and strike a bargain with the Volvo dealer before the week is out. In the interim, however, you go to a cocktail party where you announce this intention to an acquaintance. He reacts with disbelief and alarm. "A Volvo! You've got to be kidding. My brother-in-law had a Volvo. First, the fancy fuel injection computer thing went out. 250 bucks. Next he started having trouble with the rear end. Had to replace it. Then the transmission and the clutch. Finally sold it in three years for junk."[17]

The appropriate response to this cocktail-party conversation, of course, is the "calm observation that 'every now and again one does sample from the tail of the distribution.' "[18] But in the real world, the chances seem overwhelming that the prospective buyer will now shun the Volvo dealership. A little reflection suggests that there seems no good reason to expect that such inferential failings will be restricted to decisions concerning Volvos.

But surely, it may seem, any general problems that people have with inferences are going to be limited; they will be a matter of lack of focused attention, specific to certain domains, or something of the sort. After all, while many of us may indeed be tempted to make the same mistake that the erstwhile Volvo buyer is apparently going to make, it is not as though we cannot see the problem when it is brought to our attention. And aren't physicians precisely the kind of people whose basic endowments and specialized training could be trusted to make them much better than average at avoiding mistakes in inference as they reflect on their own clinical experience and presenting cases?

According to Richard Nisbett and Lee Ross, workers in the area of human inference, however, "there is *no* inferential failure that can be demonstrated with untrained undergraduates that cannot also (at least with a little ingenuity) be demonstrated in somewhat more subtle form in the highly trained scientist."[19] This theme of general skepticism has been developed perhaps most thoroughly by Amos Tversky and Daniel Kahneman. As characterized by Hilary Kornblith,

Tversky and Kahneman showed that there are patterns of inference which are extraordinarily widespread across all individuals, that these inferences are extremely resistant to change and that they violate the canons of good statistical inference. Tversky and Kahneman did not limit their subjects to clinicians, nor did their examples require the aggregation of numerous interrelated factors, as is frequently the case in clinical prediction. Important and depressing as Meehl's results were, the work of Tversky and Kahneman seemed to embody an even more important and more depressing moral: human beings have a strong natural tendency to reason very badly.[20]

Against this skepticism based on empirical investigation of how humans actually reason, I pose an epistemological orientation that also aims to be responsive to how humans actually know and reason about the world in which they live. This is a view pioneered by Willard Van Orman Quine, called *naturalized epistemology*. Naturalized epistemology regards human success in coming to know the world, as exemplified most powerfully by the development of science, as strong evidence that our psychological capacities give us significant access to the actual causal structure of the world.

As the naturalized view of human knowledge is developed in Kornblith's work, a major task is to vindicate human inferential strategies against precisely the kind of skepticism found in the work of Meehl and Tversky and Kahneman, along with other psychologists working in this area.

The approach takes two mutually supporting steps. Naturalists in epistemology typically assume that the world is such that it divides into *natural kinds.* If they are right, then at least many of the important divisions we recognize within the world—divisions such as species or elements—are not the result of the human mind or human social practices operating upon the world; they are the result of the world operating on human minds and social practices. The belief that the world has such a structure is, apparently, part of our natural endowment. Children come into the world with a strong propensity to make sense of it as sorted out into enduring kinds of things exhibiting stable clusters of properties.[21]

If the world in fact has such a structure, then what might at first appear to be rampant bad reasoning takes on a different appearance. For example, a major form of poor inference, from the perspectives of critics such as Tversky and Kahneman, is the human tendency to operate according to a "law of small numbers"—that is, to assume that small samples of some population constitute good grounds for making inferences to properties possessed by the population as a whole. From a statistical point of view, this view is completely backwards; it is large numbers that give us reasonable grounds to assign traits to populations as a whole. But if the world is in significant part a collection of natural kinds, and if human beings are naturally well adapted to recognizing which among the properties of an individual object are a matter of its being an instance of that kind, then making inferences from small samples to properties of the whole would not be an instance of epistemic failure. Indeed, it constitutes an important way to get to the truth about certain matters.

Indeed, looking at the matter in this way helps us understand the common failure in the Volvo case mentioned above. Any disinclination we may feel about buying the Volvo as a result of the cocktail-party conversation is explicable if we have thought about Volvos as constituting a natural kind, with a certain "life span" and a set of predictable weaknesses. If Volvos were natural kinds, then such inferences would indeed have some merit to them, despite their being based on a very small sample. After all, if a person inferred from one sample of copper that copper was a good conductor of electricity, he would be absolutely right, despite the smallness of the sample. But as it happens, Volvos are artifacts, not natural kinds. An artifact's properties may not cluster together quite so tightly as those of a natural kind; classical inductive reasoning might well in general be better for such things.

So, what the Volvo case indicates is not that people typically reason poorly, but that it is possible for us to misidentify the characteristics of the objects we reason about, and to mistake idiosyncratic traits for what are called "projectable" traits. We don't always separate the natural wheat from the artifactual chaff. Further, we sometimes misidentify what traits can be appropriately projected from one sample of a natural kind to another, or to the whole.

These flaws, real as they are, are not as dire as wholesale inferential unreliability.[22] And there is good reason to think that humans are typically sensitive to the presence of such natural kinds as there are, and fairly sharp at being able to distinguish projectable from nonprojectable traits.[23] The situation with clinical inference is extremely complicated, of course. While diseases would seem to fall into the category of natural kinds, the relationships between diseases and symptoms is highly complex. Figuring out how different properties relate to one another—how, for instance, the presence or absence of some observation or other is indicative of the presence or absence of some unobserved trait—is something with which human beings do seem to have considerable trouble when the manner in which the properties interact is variable.

And yet, the notion that we need to reduce reliance on professional judgment in clinical decision making as much as possible because we can't trust physicians' reasoning seems, again, overblown. The implications of the naturalized epistemology literature removes some of the sting from the Meehl-Tversky-Kahneman position and helps support the idea that clinical judgment ought to be studied as such, with an eye to its improvement, not simply replaced by outcomes-based decision making. But the guarded optimism of epistemological naturalists such as Kornblith about human judgment should be comforting to people trying to design and implement outcomes studies and clinical guidelines as well. As Murphy helps us see, judgment is required in getting useful and reliable information from studies of this sort.

But the naturalistic program in epistemology may do more than simply reduce one source of suspicion about clinical judgment. It may also suggest avenues for its improvement. A number of feminist epistemologists have been interested in broadly naturalistic approaches to understanding knowledge; however, they have insisted on the significance of the fact that human knowing emerges from the activities of and relationships within human communities, and that the various positions to know of many subjects in such communities must be taken seriously.[24] This suggests that a deepened understanding of clinical judgment may highlight the role of "communities of judgment" in the formation, employment, and improvement of that faculty. It further suggests a reorientation in the way we commonly think of judgment. Rather than some sort of privileged intuition possessed by individual doctors, clinical judgment might be thought of as a joint achievement that arises out of interactions among various involved clinicians—and even patients. To see judgment as social in this way erodes some of the suspicious stigma of excessive individualism cited earlier as a feature draining credibility from the use and study of judgment. To see judgment as interactive in this way provides a conceptual opening for the development of clinical judgment enhanced by other sorts of interaction—for example, interaction with the resources of evidence-based medicine.

The general moral to which these considerations incline is that the campaign to stamp out medical mistakes ought not try to unseat altogether the forms of perception and assessment physicians have typically used. Not only will such a strategy spur various forms of reluctance and resistance, it will also undervalue the potential for improvement in clinical judgment itself. This should not be seen as a zero-sum game. In making medicine's skies safer, randomized controlled trials, meta-analyses of studies, clinical guidelines, and the whole panoply of evidence-based medicine have an important role to play—but not an imperialist one.

ACKNOWLEDGMENTS

Susan B. Rubin and Laurie Zoloth provided very useful commentary on an earlier version of the article, as did Hilde Lindemann Nelson. I am grateful for their contributions.

NOTES

1. M.M. Weinstein, "Checking Medicine's Vital Signs," *New York Times,* 19 April 1998, 36.

2. Ibid.

3. Ibid.

4. See S. Tannenbaum, "What Physicians Know," *New England Journal of Medicine* 329 (1993): 1268-71.

5. See my discussion of clinical judgment and rules in " 'Unlike Calculating Rules?' Clinical Judgment, Formalized Decisionmaking and Wittgenstein," in *Slow Cures and Bad Philosophers,* ed. C. Elliott (Durham, N.C.: Duke University Press, forthcoming).

6. See M. Wartofsky, "Clinical Judgment, Expert Programs, and Cognitive Style: A Counter-Essay in the Logic of Diagnosis," *Journal of Medicine and Philosophy* 11 (1986): 81-92.

7. H.L. Nelson, "Knowledge at the Bedside," *The Journal of Clinical Ethics* 7, no. 1 (Spring 1996): 20-8.

8. See K.M. Hunter, "Aphorisms, Maxims and Old Saws: Narrative Rationality and the Negotiation of Clinical Choice," in *Stories and Their Limits: Narrative Approaches to Bioethics,* ed. H.L. Nelson (New York: Routledge, 1997), 215-31.

9. P.E. Meehl, *Clinical versus Statistic Prediction: A Theoretical Analysis and a Review of the Evidence* (Minneapolis, Minn.: University of Minnesota Press, 1954).

10. See, e.g., *Heuristics and Biases* (Cambridge, England: Cambridge University Press, 1982).

11. M. Schwartz et al., "Small Area Variation in Hospitalization: How Much You See Depends on How You Look," *Medical Care* 32 (1994): 189-201.

12. Ibid., 196.

13. R. Grilli and J. Lomas, "Evaluating the Message: The Relationship between Compliance Rate and the Subject of a Practice Guideline," *Medical Care* 32, no. 4 (1994): 202.

14. D.J. Murphy, "Guideline Glitches: Measurements, Money and Malpractice," in *Getting Doctors to Listen: Ethics and Outcome Data in Context,* ed. P.J. Boyle and D. Callahan (Washington, D.C.: Georgetown University Press, 1998), 100.

15. Ibid., 103.

16. P.J. Boyle and D. Callahan, "Physicians' Use of Outcomes Data: Moral Conflicts and Potential Resolutions," in *Getting Doctors to Listen: Ethics and Outcomes Data in Context,* ibid., 15-6.

17. R.E. Nisbett et al., "Popular Induction: Information Is Not Always Informative," *Cognition and Social Behavior* 2 (1976): 227-36.

18. R. Nisbett and L. Ross, *Human Inference: Strategies and Shortcomings of Social Judgment* (Englewood Cliffs, N.J.: Prentice-Hall, 1980), 15.

19. Ibid., 14.

20. H. Kornblith, *Inductive Inference and Its Natural Ground* (Cambridge, Mass.: MIT Press, 1993), 8.

21. Kornblith provides a useful review of the psychological literature on this point in his *Inductive Inference and Its Natural Ground.* Ibid., 64-70.

22. However, they can be clinically relevant. See Kornblith's discussion of the fallacious use of the "Draw a Person" psychological diagnostic device, in *Inductive Inference and Its Natural Ground.* Ibid., chap. 5.

23. Ibid., 105-7.

24. See, for example, L.H. Nelson, "Epistemological Communities," in *Feminist Epistemologies,* ed. L. Alcoff and E. Potter (New York: Routledge, 1993), 121-59.

11

How Should Ethics Consultants Respond When Careproviders Have Made or May Have Made a Mistake? Beware of Ethical Fly Paper!

Edmund G. Howe

INTRODUCTION

What should ethics consultants do when they learn that a careprovider has made or may have made a mistake? The self-evident answer would seem to be that ethics consultants should take whatever steps are necessary to ensure that the patient is informed. However, this answer may be less unequivocal than it seems. For example, if ethics consultants respond in this manner, they may alienate other members of the medical team. If ethics consultants alienate other careproviders, their colleagues may shy away from future ethics consultations or be less forthcoming with information when consultations take place.

The price of pursuing a policy of absolute truth-telling may be a reduced capacity to work well with careproviders to help other patients. For this reason and others, although full disclosure to patients seems to be self-evidently morally obligatory, the question is more complex and open to debate than it appears.

The discussion that follows explores this question in several contexts. It does not reach a conclusion about how ethics consultants ultimately should come out on this question, but it delineates in considerable detail how the relative merit of truth-telling decreases as its costs become greater.

This essay starts by identifying and discussing these categories of careproviders' mistakes: (1) nonmistakes, (2) mistakes, and (3) possible mistakes. It then presents two circumstances that may especially warrant disclosure: when a patient has undergone harm and when there is a significant potential harm to future patients.

The essay then moves on to a discussion of three more subtle concerns that may offset harms to patients and so bolster an argument for not telling the truth: (1) patients may lose the placebo effect, (2) patients may have to retain symptoms if they sue, and (3) patients may undergo trauma if they sue a care-provider they like. The essay then describe the ethics consultant's obligations to the careprovider if the consultant decides to tell a patient the truth when the careprovider will not. The essay concludes with a discussion of two important factors: our present legal context and patients' unrealistic expectations. For care-providers and ethics consultants to tell the truth and for careproviders to be treated justly, both of these factors must change.

USEFUL CATEGORIES FOR
ETHICS CONSULTANTS

When deciding what to do in these situations, it is useful for ethics consult-ants to conceptualize mistakes as falling into one of three categories: nonmistakes, mistakes, and possible mistakes. The category into which a mistake is placed should be determined by imagining how large numbers of competent clinicians would have acted in a given situation.

1. *Nonmistakes.* A clinical example helpful for illustrating this approach is that of reading a chest x-ray. Suppose that 100 radiologists view an x-ray; all except one or two see nothing on the x-ray that suggests cancer. In seeing nothing, the vast majority have not made a mistake.

2. *Mistakes.* A mistake exists when a careprovider unequivocally has been negligent. This might be the case, for example, if 100 radiologists are asked whether they see a lesion on a chest x-ray, and almost all point out the lesion. A radiologist who misses the lesion would be practicing outside and below the standard of care.

3. *Possible mistakes.* This third category lies conceptually between the first two. This category applies when competent careproviders would rea-sonably differ in concluding whether a mistake has been made. Suppose that 100 radiologists are shown an x-ray that has a barely distin-guishable early lesion that subsequently has turned out to be cancer. They are asked to read it blindly; 50 radiologists identify the lesion and 50 do not. To miss such a lesion is an example of what is referred to here as a possible mistake. This degree of disagreement is not so un-common as might be imagined. In a review of errors made in an out-patient setting, for instance, the reviewers disagreed about half of the time.[1]

In summary, these categories are decided using this hypothetical, opera-tional approach. A nonmistake occurs when almost no radiologists would iden-tify a lesion. A mistake occurs when almost all would. A possible mistake oc-curs when competent careproviders would be nearly evenly divided. The bound-ary between each of these categories is indistinct but, notwithstanding the ambi-guity of the boundaries, these categories may be extremely helpful. Each category serves to earmark key issues that ethics consultants should consider when deciding what to do when they learn that a careprovider may have made a mistake.

NONMISTAKES

Suppose that, using the operational criteria described above, a careprovider reading an x-ray made "no mistake"; six months later, cancer that was "not detectable" initially on the x-ray grows and becomes clearly detectable. At this later time, the careprovider may again review the original x-ray; now, with the hindsight of knowing where the cancer subsequently occurred, the lesion on the original x-ray may be distinguishable.

Under these circumstances, although no mistake was initially made, if even one radiologist can be found who says that he or she believes that initially he or she would have detected it, the patient could sue the radiologist who missed the lesion on the original x-ray. That is, since the lesion on the original x-ray is objectively distinguishable, even though it can be distinguished primarily only with the benefit of hindsight, a judge or jury may determine that the careprovider should have seen it initially and, thus, was negligent. This decision may be influenced by the judge or jury's knowing that a patient and his or her loved ones have suffered, and that the careprovider is insured or has "deep pockets."[2] This determination is particularly likely when a jury is involved.

The quandary this poses for ethics consultants is this: Should they disclose to patients *all* possible mistakes? There is virtually no limit to the number of situations in which patients could sue and be successful. If ethics consultants believe that they must disclose to patients all situations in which a mistake may have been made, they would have to do so even cases such as this one, in which only one out of 100 radiologists believes a mistake has been made. Further, if ethics consultants do so, they become a critical link in a chain of events that has what many (and especially careproviders) may see as an unjust result. If a successful suit, even in a case such as this, is seen as an unavoidable result of a system that is better than any other, this result might not be considered unjust, but only a negative aspect of the best result that can be achieved.

The alternative is to disclose only *some* possible mistakes. However, if ethics consultants do this, they appear to have abandoned their absolute allegiance to truth-telling; they take on the role of arbiter, judging which patient should be informed so that the patient has the option of bringing suit. If ethics consultants do this, they must also justify why they, rather than careproviders, should have this role. This burden of justification is problematic, as careproviders—at least indirectly—have been given authority to exercise this discretion by the law. Ethics consultants may, as a third option, leave the decision of disclosure totally to other careproviders. This approach may best further the consultant's capacity to continue to work with other members of the medical team to help patients.

The question arising for an ethics consultant when no mistake has been made, then, is this: Should he or she disclose facts to a patient that could be used as a basis for a lawsuit, even though it is likely that no mistake was made?

MISTAKES

What an ethics consultant should do when it is certain that a careprovider has made a mistake is generally not a difficult decision. The consultant should do what careproviders should do and what quality assurance personnel insist they do: tell patients the truth. Quality assurance personnel customarily inform careproviders that they must tell the truth and apologize. Ostensibly, this is the best approach ethically. A careprovider acknowledges his or her error by disclosing it fully and making genuine interpersonal amends.

But, for several reasons, this is not the best approach. First, it provides patients with only implicit knowledge that they could sue. Some may argue that any patient who has been informed that he or she has been harmed by a mistake could infer this knowledge. For more-sophisticated patients, this is no doubt true. But less-sophisticated patients may not make this inference; short of providing them with this specific information, expecting them to know it may be unrealistic. If careproviders are less than explicit in disclosing to patients when an unequivocal mistake has been made, only sophisticated patients will understand the implications of such a disclosure, and only they will be able to benefit from any award. This approach leads to inequity, because it discriminates between more- and less-sophisticated patients.

In addition, being less than explicit is ethically inadequate, because careproviders who do this are making less than full amends. If careproviders do *all* that they can to make up for mistakes they have made, this would include making amends to the greatest extent possible; this includes telling a patient explicitly that he or she could probably successfully sue.

Presently, careproviders indicate they have made a mistake and apologize but do not indicate that patients could sue and possibly recover monetary damages. When careproviders respond in this manner, they may actually benefit themselves much more than they benefit the patient. It is well known that whether patients sue largely depends on how they feel toward their careprovider. A bad outcome and negative feelings toward a careprovider are the *sine qua nons* for patients who initiate suits.[3] A careprovider's apology to a patient may evoke the patient's compassion. When a careprovider says, "I have erred. I am sorry," he or she acknowledges human frailty. This may elicit a patient's understanding. It may move a patient, as though the careprovider has said, "I realize that you are suffering. But I am human, too. Please don't add to the net adverse consequences by suing me."

Thus, apologizing may be both ethically optimal and, unintentionally, subtly manipulative. It is ironic that both of these features also exist when a careprovider takes the further step of telling a patient that he or she could sue. Patients may be so moved by the careprovider's caring and selflessness that they may decide not to sue. Because apologizing and telling patients that they could sue may benefit careproviders in this way, this course of action raises a Machiavellian question: Could careproviders apologize, fake genuine remorse, and tell the patient that he or she could sue to enhance this effect, in the hope that the patient would be moved and not sue? That we can even imagine this action illustrates how self-serving apologizing may be.

Legally, if careproviders withhold the truth after they make a mistake, they risk additional, punitive damages. Punitive damages are awarded to patients in addition to the damages awarded to compensate them for harm they have undergone; punitive damages are intended to punish "wrongdoers" for exceptionally offensive behavior.

The question that arises for ethics consultants when an unequivocal mistake has been made is this: Should ethics consultants go beyond ensuring that these patients are told the truth, and ensure that the patients also know that they could sue?

POSSIBLE MISTAKES

When a careprovider has made a possible mistake, an ethics consultant may believe that it should be disclosed, but the careprovider and quality assurance personnel are likely to disagree. Brody illustrates this difference in relating that a patient's internists, having made a possible mistake, "ordered the residents, intern, and medical student who were following the patient's case not to give any information about the deteriorating course and its causes to the man or his family."[4]

When careproviders only *may* have acted outside the standard of care, quality assurance personnel generally do not advise them to tell patients that a mistake may have been made.[5] There are several rationales behind this approach. First, careproviders' disclosing all possible mistakes could result in extremely large numbers of lawsuits; in many of those cases, patients otherwise would not sue because they would not know that a possible mistake had been made. Not telling the patient is more feasible when only a few careproviders know that a possible mistake has been made, because then it is less likely that the patient will find out from other sources. Instances in which only a few careproviders know that a mistake may have been made apparently are not infrequent.[6]

If a careprovider makes a disclosure and a patient does sue, the act of disclosure may work against the careprovider in court. The disclosure may be construed as the careprovider's "admission" against his or her own best interest. The law presumes that persons tend to act in their own best interest; thus, if they act against their best interest, what they say may warrant greater credibility or evidentiary weight. A judge or jury may use this same reasoning. They may presume that if a careprovider discloses a possible mistake, doing this is tantamount to "proof" that he or she has acted negligently.

The argument that follows goes against the above arguments that favor *not* disclosing possible mistakes. Society has determined by means of its legal system that judges and juries, not careproviders, should be the persons to determine whether negligence has occurred. Many considerations support this. For example, as a result of being subjected to the court process, more evidence may come to light. When careproviders do not inform patients that a possible mistake has been made, and patients thus do not know that they can sue, it is careproviders, rather than judges or juries, who determine whether negligence has occurred. Inevitably they determine that it has not.

The argument that society has decided that judges and juries, not careproviders, should determine when negligence has occurred may appear compelling on its face. In actuality, however, what society has done is more complex. The law contradicts this determination by allowing both careproviders and quality assurance personnel to make this decision. For instance, careproviders may not be required to report other careproviders who have made a possible mistake. Beiser reports, for example, that a statute in Rhode Island permits physicians to report other physicians, but does not require them to do so.[7] In contrast, careproviders are required in every state to report suspected child abuse and can be criminally prosecuted if they do not. Thus, the law could require careproviders to disclose possible mistakes just as it requires them to report child abuse. Similarly, quality assurance records generally are protected from legal discovery.[8] Thus, quality assurance personnel can investigate possible mistakes fully and, based on their own judgment, choose to remain silent.

Through its legal system, our society, allows judges and juries, not careproviders, to decide whether negligence has occurred. One the one hand, if careproviders usurp this decision-making authority indirectly by precluding patients from knowing that they could sue, this violates the dictates of society. But, on the other hand, society also allows careproviders and quality assurance personnel to make this decision by allowing them not to disclose possible mistakes to patients.

The same logic can be used to examine the obligations of ethics consultants. Ethics consultants who choose to exercise independently their own discretion usurp the decision-making discretion that the law gives, to some degree explicitly, to careproviders and quality assurance personnel. In this sense, ethics consultants who disclose possible mistakes to patients put themselves above the law.

A final argument against ethics consultants' obligation to disclose when careproviders will not is that disclosure may harm ethics consultants' capacity to help other patients. Suppose that a careprovider does not disclose a possible mistake to a patient; an ethics consultant, learning of this possible mistake, tells the patient. The consultant would be acting as the patient's advocate, but also as an adversary to the medical team. This could create such strong enmity among other careproviders toward the consultant that they no longer turn to the consultant when future ethical issues arise.

The question that arises for ethics consultants when careproviders have made possible mistakes is this: Should the consultant disclose such mistakes to the patient and, as with unequivocal mistakes, tell the patient that he or she could sue, when quality assurance personnel and careproviders would not do so?

EXCEPTIONAL CIRCUMSTANCES
THAT FAVOR DISCLOSURE

HARM TO PATIENTS

Suppose, on the basis of the above rationales, that an ethics consultant cannot decide whether to inform a patient that a careprovider has made a possible mistake (or even a nonmistake). An additional factor that the consultant may want to consider is the extent to which the patient has been harmed. The ethical ground for this is compensatory justice. Obviously, when patients have been seriously harmed, monetary gain may help offset the losses they have undergone.

POTENTIAL HARM TO FUTURE PATIENTS

A second consideration is the risk a careprovider may pose to future patients. In assessing whether future patients are at risk, ethics consultants must evaluate the kind of mistake or possible mistake that occurred.

Even unequivocal negligence may be of two types: inadvertent (and thus unavoidable) or easily anticipated (and thus avoidable). Inadvertent negligence occurs as a result of careproviders' simply having human limitations. That is, careproviders are vulnerable to innumerable factors that can result in error. Examples are extreme fatigue or severe mental distraction resulting from an exceptionally distressing event, such as the death of a loved one. These events are unavoidable. For instance, one physician states: "All doctors are, at times, distracted by family or business matters."[9] If these states of mind occur more than rarely, however, future patients will be at risk.

Other unequivocal mistakes are avoidable. These mistakes may result, for example, from careproviders' habitually behaving toward patients in a manner that is cavalier. For instance, a careprovider knows that a patient could be allergic to a drug such as penicillin, but does not take the time to call another hospital to check the patient's records in the middle of the night.

These two types of unequivocal negligence could be illustrated by how a careprovider reads x-rays. A careprovider could take sufficient time to view an x-ray but, for reasons beyond his or her control (such as lack of sleep or distraction), could simply miss a lesion he or she otherwise would detect. This could occur despite the careprovider's best effort, just as one can read and reread a typographical error without detecting that an error has been made. On the other hand, a careprovider could miss a lesion because he or she habitually takes insufficient time to read an x-ray. This is cavalier. When a patient sues a negligent careprovider, it can serve as a wake-up call and deter future negligent behavior. It may be that when a possible mistake has been made and harm has occurred, a patient should be informed so that he or she can have the opportunity to sue. If, however, a possible mistake has been made and the careprovider has acted in a cavalier manner that is habitual, the risk to future patients may be the deciding factor in the decision about how much to disclose.

MEDICAL, EMOTIONAL, AND ETHICAL MISTAKES

A further consideration ethics consultants may want to take into account when they assess a careprovider's potential danger to future patients is the type of mistake or possible mistake that the careprovider has made. Medical, emotional, and ethical mistakes particularly should be distinguished because they are likely to differ in the probability of the risk they pose to future patients.

A medical mistake may be more likely to recur than emotional or ethical mistakes, which both tend to be more self-correcting. The latter two types of mistakes may reflect not that a careprovider has been cavalier, but the opposite—that the careprovider is *too* dedicated to patients.

Medical mistakes. The first of these types of mistakes is medical. Two kinds of medical errors are discussed above: when careproviders make a mistake that is unavoidable due to human frailty, and when they make a mistake that is avoidable.

Emotional mistakes. An emotional mistake is one that results from careproviders' having an exceptionally powerful feeling that clouds their judgment. In contrast to a medical mistake that is made because a careprovider is cavalier, an emotional mistake, in and of itself, may be praiseworthy. An example, albeit one with a particularly tragic outcome, involves a little boy who was admitted to a hospital with lethargy. The careprovider suspected that the child's lethargy was due to his having ingested drugs, but this could not be definitively determined. A child welfare agency was contacted. The agency agreed to investigate the child's home situation prior to his discharge, but the agency had a long case backlog. The child recovered fully and missed his mother. Days passed. The mother pleaded with her child's physician to release him so that he could come home. The child pleaded, too. The physician, moved by concern for the child and his mother, allowed the mother to take her child home. Months later the boy died as a result of drugs he ingested. In this instance, the careprovider's mistake was, in a sense, caring too much. He had been so moved by the mother's and child's appeals that he was insufficiently suspicious to appreciate the risk posed by allowing the boy to return home.

Caring too much can take many forms. Another example involves a gynecologist who was beloved by staff and patients for the care he showed his patients. After he performed surgery on a patient, she showed signs of an intra-abdominal infection. The doctor had taken his usual extra measures to ensure that the patient's abdominal cavity would not become infected. Possibly because of these extra measures, no prior patient of his had ever had a postoperative intra-abdominal infection. He told her that none of his patients had ever experienced an intra-abdominal postoperative infection and that he believed he should operate again, in case she had developed an infection in her abdominal cavity. She pleaded with him not to subject her to a second operation unless and until the procedure was absolutely necessary. He then erred. In response to her pleading, he violated his better judgment and treated her conservatively with antibiotics. He waited too long before re-operating, and she died.

Careproviders who make emotional mistakes may, like these two physicians, be especially committed to their patients. Still, if their judgment is repeatedly clouded by emotions, they—like careproviders who make inadvertent mistakes and careproviders who are habitually cavalier—may pose a continuing risk to patients. Ethics consultants, accordingly, may wish to assess not only the type of mistake, but its likelihood of recurrence when they decide whether to disclose a mistake or possible mistake that the careprovider would not disclose.

Ethical mistakes. An ethical mistake is one in which a careprovider pursues his or her values conscientiously; although in and of themselves these values are good, due to the context or some other reason the outcome is not. The careprovider may overlook another important value in his or her ethical analysis, as in the following example. A surgeon whose patient was in an intensive care unit with a deteriorating heart condition had given consent for cardiac surgery. This surgery was his only hope for living several more years. The patient became less capable of verbalizing his reasons for wanting surgery as his condition continued to decline. Although the patient was having difficulty concentrating, the surgeon could have deemed the patient still competent (since the patient continued to be able to say "yes" or "no") or the surgeon could have operated on an emergency basis. Instead, he cancelled the surgery to obtain a surrogate decision maker because he believed that this was necessary, ethically, to respect the patient's autonomy. The window of opportunity during which the operation could have been successful was lost, and the patient died. Although the surgeon's commitment to respecting the patient's autonomy was meritorious, he failed to see this value in a wider context. It is for this reason that his judgment well might be questioned.

Another example of a possible ethical error involves a patient who had pneumonia and, due to sepsis, was incompetent. The patient was placed on a respirator. The patient had stated in an advance directive that he would not want to be kept on a respirator; presumably he had meant that he would not want to be kept on a respirator permanently, as opposed to briefly for treatment of pneumonia. Again, his careprovider was committed, above all other concerns, to the value of respecting a patient's autonomy. He felt this so strongly that he believed he had to construe this patient's advance directive literally by following it to the letter. Thus, he discontinued the respirator to respect the patient's wishes as documented in his advance directive, and the patient died.

When careproviders make ethical mistakes, this may be because they care to an exceptional degree. Further, like those who make emotional mistakes, they are highly likely to learn from their mistakes so that they never repeat them, because they care. If, on the other hand, they repeat such ethical mistakes, they—like those who make repeated emotionally driven mistakes—pose a risk to future patients.

It is not likely that careproviders will learn from their mistakes when they are cavalier. Ethics consultants may therefore want to consider this difference when deciding what they will disclose.

POSSIBLE HARMS THAT MAY RESULT
FROM DISCLOSURE

When the harm to patients is less serious, the other harms that may result from a consultant's disclosing a possible mistake may offset the harm done by the mistake, thus giving the harm from nondisclosure relatively less moral weight. Three possible harms may result from disclosure: loss of the placebo effect, worse symptoms, and trauma from becoming an adversary of a careprovider for whom the patient cares.

LOSS OF THE PLACEBO EFFECT

Even when patients have not been harmed by a possible or actual mistake, a case for disclosure still remains, because this would respect the patient by telling him or her the truth. Possibly offsetting this argument, however, is the harm that may result from disclosure. If a patient learns that the careprovider has erred, the patient may lose the benefits of the placebo effect.

Patients and careproviders may benefit greatly when patients realize that careproviders are only human and may err. Yet this may require many patients to change how they view careproviders, which may take a long time. Still, potential gains may result. For example, a patient challenged a careprovider who recommended that she undergo surgery. The patient suggested that they try a more conservative measure first, although it was much less likely to succeed. "We'll try it," the careprovider said. "Even after making decisions for 20 years, patients sometimes know better than I do." The patient felt greater respect for the careprovider because he had acknowledged that he might be wrong. (The conservative treatment, incidentally, was effective.)

The opposite effect—the loss of the placebo effect—may occur as a result of disclosure, and its magnitude may be far greater. The placebo effect is the phenomenon that patients apparently improve simply because they believe they will. This is illustrated by a passage from an article by Brody. A senior physician states, "Have you seen a patient sent for a series of diagnostic X rays, but who does not know the purpose of the X rays, and who tells the physician later how grateful he is for the relief that he has experienced as a result of the X ray treatments?"[10] If such a patient knew that the physician had made a serious mistake or possible mistake, this placebo effect may not have occurred.

A second example that does not involve negating the placebo effect, but involves negating another positive effect, occurred when I was a medical student. I was treating a child who was in a coma and was dying from cancer. He had metastases in his brain and required medication to prevent seizures. I was tired and injected excessive antiseizure medication into his intravenous line. I recognized this almost immediately and stopped the intravenous infusion at once. I did not know how much antiseizure medication I had given him. He may have received too little, not enough, or the right amount. I had no way of finding out.

I was very afraid that the antiseizure medication I had given could cause a cardiopulmonary arrest. I stayed, sitting with him and his parents in his room for the next three hours, watching him take every breath. I am sure that the parents, seeing me sitting there with them all that time, thought that I was exceptionally dedicated and caring. How else could they have made sense of my remaining there? The boy did not have a cardiopulmonary arrest, and he later died from the cancer. The parents' memory of me as an exceptionally caring medical student may have been among the best they took with them from the hospital. Should I have told them that I made this mistake? I remain ambivalent regarding my behavior under those circumstances, even today. I believe that, ethically, the best response would have been for me to own up to my mistake, tell the parents I might have given their son too much medicine, and arrange immediately to transfer him to intensive care. Yet, I was watching him intently to remove any risk to him by initiating cardiopulmonary resuscitation if he had gone into cardiopulmonary arrest. My admitting my mistake might have helped his parents learn that careproviders, like me, can err. Yet what is most important is for this transformation in patients' perception of careproviders to take place with large populations over time. Even if careproviders attempt to convey this reality to patients and their loved ones on an individual basis, it is likely that patients and their loved ones would be less able to acquire this understanding while they experienced great fear due to their own serious illness.

I tell medical students that disclosing such a mistake is the higher ethical road. Nonetheless, somewhere deep inside, I remain glad that I did not disclose my mistake, and that this family (presumably) has this memory. This awareness makes me wonder whether my ethical belief represents a view that is truly illuminated by moral reasoning, or if it is reflexive in nature—representing a blind allegiance to truth-telling and failing to take into account deeper aspects of human reality that rational scrutiny is likely to miss. In any case, my ambivalence reflects what I intended to suggest by using this example: when a possible mistake or, as in this case, an actual mistake has done no harm, the costs of disclosure may outweigh the gains.

THE HARM OF HAVING TO RETAIN SYMPTOMS TO GAIN LEGAL COMPENSATION

Patients who are told the truth may risk more than losing the placebo effect. If they choose to sue, they may suffer to an increased extent as a result of unconsciously retaining symptoms, such as pain. For reasons that are poorly understood, when patients sue, symptoms that otherwise might go away are more likely to remain.[11]

The mind appears to have the capacity to maintain and even bring about symptoms if the patient stands to benefit significantly from having these symptoms, even when the patient consciously would oppose this. If the patient is suing, it is as if the mind can know that under this circumstance, the symptom must persist for the patient to acquire greater monetary gain as a result of the court decision. This psychological phenomenon is known as "secondary gain."[12] It has resulted in the rubric, often voiced, that patients are unlikely to respond to treatment when they are engaged in litigation if they need the symptom to recover the maximum in monetary damages.

This risk is probably insufficient in and of itself to ever justify not disclosing that a possible mistake has been made, and nondisclosure on this basis probably would be unjustifiably paternalistic. Yet this information still may be important to some patients when they decide whether to sue. An ethics consultant should, therefore, inform a patient of this risk under such circumstances.

HARM FROM BECOMING AN ADVERSARY OF A CAREPROVIDER

A third significant loss patients may experience as a result of disclosure is the pain of becoming an adversary of a careprovider about whom the patient cares. Patients may experience this pain very acutely, especially if they testify against their careprovider in court. The possible negative impact of this encounter should not be underestimated. Its magnitude cannot be established empirically, but everyday experience suggests it is considerable. For instance, persons often find it difficult to talk to others after they have confronted them, and some cannot even look the other in the eyes. Levinas has discussed the significance of such face-to-face encounters. He believes that looking into another person's eyes puts one in touch with others' vulnerability more than other experiences: "The face in its nakedness as a face . . . attests the presence of . . . the whole of humanity, in the eyes that look at me."[13]

This harmful effect may be particularly great if the patient-careprovider relationship has been long-standing and close. However, the following example, taken from a short story, illustrates that patients and their relatives may come to care deeply for their careprovider because of what they have experienced together, even after only a matter of days.

A boy had been hit by a car. He was expected to do well but did not, and he died. His doctors "said it was a one-in-a-million circumstance." The boy's doctor, Dr. Francis, "was shaken." He said to the boy's mother, Ann, " 'I can't tell you how badly I feel. I'm so very sorry, I can't tell you.' " Then, "Dr. Francis guided Ann to the sofa, sat down beside her, and began to talk in a low, consoling voice. At one point he leaned over and embraced her."[14]

Since a mistake may have occurred, the boy's parents could have sued Dr. Francis. Ann would have been testifying against the same man who had said, " 'I'm so very sorry, I can't tell you,' " and who had guided her to the sofa and embraced her. How Ann's testifying against him would have affected her is left to the reader's determination, but it is hard to imagine that it could be anything other than exceedingly traumatic and painful.

MEANS BY WHICH ETHICS CONSULTANTS
CAN ATTEMPT TO REDUCE THIS HARM

The harm patients may suffer in testifying against a careprovider for whom they care should not, in and of itself, justify not disclosing a possible mistake.

Nondisclosure on this basis would be impermissibly paternalistic. The ethics consultant should, however, make patients aware of this risk so that they can consider it when deciding whether to sue. This potential harm could be reduced, and ethics consultants could tell a careprovider who would be willing to do this how to reduce this harm.

If, for the reasons previously stated, a careprovider tells a patient that he or she could sue, the careprovider could at the same time assure the patient that suing is what the careprovider would want. The careprovider could add to the credibility of this assertion by giving reasons, such as a commitment to the principle of compensatory justice and a desire that the patient receive some monetary award, unequal to his or her real loss as it may be.

A careprovider who tells a patient this may, of course, suffer adverse, retaliatory repercussions from quality assurance personnel, insurance companies, and the institution where he or she practices. Thus, potential harm may be a factor that limits the degree to which careproviders might be willing to try to reduce harm to patients. Accordingly, ethics consultants who are concerned about disclosure seem to have an obligation to discuss with careproviders not only the potential harm to patients, but also the risk to careproviders.

Careproviders who engage in such discussions may raise the following question: Should they ask the patient not to disclose that the careprovider said that the patient could sue? It is generally ethically preferable not to "game the system"; some would say that this should never be done. However, others believe that the present malpractice system is deeply flawed, because it functions as if careproviders could be perfect; it allows the award of unwarranted monetary damages when careproviders fail, and, in doing so, compounds this error as it fosters the perception that careproviders could be perfect. If this negative assessment of the present legal system is valid, the ethical ground for gaming the system may be greater. That is, gaming the system may be the only way, under the present system, that careproviders can offset an unduly harmful result. It may be the only way that they can both allow the patient to obtain some monetary compensation and protect themselves.

On the other hand, if careproviders ask patients not to disclose that careproviders have advised them to sue, this gives the patients the extra burden of having to lie. Careproviders who make this request may also increase their own risk; if their institution learns that they told the patient that he or she could sue and asked the patient not to disclose this, the institution may retaliate.

PRACTICAL IMPLICATIONS

What should ethics consultants do, then, when careproviders have made or may have made a mistake? As the previous discussion suggests, the best answer may be that it depends. Ethics consultants face conflicting values in all situations, but what they should do is most difficult to determine when careproviders have made only a possible mistake.

In all situations, however, ethics consultants have two basic options: (1) they can ignore their personal values and follow the practices of careproviders and quality assurance personnel, or (2) they can adhere to their personal beliefs and tell the absolute truth even when careproviders and quality assurance personnel would not.

Careproviders' present practice is, in general, not to disclose mistakes that are only possible mistakes.[15] When in doubt, they are expected to inform quality assurance personnel, who will assess the situation and then decide whether the mistake must be disclosed. Regardless of what careproviders do, ethics consultants may see their own ethical obligation in all situations as not the least bit problematic. They may presume that they merely need to ensure that patients are informed about whatever has occurred. Indeed, I have argued that the ethical "high road" for careproviders to take after making a mistake or possible mistake in which a patient is harmed is to fully disclose whatever has happened.[16] I would argue that this would be equally true for ethics consultants when they err. Yet in the two situations just discussed, careproviders and ethics consultants must decide whether to report mistakes that they, themselves, have made.

The situations considered here involve a critical difference. In these situations, ethics consultants must decide whether to report mistakes made by others. Ethics consultants, as a result of the nature of their profession, may believe that this difference is morally irrelevant. Disclosing mistakes and possible mistakes to patients is only honest, and doing otherwise would violate an implicit promise made by all careproviders to tell patients the truth. Ethics consultants may reason, entirely logically, that if they do not act to ensure that patients are informed under all circumstances, ethics consultants should not be called *ethics* consultants.

Yet if ethics consultants do not follow the practices of careproviders and quality assurance personnel, but insist upon disclosing mistakes and possible mistakes, their relationships with careproviders and quality assurance personnel could become very problematic. Being sued has profound emotional consequences for careproviders, not to mention the very negative effects on their careers and reputations.[17] Careproviders therefore have an overriding fear of malpractice suits. Nowhere is this exemplified more convincingly than by the screening practices used in regard to patients with prostate problems. There is a lack of scientific evidence that screening for a specific prostate antigen is beneficial. Nonetheless, a recent study reported that many primary care doctors and urologists continue to carry out this screening, and the degree to which they screen correlates with their beliefs regarding whether patients could successfully sue.[18]

If ethics consultants believe that all possible mistakes should be disclosed, what should they say to careproviders and quality assurance personnel? They have two options. (1) They could refrain from saying what they would do until the first time they learned of a possible mistake, and then disclose it; this would be implicitly deceitful, as careproviders would be caught unaware and, most likely, feel betrayed and enraged. (2) They could tell careproviders and quality assurance personnel what they would do before a first possible mistake occurred. Careproviders might then not trust them from the start, and quality assurance personnel might advise careproviders not to give the ethics consultants potentially "self-incriminating" information.

In either case, careproviders could be expected in short order to regard ethics consultants as persons outside their medical team. As a result of this isolation, ethics consultants could lose their capacity to help patients. This loss would be dear.

Whether telling the truth or meeting future patients' needs should prevail is open to dispute but, all too often, truth-telling is accepted uncritically as an absolute value. The obligation to give this value priority over all others is viewed as so compelling that competing values are not considered. Like the careproviders who gave complete allegiance to autonomy, ethics consultants who value truth-telling above all else may make a similarly unfortunate mistake.

CONCLUSION

For ethics consultants who decide not to disclose possible mistakes to patients, there is possibly a "redeeming" aspect. That is, presently, they have no choice but to violate respect for either patients or careproviders. This is because in the United States, at least, many patients have unrealistic expectations regarding careproviders. Some patients believe that careproviders can and must function perfectly and, if they do not, they are morally culpable and should pay huge monetary awards. This attitude is not new and exists elsewhere.

It is epitomized, perhaps, nowhere better than in Kafka's *A Country Doctor*. The doctor laid his head "to the boy's breast," and "confirmed what I already knew; the boy was quite sound." But as the doctor was about to leave, "I discovered . . . an open wound as big as the palm of my hand. . . . Worms, as thick and as long as my little finger . . . were wriggling . . . in . . . the wound."[19]

This doctor had made a mistake. How did those present at the bedside respond? "Strip his clothes off . . . kill him dead." One person present responded, "I'd like best . . . to scratch your eyes out."[20]

The legal system reinforces these unrealistic expectations and, as a result, fosters within patients a dehumanization of careproviders. Ambulance chasers and high monetary awards, for example, reinforce these unrealistic expectations. It may then be, as Doyal and Hurwitz argue, that patients "should not seek damages for an error that results from a lack of . . . [medical, emotional, or ethical] perfection."[21] It may be that Tan is correct in his suggestion of the direction in which we should go: "The reporting method must . . . educate, not punish: restore, not denigrate." Our "fault-based system must be replaced by a no-fault model which focuses on just compensation."[22]

The excruciating pain that careproviders often experience from being sued, even if the suit is unsuccessful, is, from an ethical perspective, exceedingly unjust for several reasons. First, most physicians are dedicated to their patients. As the preceding discussion of the careproviders who make emotional and ethical mistakes exemplifies, physicians may be highly dedicated to their patients, even when they make inadvertent mistakes. Second, careproviders may experience extraordinary suffering when treating patients, even in the absence of making mistakes. Hilfiker is speaking of this, I believe, when he states, "Our profession is difficult enough without our having to wear the yoke of perfection."[23]

For example, careproviders must sometimes witness tragic harm to patients that they, themselves, have brought about, although they have little choice if they wish to try to help patients. This unique source of suffering is illustrated in the following description by a neurosurgeon of surgery he performed. He was doing brain surgery on a patient who had had headaches and had fallen and knocked two porcelain birds off a table at her home. She said to him, jokingly, "Thank God they didn't break." He thought she could be cured and told her what he believed: "In my experience I have every reason to think that we can get you through this operation without your being harmed." She hugged her family in the holding room prior to surgery. She felt "embarrassed about not having her dentures." Her well-being was not to be. After making an incision into her brain and sending off a frozen section, "the exposed brain began to undergo a transformation. . . . It was one of those moments that can occur during surgery that is defined by alarm. . . . The blood might just as well have been descending upon a sleeping town, avalanche or mud slide, it made no difference. . . . Fragments of brain, cortex and white matter, welled up in that bleeding like victims being swept back in a torrent. . . . The patient would not survive." The surgeon, who had just talked to this woman and enjoyed her humor saw her brain disgorge before him. And he had caused it himself. He reports, "A human being lay there, now irreversibly lost . . . wife and mother undone." The suffering that work such as this surgeon's requires is outside that of most other persons. And he could not grieve immediately afterward. "I completed the closure and made my way to the waiting family."[24]

Ethics consultants who disclose to patients what careproviders would not disclose themselves do not fulfill their duty to patients but, in making this choice, do avoid acting in complicity with the injustice to careproviders wreaked by the law and patients' unrealistic expectations. To eliminate this injustice, it will be necessary to change patients' views and the law to create a context in which careproviders, quality assurance personnel, and ethics consultants can and want to tell all patients all the truth. If this could be achieved, patients could look into the eyes of careproviders who have made mistakes, and ethics consultants could adhere to their beliefs but still look into the eyes of careproviders. It is as Levinas has said: "The epiphany of the face is ethical."[25]

NOTES

1. G. Fischer et al., "Adverse Events in Primary Care Identified from a Risk-Management Database," *Journal of Family Practice* 45, no. 1 (1997): 40-6, p. 43.

2. L. Doyal and B. Hurwitz, "The Morality of Medical Mistakes," *The Practitioner* 231 (22 April 1987): 615-20.

3. W. Levinson et al., "Physician-Patient Communication: The Relationship with Malpractice Claims among Primary Care Physicians and Surgeons," *Journal of the American Medical Association*

277, no. 7 (19 February 1997): 553-9.

4. H. Brody, "The Chief of Medicine," *Hastings Center Report* 21, no. 4 (July-August 1991): 17-22, p. 17.

5. D. Short, "Learning from Our Mistakes," *British Journal of Hospital Medicine* 51, no. 5 (March 1994): 250-2, p. 250.

6. Ibid.

7. E.N. Beiser, "Reporting Physicians' Mistakes," *Rhode Island Medical Journal* 73, no. 8 (August 1990): 333-6.

8. See note 1 above, p. 45.

9. Martha, "The Man Who Never Comes Back," *Lancet* 8156 (22-29 December 1979): 1358-9.

10. See note 4 above, p. 20.

11. L.M. Binder and M.L. Rohling, "Money Matters: A Meta-Analytic Review of the Effects of Financial Incentives on Recovery after Closed-Head Injury," *American Journal of Psychiatry* 153 (January 1996): 1-10.

12. F.W. Silver, "Management of Conversion Disorder," *American Journal of Physical Medicine and Rehabilitation* 75 (1996): 134-40, p. 139.

13. E. Levinas, *Totality and Infinity,* trans. A. Lingis (Pittsburgh, Penn.: Duquesne University Press, 1969), 213.

14. R. Carver, "A Small, Good Thing," in *Where I'm Calling From: New and Selected Stories* (New York: Atlantic Monthly Press, 1988), 280-301.

15. D.H. Novack et al., "On Physicians' Attitudes Toward Using Deception to Resolve Ethical Problems," *Journal of the American Medical Association* 261, no. 20 (26 May 1989): 2980-5. In this study, a third of physicians indicated that they might not tell a patient even if a physician made a serious mistake.

16. E.G. Howe, "Possible Mistakes," *The Journal of Clinical Ethics* 8, no. 4 (Winter 1997): 323-8.

17. M. Newman, "The Emotional Impact of Mistakes on Family Physicians," *Archives of Family Medicine* 5 (1996): 71-5.

18. M.M. Collins, F.J. Fowler, Jr., and R.G. Roberts, "Medical Malpractice Implications of PSA Testing for Early Detection of Prostate Cancer," *Journal of Law, Medicine and Ethics* 25 (1997): 234-42.

19. F. Kafka, "A Country Doctor," in *The Penal Colony,* trans. W. Muir and E. Muir (New York: Schocken Books, 1961), 139-42.

20. Ibid.

21. See note 2 above, p. 616.

22. S.Y. Tan, "When Doctors Make Mistakes," *Hawaii Medical Journal* 55, no. 8 (August 1996): 135-46, p. 146.

23. D. Hilfiker, "Facing Our Mistakes," *New England Journal of Medicine* 310, no. 2 (12 January 1984): 118-22, at 122 (Hilfiker's article is reprinted in chapter 6 of this book—ED.).

24. M. Flitter, *Judith's Pavilion/The Haunting Memories of a Neurosurgeon* (South Royalton, Vt.: Steerforth Press, 1997), 3-25.

25. See note 13 above, p. 199.

12

Taking Responsibility for Medical Mistakes

Virginia A. Sharpe

INTRODUCTION

Look at the title of this chapter. For most people, it suggests the need for someone to own up to something, to shoulder the burden of having erred, to admit responsibility for something that happened. However, another interpretation can be given to the expression "taking responsibility"—taking prospective responsibility. It is this second interpretation that is put forward here as a more constructive way to think about medical error. This chapter (1) contrasts two senses of responsibility—responsibility understood retrospectively and responsibility understood prospectively, (2) examines the implications of a systems theory of causation for models of individual versus collective responsibility, and (3) argues that if continuous quality improvement systems approach (and thus a collective approach) to the safety of patients is to succeed, it must be joined by a compensation scheme that shares its prospective orientation to the question of responsibility.

TWO SENSES OF RESPONSIBILITY

Moral responsibility can be taken in a retrospective or a prospective sense. The backwards-looking or retrospective sense is linked to practices of praising and blaming and is the basis for theories of moral assessment. It is typically captured in expressions such as "She was responsible for harming the patient," or "He made a mistake and he should be held responsible for it." The forward-looking or prospective sense of responsibility, by contrast, is linked to theories and practices of goal setting and moral deliberation and, as such, is central to theories of moral reasoning. It may be expressed in phrases such as: "As a parent, I am responsible for the welfare of my child," or "Democratic citizenship involves both rights and responsibilities." In distinguishing these two senses of responsibility, it is also important to note that the backward-looking sense tends to have an *individual* as its object, while the forward-looking sense contextualizes responsibility as it relates to the particular *roles* that a person may occupy. In addition, whereas responsibility in the retrospective sense focuses on *outcomes,* prospective responsibility is oriented to the deliberative and practical *processes* involved in setting and meeting goals.

RESPONSIBILITY IN THE RETROSPECTIVE SENSE

In asking readers to look at the title of this chapter, I postulated that they would interpret it in the retrospective sense. Indeed, so potent is the practice of moral assessment and, more specifically, the practice of blaming, that it has given rise to many great institutions and intellectual edifices. The possibility of holding someone responsible for their actions is, for example, at the heart of the enduring philosophical problem of free will and determinism. More specific to our purposes, assessments of blame give rise to the practices of justification and excuse. In what follows, I discuss both of these practices and situate mistakes and errors within the domain of possible excusing conditions.

When we consider medical mistakes and particularly those that cause harm,[1] the blameworthiness of the error depends on how it squares with the obligation of due care. Due care is a legal doctrine that allows that certain individuals may inflict injury while engaged in lawful professional behavior and are liable for damages only if their conduct fails to meet a certain standard of care.[2] In moral terms, if harm results from one's legitimately risky professional conduct, one's blameworthiness depends upon a number of factors related to the reasonable standard of care due or owed. These factors are highlighted in the practices of justification and excuse.[3]

In offering a *justification,* the agent of harm admits responsibility for the harm but argues that the acts or omissions that led to it were defensible or permissible on the basis of some countervailing demand or obligation.[4] Possible justifications for medical harms include triage, where the demands of justice based on need are paramount; medical research and education and public health, where the demands of utility—or the greatest good for a population—might permit harms to particular individuals; or benefit itself to the individual who chooses to endure a harm in order to obtain a desired outcome.

In offering an *excuse,* by contrast, the alleged agent of harm denies responsibility (and thus moral agency) for an admittedly unfortunate outcome and argues that the outcome was the result of—and therefore should be excused by—certain features of the situation.[5] Possible excusing conditions include innocent ignorance, duress, lack of sufficient resources, "necessary fallibility," and errors or mistakes. It is errors or mistakes that concern us here.

A *mistake* is standardly defined as "an error in action, opinion, or judgment caused by poor reasoning, carelessness [or] insufficient knowledge."[6] As noted above, the blameworthiness or excusability of a harmful medical mistake depends on how it squares with the obligation of due care. Harms associated with recklessness, incompetence, or negligent incapacitation (such as when the practitioner is inebriated) are not genuine "mistakes," since they do not result from error *per se*, but from a disregard for due care itself. When a mistake in reasoning, judgment, or action does involve erring from standards of due care, however, it is a genuine *error* and, as such, is presumed to have occurred within a context of good faith.

Because excusing conditions are marshaled to respond to negative moral assessments (in other words, because excusing conditions emerge within the framework of responsibility understood *retrospectively*), medical mistakes—as excusing conditions—have, until recently, rarely been discussed outside of the context of a harm with which they are associated. Indeed, at least one study of medical mistakes defines a mistake in terms of its outcome as "an unanticipated negative consequence of a medical intervention."[7] Another consequence of this retrospective orientation to medical mistakes is that it presumes a model of individual agency. In other words, the practice of blaming, especially in the case of medical negligence, is premised on there being an identifiable individual who can be held accountable for poor performance. However, as we will see below, the conflation of a mistake with a harm and the emphasis on individual agency mischaracterize the nature and etiology of mistakes and serve as an obstacle to their prevention.

RESPONSIBILITY IN THE PROSPECTIVE SENSE

In its forward-looking sense, responsibility refers to the burden of obligation that accompanies certain roles and offices. When we ask "for what am I responsible?" we are asking about the substantive moral commitments that pertain to the specific practices in which we are engaged, the goals that define the practices, and the proper means of attaining them. Responsibility is forward-looking in this sense because it involves prospective reasoning about what one should do and why one should do it rather than retrospective assignment of blame.[8]

Although many theoretical discussions debate the source of medical morality—whether it resides in the fiduciary nature of the healing relationship, in a pragmatic concern to produce "patient satisfaction," or in the autonomous choices of individuals—it is commonly accepted that the healing enterprise is guided by the imperative "to help, or at least to do no harm."[9] In addressing the question of medical mistakes, it is this imperative that, above all, defines the prospective responsibility of all who are engaged in the healing enterprise.[10] Because prospective responsibility is linked to practices and roles, it applies to collectives as well as to individuals. To the extent that a group of people contribute to a practice and the goals that define it, they can be said to have collective responsibility—in the prospective sense. In healthcare, helping and avoiding harm is one of the primary bases on which physicians, nurses, and other healthcare providers find solidarity in their work.[11] Collective responsibility in this uncontroversial sense has been largely overlooked because, like most discussions of responsibility in the philosophical literature, discussions of collective responsibility have focused almost exclusively on the (retrospective) question of blame and whether collectives can properly be held accountable for harmful events.[12]

It is necessary to set this question aside in order to examine how those in healthcare might be said to have responsibility in this forward-looking sense and what its implications might be for medical mistakes. To do this, we look at recent literature on the etiology of medical mistakes.

THE ETIOLOGY OF MEDICAL MISTAKES

Traditionally, attention to medical error has focused on the evaluation of individual agency and responsibility. As Leape has pointed out, this view of error is deeply embedded in the culture of medicine.[13] Under a socialization process that emphasizes perfectibility and infallibility, mistakes are viewed as unusual, unacceptable, and indicative of flawed character.[14] Implicit in this view of error is the belief that medical quality itself is essentially a function of the competence and integrity of individuals. This belief has often been explicitly articulated in the medical literature. In 1947, G.G. Ward made the following assertion: "The product of the hospital is health, and . . . we know that it is the character of the medical staff that determines the product of the hospital."[15] In 1993, a physician-ethicist averred that "in the end, the patient's greatest guarantee of quality of care is the physician's character."[16]

Although few would deny that the physician's integrity and competence are important ingredients in the overall quality of care, the assumption that these characteristics are sufficient to guarantee quality belies the empirical evidence regarding quality failures. Physicians may strive for faultless performance, but the fact is that many aspects of patient care are simply beyond physicians' power to control. Researchers investigating iatrogenic complications have found that system failure and poor system or job design contribute significantly to harmful error by providing the conditions under which error will thrive. Although a physician may be the proximal cause of a deadly prescribing error, the underlying cause may be a dangerously heavy workload or a poor system of drug information dissemination. A harmful error in drug dispensing may have been facilitated by a system that does not adequately control for look-alike drug packaging or sound-alike drug names.

In a recent study of adverse drug events occurring in hospitals, Leape and colleagues found that system failures accounted for 78 percent of harmful errors.[17] These findings strongly suggest that, from the point of view of actual practice, the principal locus of quality is not the individual, but rather the design of systems, processes, and policies. These findings have been substantiated elsewhere. In a study by Dearden and Rutherford, institutional staffing policies played a key role in critical care management errors.[18] In particular, harmful errors were associated with staffing arrangements in which only inexperienced, junior doctors were on duty outside of regular office hours. Similarly, policies that require long working hours for residents or discourage or prevent adequate supervision of residents may be significant catalysts of harmful error. In a study by Wu and colleagues, house officers reported that job overload played a part in

65 percent of their mistakes.[19] Such system failures were also implicated in the 1984 death of Libby Zion, a college freshman who died nine hours after being admitted to New York Hospital with fever and agitation. Review of her case identified the policy of 36-hour resident shifts and the "closed-book order"—a common practice that allows only interns (those in their first year of residency training after receiving the medical degree) to write orders for patients—as factors contributing to her death.[20]

Although many of these errors were made visible only because they produced harm, empirical studies indicate that most medical errors do not result in an adverse outcome.[21] Unless there is a system in place that identifies errors before they cause harm, then harm becomes a necessary component in error prevention. Although paradoxical, given medicine's defining obligation, this is precisely the situation created by the retrospective orientation to mistakes embedded in quality assurance and medical malpractice.

QUALITY ASSURANCE AND MEDICAL MALPRACTICE: RETROSPECTIVE ORIENTATIONS TO MEDICAL MISTAKES

Quality assurance (QA) is medicine's prevailing quality management scheme. It is based on a retrospective notion of responsibility. Under this model, poor quality of care is understood to be the result of incompetent or careless individuals, or, as Berwick has described it, of "bad apples."[22] Quality is accordingly "assured" through a system of standards, inspections, and penalties that mark the boundaries of acceptable conduct. "Outliers," those whose work fails to meet established standards, are identified by sophisticated inspection and measurement techniques, and brought into line by penalty and probation. The assumption that errors and poor quality are largely if not wholly the product of individual deficiencies naturally engenders an atmosphere of defensiveness (such as the tendency to offer excuses) and evasiveness. Under the QA model, there is very little incentive to admit possible error because the mechanisms for addressing it are largely punitive. Because it discourages openness about error, leads to evasive tactics, and discourages learning opportunities, this model is counterproductive in error prevention. Likewise, because QA uses conformity to standards as a relatively static basis of performance evaluation, it does not have a built-in mechanism for review of the standards themselves.[23]

The retrospective notion of responsibility functions paradigmatically in medical malpractice law. As a species of tort law, the primary purpose of medical malpractice is to determine blame for the purposes of compensation.[24] In medical matters, the most prominent theory of tort law is that of negligence. Under the law of negligence, liability for a harm depends on the following conditions: (1) the professional must have a duty to the harmed party; (2) the professional must breach that duty; (3) the affected party must suffer a harm; and (4) the harm must be caused by the breach. Compensation depends upon the identification of an individual agent who, in failing to abide by established standards, caused harm to a patient. As in QA, medical malpractice's emphasis on individual agency disregards the system dimensions of patient harm. Likewise, its emphasis on individual fault stands as one of the most powerful disincentives to error reporting. Finally, given that malpractice is concerned with mistakes only when they cause harm, it diverts attention from the majority of mistakes that occur in the process of healthcare decision making.

In recent years, the call for tort reform has emphasized the promise of a no-fault compensation scheme for medical injuries. One rationale for such a scheme is that, by deemphasizing individual agency and removing the contributory fault condition for liability, it may encourage quality improvement programs that focus on the complex, system-related causes of patient harm.

CONTINUOUS QUALITY IMPROVEMENT AND NO-FAULT LIABILITY: PROSPECTIVE ORIENTATIONS TO MEDICAL MISTAKES

Patient care, especially in an institutional setting, involves coordination among an array of providers. Likewise, it involves multiple complex interactions with technology. At every juncture there is the possibility for error. Continuous quality improvement (CQI) is a quality management scheme that is designed with this in mind.[25] CQI is premised on a "systems theory of causation." A system is "an interdependent group of items, people or processes with a common purpose."[26] As stated above, the purpose of healthcare is patient benefit and the avoidance of harm. Responding to data from industry and healthcare that as many as 75 percent of errors can be traced to system deficiencies,[27] CQI identifies a number of subsidiary goals—instrumental to the general goal of the patient's welfare—that are specific to the system dimensions of care. They include a focus on processes (rather than individuals) as objects of improvement, elimination of unnecessary variation and complexity, improved communication, and respect for human limitations in the design of tasks and work systems.[28] This broader description of prospective responsibilities correspondingly expands the scope of the "collective" that bears them.

Traditionally, role-specific obligations in healthcare have been associated exclusively with clinicians—those who have a direct relationship with patients. In part, this is a function of the history of healing, that—up until the emergence of the modern hospital—was largely performed by solitary practitioners. Given the complexity in the financing and delivery of today's healthcare in the United States, a strong case can be made that obligations specific to the practice of healthcare should also be extended to those who have indirect but, nonetheless, significant control over decision making that affects patient welfare. This includes hospital and healthcare plan managers and administrators. At present, the backlash against managed care in this country constitutes somewhat of a referendum on this issue. What is the proper relationship between the values of the marketplace and the values of healing? Should a patient's welfare be compromised in the name of cost control? Is healthcare a unique social good or a commodity? Is the healing relationship a fiduciary or a contractual one? I have argued elsewhere that the vulnerability of the patient and the consequent power differential between the patient and healthcare providers give rise to a legitimate expectation that medicine will serve the patient's welfare.[29] This, coupled with the growing body of evidence regarding the administrative dimensions of quality and quality failure, suggests that it would be inappropriate and impractical to exclude managers and administrators from the collective whose responsibilities involve continuous improvement.

Continuous improvement, after all, requires continuous attention to all of the processes that contribute to the healthcare enterprise. If, for example, there are no sinks available near an intensive care unit, it will require more effort for clinicians to wash their hands. Without a policy of "unit dosing" in hospital pharmacies, there is a greater likelihood for error when nurses must calculate doses or draw doses from multiple-use vials. Without computerized drug ordering, potentially harmful drug interactions might not be detected in time. Staff cutbacks or poor staffing arrangements might lead to errors in the management of patients. All of these issues are based in part on administrative policies. Quality improvement requires a concerted and systematic effort on the part of practitioners, administrators, and managers to identify and anticipate such failures and to implement processes that make them less likely. Collective responsibility, in the forward-looking sense, thus extends to all of these healthcare decision makers.

Because one of the central conditions for quality improvement is the identification of errors and quality failures, it has been argued that under the current tort system, the success of quality management programs depends upon the guarantee of confidentiality and immunity from punitive action.[30] Under the existing fault-based compensation system, however, confidentiality and immunity are achieved largely at the expense of the injured patient.[31] Through the doctrine of legal privilege, patients are prevented access to in-house information on harmful quality failures associated with their care. Likewise, disclosure of errors to patients is discouraged by in-house counsel.

Many believe that the most comprehensive way to overcome such concerns about confidentiality and immunity—and to do so in a way that does not compromise the interests of the individual patient—is through a no-fault compensation scheme for medical injuries. No-fault, also known as "strict liability," is a theory found in contract and tort law where, because of the high risk of hazard in a particular industry, absolute liability is assigned in advance regardless of contributory fault.[32] It has been suggested that a no-fault scheme could be implemented through the mechanism of a patient compensation fund much like workers' compensation, which also operates on the basis of this theory.[33] Such a fund could be financed through taxation or a health insurance surcharge. Although a no-fault scheme would have a number of desirable benefits, the one most central to the prevention of medical mistakes is that, because strict liability ignores fault, this compensation scheme provides the necessary background conditions for the reporting of mistakes and quality failures.

Although a no-fault scheme has this and other potential advantages, it also raises important questions regarding responsibility and deterrence. How, in a no-fault scheme for medical injury compensation, would it be possible to sustain an ethos of individual responsibility? And what, in such a system, would be the motivation for individuals to avoid poor performance? To respond to these questions, we need to take another look at the notion of collective responsibility in the theory of CQI.

As we have said, CQI is premised on a systems theory of causation—mistakes and quality failures result from the inevitable complexity of overlapping domains and processes involving multiple individuals. The hospitalized patient's receipt of the correct drug at the correct time and in the correct dose depends upon reliable systems of drug information dissemination, ordering and transcribing, and drug delivery. Similarly, the prevention of nosocomial infection involves reliable systems for sterilization and handwashing, wound dressing, catheter replacement, prevention of antibiotic resistance, and reduction of the susceptibility to infection through, for example, the maintenance of a patient's body temperature during surgery.[34] Although the application of CQI in healthcare delivery is fairly new, researchers have reported some important successes with the approach.[35]

The systems theory of causation in CQI is accompanied by an ethos of collective responsibility. Attributions of moral responsibility are not abandoned in the theory of CQI; they are prospectively oriented to meeting the goals of patients' welfare rather than retrospectively oriented to blame. In essence, quality improvement is seen to depend on cooperation and collaboration both in the achievement of primary outcomes and in the ongoing or continuous improvement of processes and outcomes. This is accomplished through supportive teamwork, error reporting, and statistical feedback. Individuals are encouraged to improve performance constantly, not simply in response to complaints or crises.[36] In a system where everyone involved in the processes of care is accountable to everyone else in the services of the ultimate end of patients' wellbeing, the potential for "free riding"—that is, the potential for individuals to perform poorly without consequence—is limited. Collective responsibility does not entail a dissipation or diminution of individual responsibility; rather, every participant in a process is morally responsible. In CQI, "free-riding" is inconsistent with the moral demands of collective effort. As those working in the field of medical quality improvement have noted, the success and staying power of an ethos of CQI depends in large part on the willingness of leadership in healthcare institutions and organizations to abandon the practice of finger-pointing in favor of supportive and cooperative goal setting. In such a context, the incentive system will be oriented to rewards for cooperation rather than penalties for noncompliance.[37]

CONCLUSION

In the 18th and 19th centuries, the ethos of personal responsibility held that for the physician confronted with the consequences of error, there was "no tribunal, other than his own conscience."[38] In medicine today, the potential for error extends far beyond individual conduct to the design of systems, policies, and processes. In the face of the complex and collective efforts that comprise healthcare today, individual practitioners can no longer plausibly argue that they are accountable only to themselves. Likewise, it is no longer plausible to argue that errors and quality failures result from individual agency alone.

CQI and the doctrine of no-fault liability are powerful and constructive frameworks for approaching the prevention of medical error, because they share a prospective orientation to responsibility that can encompass the system dimensions of medical error. On that score, there seems to be no better evidence of the breadth of the system than the degree to which the current models of quality assurance and malpractice discourage and obstruct positive approaches to error prevention. As a small but important step in reorienting our thinking in this regard, we should consider redefining the term mistake as an error in action, opinion, or judgment caused by poor reasoning, carelessness, insufficient knowledge, or poor system design.

NOTES

1. The ethos of infallibility is so powerful in medicine that mistakes themselves, regardless of whether they result in adverse outcomes, engender feelings of guilt and responsibility on the part of physicians. See J.F. Christensen, W. Levinson, and P.M. Dunn, "The Heart of Darkness: The Impact of Perceived Mistakes on Physicians," *Journal of General Internal Medicine* 7 (1992): 424-31.

2. C.B. Chapman, *Physicians, Law, and Ethics* (New York: New York University Press, 1984), 54, 59.

3. When I wrote on these issues in *Medical Harm*, I was not yet clear on these two orientations to the notion of responsibility. As a result, I privileged the discussion of justification and excuse. This essay, although drawn from chapter 6 of the book, is a rethinking of the issues. See V.A. Sharpe and A.I. Faden, *Medical Harm: Historical, Conceptual and Ethical Dimensions of Iatrogenic Illness* (New York: Cambridge University Press, 1998).

4. J. Feinberg, *Harm to Others: The Moral Limits of the Criminal Law* (New York: Oxford University Press, 1984), 1: 108.

5. Ibid.

6. *Websters College Dictionary* (New York: Random House, 1991): 867-8.

7. T. Mizrahi, "Managing Medical Mistakes: Ideology, Insularity and Responsibility among Internists-in-Training," *Social Science & Medicine* 19, no. 2 (1984): 135.

8. Of course, it is true that when one fails to fulfill a (prospective) obligation, one can be (retrospectively) blamed. This fact is often the justification given for ignoring the one sense in favor of the other. See, for example, M. Klein, "Responsibility," in *The Oxford Companion to Philosophy,* ed. T. Honderich (Oxford, England: Oxford University Press, 1995), 771-2. "These two notions of moral responsibility are linked, in that one can be deemed blameworthy for failing to fulfil a moral obligation. (In what follows 'moral responsibility' will be used in its blame-deserving sense)."

9. Hippocrates, "Epidemics I," in *Hippocrates,* trans. W.H.S. Jones (Cambridge, Mass.: Harvard University Press, 1923, 1988), 165.

10. Some have argued that there is nothing morally distinctive about healthcare and that the norms governing it, therefore, are no different than those governing the exchange of other goods and services in the marketplace. From this vantage point, the obligation "to help" would be absent but the obligation "to do no harm" would be operative as the general principle of noninterference. For a fuller discussion, see V.A. Sharpe, "Why Do No Harm?" *Theoretical Medicine* 18 (1997): 197-215.

11. As pointed out later in the chapter, the "collective" includes healthcare managers and administrators.

12. See L. May and S. Hoffman, ed., *Collective Responsibility: Five Decades of Debate in Theoretical and Applied Ethics* (Savage, Md.: Rowman and Littlefield, 1991).

13. L.L. Leape, "Error in Medicine," *Journal of the American Medical Association* 272 (1994): 1851-7. [Leape's article is reprinted as chapter 7 of this book—*Ed.*]

14. For a more fine-grained account of the evaluation of medical error, see C. Bosk, "Professional Responsibility and Medical Error," in *Applications of Social Science to Clinical Medicine and Health Policy,* ed. L. Aiken and D. Mechanic (Rutgers, N.J.: Rutgers University Press, 1986), 460-77; C. Bosk, *Forgive and Remember: Managing Medical Failure* (Chicago: University of Chicago Press, 1979).

15. G.G. Ward, "Audits Measure Our Results," *Modern Hospital* 69 (1947): 86-8.

16. P. Dans, "Clinical Peer Review: Burnishing a Tarnished Icon," *Annals of Internal Medicine* 118 (1993): 566-8.

17. L.L. Leape et al., for the ADE Prevention Study Group, "Systems Analysis of Adverse Drug Events," *Journal of the American Medical Association* 274 (1995): 35-43.

18. C.H. Dearden and W.H. Rutherford, "The Resuscitation of the Severely Injured in the Accident and Emergency Department: A Medical Audit," *Injury* 16 (1985): 249-52.

19. A.W. Wu et al., "Do House Officers Learn from Their Mistakes?" *Journal of the American Medical Association* 265 (1991): 2089-94.

20. N. Robins, *The Girl Who Died Twice: Every Patient's Nightmare: The Libby Zion Case and the Hidden Hazards of Hospitals* (New York: Delacorte Press, 1995), 101-3.

21. D.W. Bates et al., "Relationship between Medication Errors and Adverse Drug Events," *Journal of General Internal Medicine* 10 (1995): 199-205.

22. D. Berwick, "Continuous Improvement as an Ideal in Health Care," *New England Journal of Medicine* 320 (1989): 53-6.

23. D. Laffel and D. Blumenthal, "The Case for Using Industrial Quality Management Science in Health Care Organizations," *Journal of the American Medical Association* 83 (1989): 1031-7.

24. P. Keeton et al., *Tort and Accident Law* (St. Paul, Minn.: West, 1983), 1.

25. See note 22 above.

26. See note 17 above.

27. W.E. Deming, *Out of the Crisis* (Cambridge, Mass.: MIT Center for Applied Engineering Studies, 1986).

28. These subsidiary goals are discussed in more detail in Laffel and Blumenthal, see note 23 above; and M. Crane, "How Good Doctors Can Avoid Bad Errors," *Medical Economics* 74 (28 April 1997): 36-43.

29. V.A. Sharpe, "Justice and Care: The Implications of the Kohlberg-Gilligan Debate for Medical Ethics," *Theoretical Medicine* 13 (1992): 295-318; see note 3 above.

30. See note 17 above.

31. E. Vogel and R. Delgado, "To Tell the Truth: Physicians' Duty to Disclose Medical Mistakes," *UCLA Law Review* 28 (1980): 52-94; T.R. LeBlang and J.L. King, "Tort Liability for Nondisclosure: The Physician's Legal Obligation to Disclose Patient Illness and Injury," *Dickinson Law Review* 89 (1984): 1-52.

32. J. Feinberg, "Collective Responsibility," in *Collective Responsibility: Five Decades of Debate in Theoretical and Applied Ethics,* see note 12 above, pp. 54-5.

33. B.M. Manuel, "Professional Liability: A No-Fault Solution," *New England Journal of Medicine* 322, no. 9 (1990): 627-31.

34. A. Kurz et al., "Perioperative Normothermia to Reduce the Incidence of Surgical-Wound Infection and Shorten Hospitalization," *New England Journal of Medicine* 334 (1996): 1209-15.

35. L.I. Solberg et al., "Using Continuous Quality Improvement to Improve Diabetes Care in Populations: The IDEAL Model. Improving Care for Diabetics through Empowerment Active Collaboration and Leadership," *Journal of Quality Improvement* 11 (1997): 581-92; D. Blumenthal and C.M. Kilo, "A Report Card on Continuous Quality Improvement," *Milbank Quarterly* 76 (1998): 625-48.

36. C.P. McLaughlin and A.D. Kaluzny, "Total Quality Management in Health: Making It Work," *Health Care Management Review* 15 (1990): 7-14.

37. D. Smith, "Medicine's Need for Kaizen," *British Medical Journal* 301 (1990): 679-80.

38. American Medical Association, *Code of Medical Ethics,* 1st ed. (New York: William Wood, 1847), 3.

Part 3

Error in Ethics Consultation

13

Dead Wrong:
Error in Clinical Ethics Consultation

Susan B. Rubin and Laurie Zoloth

INTRODUCTION

Ethical judgment is by nature an act of discernment, a single moral gesture chosen against a horizon of possible choice. To work as an ethicist in the clinical context is to be surrounded by an acute awareness of both the power and the fragility of this gesture, and of its paradoxical tenacity, of all that we yearn to control, and of all that can go terribly wrong. It is our reflection on this reality and our shared experience of engaging in the work of ethics consultation that has led to this chapter and to this book.

In our practice we have come to expect mistakes as an inevitable and unavoidable element of clinical medicine, and we have been consistently moved by the complex tragedy of errors that abound. As ethicists, we are frequently asked to reflect on the moral meaning and appropriate management of clinical mistakes when they arise. For example, we have been asked to offer advice on how mistakes should be handled, who should be informed and under what conditions, and how concerns about accountability and prevention can best be addressed. The relationship we are asked to assume with the world of mistakes is both familiar and supported by the ethics discourse and literature on mistakes. As ethicists, we are invited to focus as bystanders on the mistakes of others and the dilemmas they face. In fact, a large portion of bioethics is riddled with the covert presupposition that the ethicist, as outsider, can offer a helpful, critical perspective to those who are struggling more directly with the ethical dilemmas that arise in clinical practice.

But our clinical experience has led us to pursue a different orientation to the problem of mistakes and ethical dilemmas. When we have turned to one another as colleagues to reflect frankly on the cases that we have faced in our own practice, and when we have applied the same degree of critical scrutiny to our own work that we apply to the work of our clinical colleagues, we have often found ourselves captivated by a string of simple but provocative questions. What if we overlooked or misapprehended some key element in a case? What if we were mistaken? What if we were, in the starkest terms, dead wrong in our assessment, analysis, and response to the ethical dilemmas presented to us?

In pursuing this self-reflective inquiry, we have noted the difficulty of framing and responding to our own critical concerns. Mistakes are a real and endemic feature of any human enterprise, including medicine.[1] But what is the nature, meaning, and ramification of this truth for the practice of ethics consultation? It is striking how little attention has been paid to the fact that the inevitability of error is as much an intrinsic part of ethics consultation as it is of medicine. It is our intention in pursuing this project to stimulate a new line of critical inquiry by drawing attention to this reality and inviting careful discussion of it by theorists and practitioners in the field. It is an inquiry that we hope will broaden debate about the meaning and scope of bioethics as it is taught and practiced as a clinical discipline. Further, directing our collective attention as ethicists to the reality of mistakes in our work will hopefully help make the occurrence of our errors more transparently recognizable and even lead to consideration of what mechanisms of review, prevention (insofar as possible), or correction we would want to develop as a field.

As scholars and practitioners in the field, our interest in the problem of mistakes in ethics consultation is twofold. On the one hand, we are interested in the theoretical problem of what it might mean to make an error in evaluative or normative judgment. On the other hand, we are interested in how the pragmatic details of clinical consultation might create unique opportunities for mistakes. While the second issue—the pragmatic one—is often the direction in which articles on mistakes lead us, it is the first problem—the challenge of applying the concept of mistakes to bioethics and offering a preliminary framework for understanding and categorizing the kinds of mistakes that might be made in bioethics consultation—that is the starting place for this intellectual project.

As cofounders of an active clinical ethics practice, we have long been captivated by the ongoing discussion of mistakes in medicine. We have learned much from theorists from a range of disciplines who have helped to deconstruct the nature of mistakes as they arise in clinical practice and who have put forth various proposals for how we ought to respond to such mistakes at both the individual and systems levels.[2] And we have been drawn to ask a number of questions. What is the meaning of this discourse for our own work? What is it that is peculiar to the practice of bioethics itself that might potentiate our capacity for inevitable human error? What of the rich and growing literature on medical mistakes is applicable to bioethics consultation? On what points might there be a need to develop new theories and new approaches to the problem of mistakes, given the unique structure and foundation of bioethics consultation? In other words, can and ought the discussion of mistakes in bioethics consultation take place simply on a parallel track with the discussion of mistakes in medicine, or are mistakes in bioethics consultation actually mistakes of a qualitatively different kind in need of a different analysis and response?

THE CHALLENGE

We first formally explored these questions in a workshop we presented several years ago at a joint annual meeting of the Society for Health and Human Values and the Society for Bioethics Consultation.[3] We began the session by asking a crowded room of colleagues whether they had ever made a mistake in bioethics consultation and what it would mean to make a mistake in such a context. Not surprisingly, the question elicited a lively discussion, largely because there was no clear agreement regarding either the definition of a bioethics consultation mistake, or the criteria by which we could judge what actions or recommendations might in fact constitute a mistake. Examples of seemingly obvious mistakes in medicine such as giving the wrong dose of a medication, amputating the wrong leg, or unintentionally aborting a live fetus seemed to have no easy analogues when it came to bioethics consultation. Yet, at the same time, colleagues had no trouble at all recounting times when they personally felt that they had in some way erred—times when the judgments that they had made, in hindsight, had clearly led to avoidable disasters. Easier still to recall were the stories of the errors of others that they had witnessed. But how did we "know" that some of these stories were the result of mistakes and not the tragic enterprise of medicine itself?[4] Intuitively, participants in the workshop agreed that we each had experienced a sense of failure and of making a mistake, of things having gone wrong in our work. Yet was our experience of loss derived from our own error or failing, or was it rather an apprehension of that which is essentially tragic in our work, of our limited ability to fix it, and of our acute sense that we are the ones who are often looked to in order to give a moral account of loss itself?

A basic problem in pursuing a discussion of mistakes in bioethics consultation is that there are still no readily definable, consensually agreed-upon standards according to which consultants are expected to function and against which they could be judged.[5] This is as true at the procedural level as it is at the substantive level. There is still a lively debate about the best procedural approach to bioethics consultation, and the nature of the theoretical grounds upon which we can construct the essential premise of an intervention. The procedural issues are not the only issues debated. When bioethics consultants are called in to consult on a case, the substantive questions they are asked to reflect on are questions about which reasonable people (and other ethicists)[6] can and do disagree. Ethicists have publicly and prominently disagreed about such basic issues as the definition and criteria of death, the legitimacy of physician-assisted suicide, and the limits of basic genetic research. On such landmark cases as the *Baby K* case in Virginia, in which an anencephalic child was maintained on life support, leading bioethicists in the field took opposing views as expert witnesses.[7] Given the range and diversity of opinions represented in the field, it seems peculiarly difficult to find credible grounds on which to judge persuasively individual acts, or even entire ventures in bioethics consultation, to be unequivocally wrong or mistaken. In considering the problem of mistakes in bioethics consultation, then, we are faced with a challenge. On the one hand, we have all had an intuitive sense of cases in which we or our colleagues have made mistakes. On the other hand, we may have difficulty articulating or defending the basis of that judgment.

WHAT DOES IT MEAN
TO "MAKE A MISTAKE"?

Significantly, we find embedded in the origins of the word "mis-take" a powerful normative judgment. To make a mistake, or *mistaka*, means to have taken the wrong path, to have been led astray. Similarly, to make an error, or *err-are*, means to wander about or to go astray. If making a mistake means taking the wrong path, this presumes not only that there is a standard, appropriate, and correct path to follow, but that we can reliably identify and judge the steps we take and the direction we go against that standard. Given the nature of bioethics consultation, these are at best controversial metaphysical and epistemological assumptions, making the question of what would constitute a mistake much more difficult to answer.

Hence, having a sense of surety of what constitutes the right path on a particular well-mapped terrain would be critical. Only then, so goes the etymological clue noted above, can one have a sense of going "astray." But the search for the emulative path is elusive. On the procedural level, persistent lack of agreement on the philosophical and methodological underpinnings of bioethics consultation makes the very discussion of mistaken paths difficult. Vigorous debate continues about a range of procedural questions that ought to frame the essential mapping process. Indeed, ethics consultation is difficult to teach formally, because the work as practiced ranges from a vaguely defined "listening with the third ear" to troubling cases and moral upset, to formal committees with chairs, minutes, and elaborate processes aimed at achieving consensus on a chosen path. Ethicists argue about whether consults should be conducted by individual consultations, small subcommittees or teams, or full bioethics committees; whether and to what extent patients and family members should be invited to participate in consultation meetings and whether their consent is necessary for a consultation to take place; whether the attending physician's consent and participation is necessary for a consultation to take place; whether it is necessary to use a consistent methodology for each case, and if so, which one; whether "curbside consultations" are acceptable or appropriate; and the list goes on.

There is ambivalence, too, regarding the appropriate goal of bioethics consultation. Some ethicists believe that the goal of bioethics consultation is to provide a forum for discussion in which awareness of the nature, source, and extent of conflict is heightened;[8] others, drawing on techniques of alternative dispute resolution, favor a focus on mediation and conflict resolution.[9] Some ethicists view themselves as primarily teachers and facilitators and would resist what they might perceive as the misguided temptation to give advice;[10] others believe that they have a responsibility to offer their own considered reflections and to make concrete recommendations.[11] While different schools of thought have emerged in response to each of these questions, bioethics as a field has resisted the idea that there is only one right procedural path and has instead accommodated a variety of approaches and perspectives. As such, it is clear that we are not on one road; we are in a geography of many possibilities.

On the substantive level, part of the difficulty of identifying a mistake lies with the nature of the work itself. The dilemmas that come to the attention of bioethics consultants are dilemmas precisely because there is disagreement about the best course of action; the goals worth pursuing; the means necessary or appropriate to employ in pursuit of a goal; even the meaning, nature, and experience of taking one path as opposed to another. If there were only one path, or if patients, families, and caregivers were always in agreement on the one best path in every circumstance, they would cheerily agree on a course of medical intervention and bioethicists would not be consulted. Dilemmas arise in the clinical arena precisely because there are a multitude of paths one could choose, each with its own moral appeal and ultimate justification, and each with its share of proponents and critics. Dilemmas are disagreements in the margins of cultural certainty, in contested terrain, or in cultural or religious border wars. Americans are divided on these substantive issues, and bioethics consultants see the struggle replicated and potentiated in the clinic. The very gesture of turning to an ethicist for consultation represents the turn to a navigator who can guide those in conflict through troubled and sometimes uncharted waters.[12]

To complicate matters, it is a basic postmodern presumption of the discipline of ethics that not only is there no uniform agreement about the universal "right" or "good" act, but also that a "view from nowhere" from which to judge the essential rightness or goodness, as well as the wrongness or badness of potential paths, does not exist. There is no absolute or objective standard; the navigator takes his or her flawed sextant and particular map, which inevitably includes some details and leaves out others. In postmodern ethics, we have a range of moral sensibilities and a host of better or worse arguments that call out to be heard and taken into account. In the end, we bring to bear not the authority of our particular perspective, but the power of our reflection and argumentation.

In ethics, we are taught that it is not enough simply to assert one's position, or claim the superiority of one path over another; one must defend one's judgment in terms accessible and intelligible even to those who do not necessarily share one's moral perspective. But, particularly in current ethical discourse, with heightened attention to the dynamics of power and language, we tend to stop short of claiming that successfully convincing someone means that one is absolutely and positively right, or that one has identified the only right and true path. Accordingly, most ethicists eschew the role of self-appointed or hospital-appointed moralist, because that would give the misimpression that they somehow had privileged access to the essential truth and their role was merely to interpret and apply it.

So there is an element of humility in the pursuit and practice of ethics that makes the naming and locating of the single right path problematic. And there is a temporality attached to it as well. Questions emerge and positions are formulated in relation to the circumstances of history, the state of the discourse, the accepted body of knowledge at the time, and the accepted or emerging norms. This makes the problem of locating instances of error, or straying from the path, even more problematic. What is at stake is the selection of a defensible reference point. Paths that are traversed today might have been unimaginable or impossible to navigate before. Consider the dilemma of whether to pursue selective reduction of multiple embryos: this question exists only by virtue of dramatic advances in reproductive technologies. Or consider the attendant treatment dilemmas for patients in a persistent vegetative state, a condition that was created by developments in critical care technology that allowed us to keep such neurologically compromised individuals alive.

Similarly, paths that may be considered unthinkable and mistaken today might have been embraced wholeheartedly in the past. For instance, there are notable historical examples over the last two decades in which ethicists have reconsidered and suggested recompense for what were once considered acceptable medical experiments or medical interventions. Consider the legacies of Tuskegee,[13] the DES (diethylstilbestrol) or thalidomide research, or more recently the experiments uncovered by the U.S. Advisory Committee on Human Radiation Experiments.[14] That we see these as instances of ethical failure is a judgment made possible by critical inquiry and powerful social movements. And because we are, as a field, clever at the articulation of trouble, we cannot help but note that the entire enterprise of consultation is heavily shaped by first questions that are outside our control: who has access to healthcare, who owns what, what class biases shape the very medical encounter we are called to offer guidance in, and, finally, that even such insights are only accessible to us because of our particular social and intellectual stance.

CORE CATEGORIES OF MISTAKES

In calling for discourse about the possible existence and nature of the path of bioethics from which we might stray, we need to move beyond the troubling sense of the intuitive to the development of at least a common language and a common taxonomy. One way of categorizing the kinds of mistakes an ethicist might make is to appeal to the standard categories of ethical analysis. Borrowing from the perspectives of consequentialism, deontology, and virtue theory, we might judge a particular instance of bioethics consultation to be mistaken if the consequences of the consultation have been divisive or harmful, if human suffering is potentiated rather than relieved; if essential duties are violated or abandoned, if questionable motives or intentions have been operative; or if key virtues or moral character are compromised or damaged. To some extent, these categories offer helpful templates. But they are not self-evident, they may be contradictory, and they may be incomplete. For example, even holding aside the obvious question of what counts as "happiness," should it really be the goal of bioethics consultation to make people happy and produce pleasant results? We have all taught introductory ethics in which seemingly paradoxical possibilities are considered, like doing the right thing and still harming oneself or others, or doing the right thing for the wrong reasons, or being an evil or morally bankrupt person and still doing the right or good thing. Because these are questions that have the deepest of historical debates in philosophy at their core, they are hardly likely to find facile resolution in the context of bioethics consultation. Hence the application of these standard categories of ethical analysis to the problem at hand is provisional at best. They may point to important categories of concern, but they are not themselves ultimately definitive. Certainly resorting to them or relying on them alone advances us but a little.

What other categories might be helpful then? Different explanatory categories have been offered by scholars who have examined the problem of mistakes more broadly. For example, there is a long and persuasive history of defining mistakes as routine occurrences in professional life.[15] Rather than viewing mistakes as the exception, those who follow this tradition frame mistakes as the expected norm. Some theorists have qualified this standard approach by making a distinction between what they describe as normal, excusable mistakes and deviant, culpable mistakes.[16] In the context of medicine, this distinction is traditionally perceived to be an important one. Most clinicians, for example, can imagine making what they describe to investigators as so-called innocent mistakes—that is, mistakes based on the inevitably precarious process of applying general scientific knowledge to particular patients in a context of imperfect information and unavoidable uncertainty. But for the most part, clinicians sharply distinguish mistakes that arise in that context from mistakes made on the basis of frank negligence, incompetence, or suspect motives. This distinction separates out actions that are considered understandable and forgivable from those that are not.

But such stark categorizations are difficult to defend, as much in medicine as in the field of bioethics consultation. And part of the problem is, as Bosk notes in his classic book, *Forgive and Remember*,[17] that the very concept of mistakes is itself an "essentially contested idea." In contrast to the sociological literature on mistakes, which assumes a shared definition of error, Bosk argues that the grounds for defining and identifying error in medicine are always arguable. One cannot assume a categorical view of error and should not give error "an equivocal ontological status." Error, Bosk contends, is ultimately a socially constructed category, and the specification of its nature and contours will always be subject to debate. This insight is instructive for our own inquiry. Just as the surgeons in Bosk's classic study had their own definitions of error, so too might we as a field have a preliminary sense, however inchoate, of what might count as straying from an acceptable path.

INTUITIONS OF ERROR

It is precisely this intuitive sense that emerged in our workshop[18] that interested us and offers a first way out of the essential problems of foreground and background struggled with above. Hence an important step in the analysis of mistakes in bioethics consultation is an accounting of the way mistakes are actually conceived and constructed by practitioners in the field, and a specifying of the terrain that remains contested.

Reflecting on our own experience of sensing that we or our colleagues have made mistakes, we note that sometimes the basis of our concern is with how the consultation was actually conducted, and other times the basis of our concern is with what was ultimately concluded and recommended. For the purposes of this analysis, then, the comments that follow are organized according to the rough and somewhat loose distinction between mistakes of process and mistakes of substance. While this division helps organize the range of our concerns, it does not resolve the difficult definitional challenge of specifying what ought and ought not be counted as a mistake. These are contested questions in need of more deliberate discussion by the field at large. Furthermore, not all mistakes can be neatly divided into the two stark categories of procedural and substantive mistakes. In fact the categories themselves are inextricably linked in reality. Nonetheless, the categories are useful in describing what actually takes place in every bioethics consultation: the epistemiological task of identifying what is the case, and the normative task of suggesting what might be or ought to be the case. By reflecting on how consultations are actually conducted and what kinds of recommendations they lead to, we will develop a better appreciation of the range of mistakes that might be made and ought to be considered.

THE VIEW FROM SOMEWHERE:
THE EXPERIENCE OF CONSULTATION

To a significant degree, the very context of the work of bioethics consultation, like the nature of medicine, makes error inevitable. In practice, bioethics is often a kind of "secondary text" work, in that the ethicist must rely at least to some degree on the perceptions of others that there is a need for the consultation in the first place. Aside from our role as educators, to the degree that we reject the role of moralist or morals police, when it comes to case consultation we wait, as ethicists, to be consulted by those who have a concern or question. The very construction of our role as consultants marks us as ancillary and supportive in significant ways. When we are called into the discursive dilemma, it is because some other person involved in the case—be it the patient, the family, or a member of the care team—has found the situation to be morally challenging or disturbing. Typically the request for bioethics consultation is made because someone thinks that what is occurring or has occurred is wrong, and further that the consultant can do something about it. At the initial level, then, one must be skilled in discerning whether the request for consultation is appropriate. Judging the nature and appropriateness of the request is a task prone to errors, in large part due to the context of bioethics in most healthcare institutions.

Ironically, bioethics consultation is probably equally at risk of being underused as it is of being overused in today's healthcare environment. On the one hand, despite the Joint Commission on Accreditation of Healthcare Organizations' (JCAHO's) ever-expanding emphasis on ethics, most hospitals fail to adequately or genuinely integrate ethics into daily clinical practice. For this reason, the work of the ethicist or bioethics committee is always at risk of being marginalized and viewed as extraneous to the reality of the front lines. For example, a common misperception is that, if the ethicist or bioethics committee have not received requests for consults, there simply are not any ethical dilemmas. What we have consistently found upon more careful examination is that the very real and inevitably present ethical dilemmas are simply not finding their way to the ethicist or committee. The enterprise of ethics works clinically only if there is genuine support for it and an expectation of active, ongoing engagement with issues of ethical concern at every level of decision making. Although healthcare professionals can develop the skill of identifying and approaching ethical dilemmas, the dilemmas themselves do not go away. In fact, familiar dilemmas often become more complex over time, and new dilemmas are forever emerging. We think it is a mistake, therefore, to set up the expectation that the successful ethicist is one who will "work himself or herself out of business." Given the nature of healthcare and the diversity of moral perspectives that will always be brought to bear on core beliefs about sickness and health, life and death, and pain and suffering, we choose rather to expect and welcome ethical dilemmas as an inevitable and unavoidable feature of clinical life. In our practice we structure programs of ethics consultation around that expectation. This means an ongoing and deepening rather than ever-diminishing presence of ethics in the institution.

But if an ethicist or bioethics committee achieves sufficient visibility and stature in an institution, there is the different risk that they will become the repositories of every difficult and politically freighted problem.[19] Choosing the right path for the development of a viable, credible ethics program is fraught with challenges that can be met well or poorly. In an effort to establish the worthiness of the enterprise, it might be tempting to stretch the mission of the ethics program to accommodate even the most inappropriate requests, particularly when they come from powerful people or committees in the institution. For example, it might be tempting, but we think ultimately misguided, to allow the ethicist or ethics committee to become an arm of quality assurance or risk management, or to agree to grant perfunctory stamps of ethical approval to individual or institutional plans. It is always necessary to balance the need to be well integrated into the day-to-day operations of a medical center, with the ever-tempting problem of "going native" and losing the very outsider/outlaw status that makes the ethicist useful in the first place.[20]

Once the gatekeeping has taken place and a request for consultation has been accepted, there are arrays of potential interpretive errors to consider. One clear source of errors in this context is the ethicist's inevitable and substantial reliance on others for information. Here is where the sense of bioethics as "secondary text" work becomes even more vivid. An ethicist comes to know the details and contours of each case through the perspectives of those who are involved first-hand in the dilemma. But each participant inevitably sees the case in a different way and, based on his or her own knowledge and experience of the case, may highlight certain features as salient while discounting others. It is the rare exception, and far from the normative rule, to have even the most basic facts of a case described the same by each person directly involved in the case. A large part of the ethicist's task then becomes gathering and sorting through an array of divergent and often contradictory information.

How an ethicist hears the story of each case then, in whose voice, and from whose perspective, will shape his or her understanding of the problem and vision of the best path to recommend. In our practice we have a commitment to an inclusive, nonhierarchical process of bioethics consultation in which every involved person's perspective is equally valued and sought out. And yet bio- ethics consultation does not take place in a vacuum. What consultants hear and what they are told is filtered through complex relationships, some of which are long-standing, and others of which have yet to be forged. In addition, the extent to which those involved genuinely participate in the process may often involve highly nuanced social, political, and emotional calculations on their part. No case can be given to the ethicist in its entirety by any one participant in the drama, and no single participant comes to the process wholly objective, disin- terested, or unencumbered. Ethics consultants are left ultimately with the chal- lenge of reconstructing a story based on partial threads shared with them by a variety of individuals, each with his or her own history, perspective, and stake.

Even if the ethicist aims to hear and credit the claims of each party with distinction, it is impossible to entirely avoid being influenced even unconsciously by a variety of factors. If the ethicist has a long-standing relationship of trust and fidelity with a clinical colleague, the ethicist might hear and weigh the colleague's story differently. If, for example, the colleague tells the ethicist that this is one of the worst cases she has ever seen, or that she has met repeatedly with the family but to no avail, on some level the ethicist cannot avoid inter- preting this information through the perspective of what he or she already knows to be true about this colleague as a caring person and dedicated clinician. The same can be said of patients or family members who impress the ethicist in a particular way and therefore shape the way the ethicist hears and understands their perspective. If we as ethicists perceive the family to be devoted and consci- entious, we are likely to interpret their statements about their loved one's pref- erences for treatment differently than if we view them as self-interested or ma- nipulative. Part of the skill involved in gathering and sorting through informa- tion then is the skill of discernment. But our ability as outsiders to discern the truth is imperfect at best and we can be grossly mistaken in our analysis of a situation.

THE DUPED ETHICIST

As ethicists, our necessary reliance on others for information often proves to be a source of significant error. We can mistakenly adopt as normative the potentially skewed perspective of any participant in the process. We can be told by the day-shift nursing staff, for example, that the family is difficult or absent, only to learn later that they have an excellent rapport with the social worker or that they visit faithfully every evening. And we can all too easily be duped or taken in by a convincing or heartfelt story. A long-estranged family member can appear on the scene and present himself as intimately familiar with the patient's greatest hopes and fears. In all instances, although the information we are forced to rely on may be presented in a thoroughly credible and even well- intentioned fashion, it may turn out to be absolutely false.

Constructing a coherent narrative about any given case is a multifaceted, many-layered enterprise. In practice, this means that it is incredibly difficult to get the full, straight story about any given case. On some ultimate level, as ethicists we have come to understand that "the real truth" about even the most carefully investigated case can never be completely or absolutely known to us. The power of this possibility haunts our thoughts about even the best known and most widely referenced cases in the field of bioethics including *Quinlan, Barber, Bouvia, Bartling,* and *Cruzan.*[21] In the course of our practice as ethicists, we have learned counter stories about each of these cases from healthcare professionals who were involved first-hand that have made the universally accepted truth presented in the standard accounts apocryphal at best. We have struggled with what to make of the conflicting stories we have heard, particularly knowing that even if we were to re-interview every single person involved in each of these cases that discrepancies would remain. At some point then, with classic cases reported in the literature, as well as with cases in which the ethicist is personally involved, anyone who does clinical ethics will have to be willing to trust some portion of the information gathered from secondary sources, while at the same time recognizing that even in the absence of malicious intent, the perceptions of these sources will inevitably be incomplete or mistaken.

It is important to note though that our resulting interpretations can be far more than innocently mistaken; they can be the result of evildoing. In the high-stakes game of medicine, especially in the highly charged atmosphere that often accompanies a bioethics consultation, in which staff and families have come to see the normative routine as seriously challenged—there is always the risk that some participants in the situation will have strong incentives to deliberately deceive and mislead the ethicist. Since the ethicist's approval is useful, it can be commodified and, hence, bargained for and manipulated. As patients can be excluded from the fullness of the truthful narrative by physicians with bad motives, ethicists too can be excluded—by pride, by fear of legal ramifications, or by political pressure to withhold the truth. Any of these can set the entire process down the wrong path, a mistake that in some situations can be irrevocable. The task of interpreting the available information must therefore be bound by the knowledge that the accuracy of our personal acts of interpretation will never be foolproof.

THE PROBLEM OF A
MUTABLE KNOWLEDGE BASE

Not only do bioethicists have an unavoidable reliance on others for information, but they must also rely on an inconstant and mutable knowledge base for their essential framing of the problem itself. Here there are two problems: not only will the prognosis, and in some cases even the diagnosis, be deeply uncertain and fundamentally unpredictable, but clinical claims made with certainty and widespread approval today may be disproved tomorrow. It is a humbling reality to note that our ethical analyses are inevitably based on clinical information that may turn out to be erroneous.

We can recount a number of stark examples of this in recent history. For example, early in the acquired immunodeficiency syndrome (AIDS) epidemic, it was commonly held that a second bout with *Pneumocystis carinii* pneumonia was a clear indicator that the patient would certainly not survive. As the years went on, AIDS patients began to survive greater numbers of infections all the time. More recently, although it had always been thought that AIDS was a universally fatal disease, with the advent of protease inhibitors and other treatments, AIDS has been reframed as a chronic illness, and more and more AIDS patients have returned to work. Peptic ulcer is a second example. Until just a few short years ago, it was classically described in medical textbooks as the quintessential psychosomatic illness, brought on by a patient's inability to cope effectively with stress. It is now commonly known that the bacteria *H. pylori* causes most peptic ulcers and that a simple course of antibiotics will result in cure, regardless of a patient's response to stress. In our own clinical practice we were recently drawn into protracted debates about the ethical issues surrounding the appropriateness of prescribing fenfluramine and phentermine (fen-phen) and including it in health plan benefits packages, only to find it being withdrawn from the market out of concerns for its safety. But concern for safety had not even been primarily at stake in our deliberations. We were preoccupied rather with the moral considerations involved in offering or not offering a diet drug, such as whether it was a legitimate therapeutic option for a real health problem or a quick fix for Americans' cultural obsession with unwanted fat. It is a humbling reality to note that our ethical analyses are inevitably based on clinical information that may turn out to be erroneous.

GETTING IT WRONG

In addition to relying on others for information and relying on a mutable base of information, the inevitable fact is that sometimes ethicists simply "get it wrong." Not only can ethicists misinterpret the information that they uncover or are given, but they can also err in their analysis of the information. Ethicists can simply misinterpret the clinical data right along with the medical team, or they can miss some crucial background fact that others either assume the ethicists know or may have missed themselves as well. And even armed with a strong clinical grasp of the salient facts, ethics consultants can misinterpret what is grounding or motivating people's beliefs and what the actual source of conflict really is. For example, if a bioethicist is unfamiliar with the particular aspects of a patient's religious or faith or cultural belief system, he or she may mistakenly ascribe certain beliefs and motivations to the patient, missing the vast terrain of moral complexity underlying the conflict.

Some of these mistakes are exacerbated by the frames of reference with which ethicists as individuals are accustomed and to which they habitually appeal. If an ethicist has an unconscious bias toward patients or families or staff, this will inevitably influence his or her perspectives. We all have or learn affinities toward or against certain kinds of families. It is not uncommon then to, on some level, favor families "like us" or like we imagine ourselves to be (nice, caring, frequent visitors, involved in the community, and so on) and to distance ourselves from the experience and perspective of families "not like us" (families who abuse drugs or are gang members). If an ethicist has particular sensitivity and concern for the disempowered and marginalized, this may paradoxically lead him or her to have less rather than more discernment about these families, or to uncritically favor such families in the face of conflicts about them. An ethicist may teach sensitivity to the issues of race, class, gender and able-bodiness, but may forget that this concern itself may predispose the ethicist to a particular and partisan stance. An ethicist may give greater weight to religiously motivated treatment refusals than ones that appear to be "idiosyncratic" or personally based. And an ethicist may tend to favor mainstream, normative religions over marginalized ones that might strike him or her as oddly constructed.

OUR HABITS OF RESPONSE

As ethicists, we confront the cases before us with more than unconscious bias. We have a habit of approach, and indeed a method, that we construct to analyze each case. In the name of procedural justice, in our practice we are serious about the consistent use of a carefully constructed methodology. Yet this very safeguard against error might lead us to essential philosophic errors. In the selection of a method and standard categories of inquiry, we know that on some level we find what we look for and expect to see. We are cognizant that how we frame the issues and the discourse surrounding them inevitably influences what we end up focusing on in the consultation. We impose our own patterns of analysis and then we see them again and again, hence confirming our own hypotheses with regularity, and being struck by the way in which they seem to repeat. We have often commented to each other about the "fictionalized" or narrative quality of the work: here is the classic surgeon, acting like a surgeon, the nurse in a stereotypical pose. We "see" classic conflicts, such as those between the nurse and the physician, repeatedly and almost formulaically. In part, this is reflective of good social observation and sociological insight, and it is why popular medical fiction and television work so well. The roles and conflicts are recognizable. In most cases this is a concomitant fact of the process of practical wisdom itself.

But there is something more; our memory of cases and the impact that they have on us and the challenge of having a more nuanced appreciation of differing cases certifies our use of this casuistic method. Yet it also allows us the fallacy of seeing cases in precisely the same light over and over. We have often seen ethicists in the principalist school adhere with excessive rigidity to certain principles or standards without attending to the particulars of the case at hand. And the same can be said of the methodology of casuistry. But not everything is about autonomy versus beneficence, not everything is Dax Cowert in Texas or Karen Ann Quinlan in New Jersey: each case is both like and not like, each principle newly challenged and each framing narrative haunted by particularity.[22]

THE PROBLEM OF
THE MISTAKEN PATH

Given the intuitive sense that so deeply inhabits the talk of error in professional circles, we have struggled in pursuing this line of inquiry with how we might define the problem for reflective analysis. Perhaps the questioning that accompanies ongoing public discourse about cases is a mark or even a construct of the field itself. But the discourse about errors is also shaped by some powerful and prevalent liberal presuppositions, particularly our notion of the freely chosen action. In our almost habitual reification of the act of choice itself, we can forget that we make all moral gestures against a horizon of possibilities that are not all equal. The mere fact that we "can" choose them or that a well-mannered and well-functioning committee "can" see them is not enough. For not all medical/moral decisions are of equal worth. Classic examples of historical struggle in the field of bioethics revolve around the withdrawal of life support. Here, the standard line is to reify the autonomy of the patient and his or her freedom to take any path. The moral glory is reserved for the least inhibited choice, the most fully informed choice, the Ralph Nader model of intelligent, rational self as an educated (and rather picky) consumer. But against what horizon can we count such routings to be the same as the appropriate or best *telos* of the journey?

Some ideas about how this might be constructed are drawn from the social-contract theories of Charles Taylor or the work of Jeffrey Stout.[23] Taylor's contribution is to recall the role of a shared moral horizon in a participatory social world, in which every object, gesture, and being exists within a hierarchy of meaning. Our hierarchy gives a visual and social form to the world that makes it interpretable. Such order restricts us, but it also contains us, allowing us to give weight, judgment, and meaning to the activities of social life.[24] Taylor speaks of this as a universal with a chain of being, by which he means the interpretive order of norm, ritual, and relationships. Hence, all the notions ethicists put forward in the clinical consultation are bounded not only by the history and the established medical parameters of the time but also by the deeper structures of social meaning that create the backdrop of possibilities from which ethicists can choose. Being "wrong" in this sense can thus mean being "out of place" or failing to grasp the idea that there is a "placefulness" in the path chosen. Understood in this way, the emphasis on the free, well-reasoned choice becomes itself a contingent preference.

But it is a delusion, suggests Taylor, to see "freedom" or "choice" as essential grounds. For these too are social constructs. The idea that the act of choice itself and not the content of the choice is what is essential is merely another cultural assumption of which bioethics has enthusiastically partaken. "Self-determining freedom has been an idea of immense power in our political life," reminds Taylor.[25] It has been a powerful idea in clinical life as well. Bioethics becomes then a kind of foreign policy that has focused on the social contract between hostile foreign nations. Note the field's preoccupation with documents like consent forms and durable power of attorney for healthcare forms to protect erroneous violations of this contract. Clinical ethicists are often called in to defend the idea that the authenticity of free choice must be maintained, whatever the content of the choice may be. It is getting this essential idea correct that nearly mesmerizes the field.

What bearing does this have on our approach to error? It brings new perspective to our belief that not all choices are equally valid. We in this culture value some choices, in the dialogical and continual assessment that all culture creates, more than other cultures do. We have, at least in the clinical arena of Western medical discourse, a "shared horizon—developing and nursing the commonalties of value between us" that becomes important in sharing a participatory moral life in medicine.[26]

This discussion of free choice is but one example of the social construction of our very perspectives and should give us pause when we attempt to mark the terrain of error. In fact, it is the very quality of the development of a shared moral life that makes the concept of error have any meaning at all. This is not to say that differences among bioethicists are not significant. Otherwise, as Taylor says, we could not recognize foreigners.[27] But it is to note that the problem of what constitutes an error is one that will develop as the field of bioethics begins to organize its own categories within the larger shared social ones.

Niebuhr reminds us that, in pursuing this idea of community and community standards, responsive and responding communities are not randomly constructed.[28] As bioethicists, we are a field that sees the errors of the past and attempts to make meaning from them by changing our behaviors in the future. Seeing error and insisting on its moral meaning is in part how the field was envisioned. It is the work of collective discourse, in large part to create aspirational goals in advance of our collective ability to achieve them. It was precisely because we could understand that new issues called out for new debates and that older sources of values had lost universal and truimphalist power that we understood the centrality of discourse and disagreement. But new ideas about justice and the meaning of human flourishing are not mere preferences: they are as contended as the new science that surrounds them. It is against this backdrop of disagreement, ambiguity, and irony, at both the procedural and substantive levels, that we must begin in understanding the implication and meaning of making a mistake in bioethics consultation.

In saying this, we are acutely aware of the problems in the construction of shared values, and hence shared normative judgments, that are not ultimately reducible to procedural issues. We have been deeply influenced by the work of Donna Haraway, Valeri Hartouni, Helen Longino,[29] and others, who understand that epistemological and ontological assumptions are all constructs of the particulars of ways of life that in turn shape the seeing of the option, and their judgments.[30] But we have come to understand that differences in cultural perception, gender, or class do not account for all of the variant choices that are defended; some paths are wrong, and not merely a curiosity, and some do violence or harm to the ethical constructs that we can speak of in common. It is our contention that the language of our work and of the conversation that it entails is translatable.

MISTAKES OF SUBSTANCE

So, even beyond all of the mistakes one can make in gathering and interpreting relevant information, there are also mistakes of substance—that is, mistakes in the normative conclusion one reaches upon review of the salient facts in any given case. But this is a harder category of mistakes to make sense of. With respect to substantive errors, given the range of moral perspectives that inevitably are brought to bear on any dilemma, it is difficult at best to persuasively distinguish what might be considered a mistaken judgment from a frank or principled disagreement. In other words, if two ethicists review a case and come to radically different normative judgments, does that necessarily mean that one of them is mistaken? We know, for example, that it is possible that two radically different perspectives could be equally defensible and that neither is necessarily mistaken.

And of what significance is the evolving and dynamic nature of the discipline? The knowledge base on which ethicists rely for their analysis and recommendations consists of not only the state of medical knowledge at any given time, but also the central tenets of the field. But these have evolved, and no doubt will continue to evolve, over time. For example, the collective understanding and hence bioethicists' use of the concept and definition of death has shifted and evolved. With the advent of neurological criteria for brain death, bioethicists began to teach with certainty that, in the common vernacular, "brain death was dead-dead." In the face of the utter confusion of healthcare professionals concerning brain death—even those involved in the clinical determination of death and organ transplantation[31]—and despite debate about the scope of the definition, in practice most ethicists accept its validity. But ethicists find the definition challenged and the debate about it shifting year after year.[32] Is it a mistake for ethicists to continue to use the concept as currently defined and to base ethical analysis in specific cases on it?

There has been evolution in other salient areas as well, such as the understanding of the role of surrogate decision makers, the relative weight and authority accorded to families and their particular interests, the power of the autonomous patient's wishes, and the weight according to the patient's wishes at all—particularly with the advent of a new generation of managed care.

Bioethicists have long relied upon family members and other close intimates to represent accurately the wishes of their loved ones when they turn to these individuals in their capacity as surrogate decision makers. But recent empirical studies suggest that the ability of surrogates to predict accurately the wishes of patients is precarious at best.[33] In the face of this evidence, is it a mistake to continue to rely on the notion or possibility of substituted judgment?

Traditionally bioethicists have turned to family members and other close intimates in an almost instrumental fashion, using them in some critical way to learn more about who the incapacitated patient was; what their values, goals, and priorities might be; and what they would most want to express if they were able. But it has increasingly been suggested that it is a mistake to assume that family members have no legitimate interests of their own, or that their interests ought to be automatically subordinated to the interests of the patient.[34] Is it a mistake then for us to be focused on patients, rather than their families, in our review of difficult cases? How ought we approach and prioritize the sometimes competing claims of patients and families when they are presented?

Until recently the paradigm conflict over care at the end of life came in the form represented by a long line of classic, precedent-setting cases in which patients or their surrogates fought to win the right to say no to unwanted medical interventions. At stake in part was who should be accorded the ultimate authority to make decisions about medical treatment. And when the wishes of autonomous patients, or surrogates on behalf of incapacitated patients, were held up against the beneficent wishes of well-intentioned healthcare professionals, the courts and the bioethics community overwhelmingly supported the right of patients to self-determination, privacy, and more recently, liberty. But with the advent of the futility debate,[35] the tables have been turned and healthcare professionals are increasingly wanting to assert their own right to say no to the wishes of patients. How might an ethicist either correctly or mistakenly respond to so-called futility cases given the unresolved nature of the current debate?

Other foundational concepts have been critically reexamined in light of recent challenges. The physician-assisted suicide debate has brought a renewed focus on the viability of concepts fought for much earlier, and, until recently, taken as reliable benchmarks. For years ethicists taught in classrooms around the country that there was a bright-line distinction between forgoing life-sustaining treatment and physician-assisted suicide or active killing, and further that there was a difference between giving patients enough medication to treat their pain—knowing it would likely depress their respirations—and intentionally giving patients an overdose of pain medication to cause their deaths. As the U.S. Supreme Court was considering the appellate court's arguments in *Washington v. Glucksberg* and *Vacco v. Quill,* the bioethics community waited with baited breath to see whether the Court would uphold these carefully constructed distinctions.[36]

On a related matter, although ethicists have confidently taught for many years that there was no legally or morally relevant difference between withholding and withdrawing treatment, and that artificial nutrition and hydration can be forgone like any other medical treatment, time and time again we face practitioners whose lived experience teaches them otherwise. Although they may accept the theory on an intellectual level, emotionally, physically, and, for some, spiritually, there are profound differences that are missed or obscured by these neat analytic concepts. How ought ethicists act in the face of changing conceptions of the nature and justification of these treatment decisions? When is it a mistake to cling to the bright lines the field has drawn or, alternatively, when is it a mistake to blur them?

LIFE IN THE MEDICAL MARKETPLACE: THE FRAME AROUND THE FRAME

Finally, the field of ethics consultation and hence each ethics consultation takes place within the changing constraints of the medical marketplace—a marketplace that is changing with rapidity and potency, shifting both the pace of reflective activity in medicine and the scope of resources available for the activity itself. For example, our practice of ethics consultation began in an era of relative prosperity in healthcare. The professional staff with whom we worked had the flexibility and institutional support to participate actively in a range of activities, including educational programs and committee functions. There was generally substantial budgetary support for ongoing ethics consultation services, extensive staff education, off-site retreats, and conferences. Union contracts for nurses, for example, even featured funded release time and allowed for extensive ethics education and multiple course offerings. But under new financial constraints in an increasingly competitive and "lean" healthcare marketplace, much of this has been eliminated.

In managed care and fee-for-service venues, and in nonprofit and for-profit systems, the focus on the bottom line has become a predominant theme. Ethics consultation as a clinical activity does not generate dollars and, despite its compassionate premise, it can be costly to an institution in terms of staff time. To complicate matters, to accomplish the task at hand skillfully and appropriately involves a considerable investment in resources. And this reality has raised a pressing concern for ethics consultants. In the literature on industrial accidents, an often-cited problem is "speed-up" and workplace stress; surely the work of ethics consultation is no exception. It should not be surprising that ethics consultations done more quickly, by fewer people, and in a shorter time inevitably have a higher rate of error, as surely as in any other industry.

Not only have time and resources been challenged by the new scarcity, but certain critical artifices of medicine have vanished. The very language and premise of our field's preoccupation with informed consent are nearly humorous in the context of a seven-minute office visit. The idea that there will be a primary care physician or a primary care nurse to speak with authority and direct knowledge about the cases ethicists are called in to consult on has ceased to be possible in a number of venues. In fact, more power is shifting to anonymous third parties in the process of decision making, parties who will never come to the table where the ethical conflict can be named and reflected upon. Many of the cases that ethicists are asked to address revolve nearly in their entirety around the weight given to profit and the primacy of the profit motive. It is significant that ethics consults can prolong hospital stays as easily as they can shorten them. How ethicists will be used, by whom, and for what purpose are all critically important questions to ask.

OTHER QUESTIONS TO CONSIDER

These questions are not the last ones in our consideration of identifying the right path and its alternatives, but they offer a sample of the ground that needs to be explored. In doing research for this chapter and deepening our own exploration of the problem of error in ethics consultation, we have identified further categories of concern worthy of consideration and debate by practitioners in the field. We offer some primary questions and preliminary reflections here in the spirit of stimulating ongoing self-reflection and debate.

In considering the kinds of choices we each make and have observed others make in our work as ethicists, we wonder about the problem of motivation. We note that, apart from a consideration of potential outcomes, some errors in consultation have their source in an utterly mistaken intention. An ethicist might choose an incorrect *telos* for his or her work, for example, such as acting in ways that are primarily self-serving, job preserving, or relationship preserving, or in ways indicative of a weakness of will or compromise of integrity. What account can we offer of the role of intention, motivation, and duty in the performance of the ethicist's work?

Others in this volume have addressed the problem of setting standards for ethics consultation. We have been struck as well, though, by the frank reality of incompetence. What are we to make of errors that seem to have their source simply in an ethicist's incompetence? It is ironic that we expect new medical students to make errors and have developed safeguards to address them, but that no similar recognition or precaution seems to exist for ethicists. Further work on this topic must be done as the field develops, since ethics consultation—like all clinical activities—has a learning curve. The field will need to find ways to protect patients from such errors of both *techne* and *phronesis* that will be made in the early stages of careers, and we must develop some sort of peer review mechanism to assess the work of long-time practitioners. Of course making this claim implies that we believe that there is a body of knowledge to master and a skill that takes time to acquire and develop, a claim that may not be universally shared by those who aspire to practice as ethics consultants.

In thinking about the particular cases we have confronted in our own clinical practice, and in thinking about the narratives that we have heard from colleagues, we have been led to wonder further about errors in style. Are some ethicists better simply because they are better listeners or have a more tender intuitive sense? What is the role of bedside manner? And what of the role of individual personalities? Clearly neither uncommunicative brusqueness nor cautious timidity would serve the work of clinical consultation well, but can such behavioral styles be characterized as "in error"?

We have wondered too about the possibility of developing a theory about and approach to the prevention of mistakes in ethics consultation. Here we have grappled with the question of whether errors in ethics consultation can only be known retrospectively. We are concerned of course about bad outcomes. But an account of mistakes that was exclusively consequentialist would seem terribly incomplete. Sometimes, for example, one might judge the outcome of a consultation to be bad, but the process to be exemplary. Mistakes are judged according to a chosen frame of reference, and clarifying as a field which frames of reference are most important will be imperative. It would seem necessary then for the field to develop clear parameters for its practitioners. Among the issues to be considered will be what would constitute "a disaster," or frank negligence in consultative practice, and what might constitute a basic decent minimum standard for competency.[37]

We have struggled too with problems of character and conscience. Is it possible to be an evil person and still be an excellent clinical ethicist? At what point should we name an act as frankly evil or as suspect because of what we know about the actor? This raises profound questions about the relationship between our public and private selves. Ought an ethicist be held accountable publicly for his or her private straying from the honorable path? And what ought our response be as witnesses to such a charade? An important question for the field to consider is what our collective response should be to the challenge of establishing and maintaining a sense of accountability. These are among the questions in need of further consideration and debate.

CONCLUSION

In this chapter, we have focused on the phenomenon of error in bioethics, reflecting on the nature, meaning, and normative implications of mistakes in bioethics consultation, and calling for more widespread discussion of the problem. The careful collective naming of and facing our mistakes is a necessary exercise for any profession, particularly one still considering its own borders. Thinking about the problem of errors, frailty, and loss rather than the task of building the triumphalist narrative in which our heroization and rescue of medicine figures prominently is the very way we hope to strengthen the profession of bioethics and deepen our shared sense of the discipline's purpose, past, and future.

We have found that the stance of the ethicist in such a context is both imperiled and empowered—a classic double-edged sword.[38] As philosophers and theologians invited into the moral world of the clinic (what Hauerwas reminds us is one of the few truly moral enterprises in our society),[39] it was a privilege to stand as observer, seeing what might be missed, commenting on the margins. The pioneers entered as anthropologists would begin: as the listening outsider. But, two decades later, clinical ethicists are surely asked for far more. Not only are we asked to frame the epistemological and ontological problems, but we are asked to frame and, in some cases, decide the normative course. And as we become more deeply engaged in the clinical world, we are not immune to the lure of the medical story itself. Like all who dwell in the modern world, we are tremendously influenced by the received wisdom of science. We are given the case history; we hear the diagnosis, the prognosis, and the treatment plans among which we will select.

But we know empirically that this is far from the entirety of the story. As ethicists, we rely on an inconstant and mutable knowledge base—a frail and particular way of hearing any story—and base our recommendation on the very science that shifts its ground beneath us. Knowing all of this, the task now is to be sure that the evolution, growth, and modification of beliefs and fact claims can serve also as a map of our mistakes and errors. If the idea of a responsive community is to have meaning, we must develop mechanisms for the family and staff with whom we consult to review and evaluate our work. We need to develop a similar process with one another as colleagues in the field. We must also develop a process to allow colleagues to report cases that they believe are mismanaged so that we can, as a field, debate the meaning and implications of such claims. Finally, we need to develop the rarest of all virtues—an open humility about the very expertise that makes us, paradoxically, so valuable. Like everyone at the table of decision, we will come to a moment when we will turn and look, and see that we have gone wrong. If the field is to achieve maturity, we will have to find the wisdom to go back to the path, and the humility to forgive our mistakenness.

NOTES

1. See E.C. Hughes, "Mistakes at Work," in *The Sociological Eye: Selected Papers on Work, Self, and Society* (Chicago: Aldine-Atherton, 1951, 1971), 316-25; S. Gorovitz and A. MacIntryre, "Toward a Theory of Medical Fallibility," *Journal of Medicine and Philosophy* 1 (1976): 51-71; M.A. Paget, *The Unity of Mistakes: A Phenomenological Interpretation of Medical Work* (Philadelphia: Temple University Press, 1988.)

2. L.L. Leape, "Error in Medicine," *Journal of the American Medical Association* 272 (1994): 1851-7 [reprinted as chapter 7 of this volume—ED.]; D. Hilfiker, *Healing the Wounds: A Physician Looks at His Work* (Omaha, Neb.: Creighton University Press, 1998); C. Bosk, *Forgive and Remember* (Chicago: University of Chicago Press, 1979); M. Millman, *The Unkindest Cut* (New York: Morrow Quill Paperbacks, 1976); S.M. Gilbert, *Wrongful Death: A Medical Tragedy* (New York: W.W. Norton, 1995); A.W. Wu et al., "Do House Officers Learn From Their Mistakes?" *Journal of the American Medical Association* 265 (24 April 1991): 2089-94.

3. "Dead Wrong: Error in Clinical Ethics Consultation," (Workshop presented at the Joint Meeting of the Society for Health and Human Values and the Society for Bioethics Consultation, Cleveland, October 1996).

4. S. Hauerwas, *Dispatches from the Front* (Durham, N.C.: Duke University Press, 1996).

5. Society for Health and Human Values-Society for Bioethics Consultation Task Force on Standards for Bioethics Consultation, *Core Competencies for Health Care Ethics Consultation* (Glenview, Ill.: American Society for Bioethics and Humanities, 1998.)

6. In a study about what ethics consultants in the field, for example, would recommend with respect to the treatment of patients in a persistence vegetative state, investigators found a wide range of opinions. See E. Fox and C. Stocking, "Ethics Consultants' Recommendations for Life-Prolonging Treatment of Patients in a Persistent Vegetative State," *Journal of the American Medical Association* 270 (1 December 1993): 2578-82.

7. *In Re Baby K,* 832 F. Supp. 1022 (E.D. Va. 1993); *In Re Baby K,* 16 F.3d 590 (4th Cir. 1994).

8. See S. Rubin and L. Zoloth-Dorfman, "First Person Plural: Community and Method in Ethics Consultation," *The Journal of Clinical Ethics* 5, no. 1 (Spring 1994): 49-54; S. Rubin and L. Zoloth-Dorfman, "Navigators and Captains: Expertise in Clinical Ethics Consultation," *Theoretical Medicine* 18 (1997): 421-32.

9. One such place is the Center for Medical Ethics and Mediation. See M.B. West and J.M. Gibson, "Facilitating Medical Ethics Case Review: What Ethics Committees Can Learn From Mediation and Facilitation Techniques," *Cambridge Quarterly of Healthcare Ethics* 1 (1992): 63-74.

10. See Fletcher, R.J. Boyle, and E.M. Spencer, "Errors in Ethics Consultation," chapter 21 of this volume.

11. Rubin and Zoloth-Dorfman, "Navigators and Captains," see note 8 above.

12. In fact, it was this image that led us to construct the role itself as primarily navigational in character. Ibid.

13. J.H. Jones, *Bad Blood: The Tuskegee Syphilis Experiment* (New York: Free Press, 1992).

14. R. Faden, ed., *The Human Radiation Experiments: Final Report of the Advisory Committee on Human Radiation Experiments* (Cambridge: Oxford University Press, 1996).

15. Hughes introduced this notion in the sociological literature. See note 1 above.

16. E. Freidson, *Doctoring Together: A Study of Professional Social Control* (New York: Elsevier, 1975).

17. Bosk, *Forgive and Remember,* see note 2 above.

18. See note 3 above.

19. Rubin and Zoloth-Dorfman, "First Person Plural," see note 8 above.

20. Rubin and Zoloth-Dorfman, "Navigators and Captains," see note 8 above.

21. *In Re Quinlan,* 70 N.J. 10, 355 A.2d 647, cert. denied, 429 U.S. 922 (1976); *Barber v. Superior Court,* 147 Cal.App.3d. 1006, 195 Cal.Rptr. 484 (1983); *Bouvia v. Superior Court,* 179 Cal.App.3d 1127, 225 Cal.Rptr. 297 (1986); *Bartling v. Superior Court,* 163 Cal.App.3d 186, 209 Cal.Rptr. 220

(1984); *Cruzan v. Director, Missouri Department of Health*, 497 U.S. 261 1990).

22. *In Re Quinlan*, see note 22 above; L.D. Kliever, ed., *Dax's Case: Essays in Medical Ethics and Human Meaning* (Dallas, Tex.: Southern Methodist University Press, 1989).

23. See, for example, J. Stout, *Ethics After Babel: Language of Morals and Their Discontents* (Boston: Beacon, 1990); C. Taylor, *The Ethics of Authenticity* (Oxford: University Press 1996).

24. Ibid, 3.

25. Ibid., 23.

26. Ibid., 53.

27. Ibid., 52.

28. H.R. Niebuhr, *The Responsible Self* (New York: Harper Collins, 1963).

29. H.E. Longino, *Science as Social Knowledge: Values and Objectivity in Scientific Inquiry* (Princeton, N.J.: Princeton University Press, 1990.)

30. V. Hartouni, *Cultural Conceptions on Reproductive Technologies and the Remaking of Life* (Minneapolis: University of Minnesota Press, 1997), 15.

31. S.J. Youngner et al., "Brain Death and Organ Retrieval: A Cross-Sectional Survey of Knowledge and Concepts among Health Professionals," *Journal of the American Medical Association* 261 (21 April 1989): 2205-10.

32. President's Commission for the Study of Ethical Problems in Medicine and Biomedical and Behavioral Research, *Defining Death: Medical, Legal, and Ethical Issues in the Definition of Death* (Washington, D.C.: U.S. Government Printing Office, 1981); R.M. Veatch, "The Impending Collapse of the Whole-Brain Definition of Death," *Hastings Center Report* 23 (July-August 1993): 18-24; A. Halevy and B. Brody, "Brain Death: Reconciling Definitions, Criteria, and Tests," *Annals of Internal Medicine* 119 (15 September 1993): 519-25; R.D. Truog, "Is It Time to Abandon Brain Death?" *Hastings Center Report* 27 (January-February 1997): 29-37.

33. R.F. Uhlmann, R.A. Pearlman, and K.C. Cain, "Physicians' and Spouses' Predictions of Elderly Patients' Resuscitation Preferences," *Journal of Gerontology* 43 (September 1988): 115-21; R.A. Pearlman, R.F. Uhlmann, and N.S. Jecker, "Spousal Understanding of Patient Quality of Life: Implications of Surrogate Decisions," *The Journal of Clinical Ethics* 3, no. 2 (Summer 1992): 114-21.

34. J.R. Hardwig, "What About the Family? The Role of Family Interests in Medical Treatment Decisions," *Hastings Center Report* 20 (March-April 1990): 5-10; J.L. Nelson, "Taking Families Seriously," *Hastings Center Report* 22 (July-August 1992): 6-12; H.L. Nelson and J.L. Nelson, *The Patient in the Family: An Ethics of Medicine and Families* (New York: Routledge, 1995).

35. L.J. Schneiderman, N.S. Jecker, and A.R. Jonsen, "Medical Futility: Its Meaning and Ethical Implications," *Annals of Internal Medicine* 112 (15 June 1990): 949-54; R.D. Truog, A.S. Brett, and J. Frader, "The Problem with Futility," *New England Journal of Medicine* 326 (4 June 1992): 1560-3; L.J. Schneiderman and N.S. Jecker, *Wrong Medicine: Doctors, Patients, and Futile Treatment* (Baltimore, Md.: Johns Hopkins University Press, 1995); S.B. Rubin, *When Doctors Say No: The Battleground of Medical Futility* (Bloomington, Ind.: Indiana University Press, 1998.)

36. *Washington v. Glucksberg*, 117 S.Ct. 2258 (1997); *Vacco v. Quill*, 117 S.Ct. 2293 (1997).

37. In the field, we might have to begin with minimal standards partly because we disagree. There are people who would think the authors of this chapter are seriously mistaken in our work because we have taken strong stands on the issue of medical futility or about having 20 people in the room for a case, or using a committee and not a sole consultant model.

38. Rubin and Zoloth-Dorfman, "Navigators and Captains," see note 8 above.

39. S. Hauerwas, speech presented at the "Birth of Bioethics" Conference, Seattle, Wash., 1992.

14

Moral Residue

George C. Webster and Françoise E. Baylis

INTRODUCTION

Difficult ethical problems in healthcare, more often than not, are framed as either practical problems (challenging puzzles) or moral dilemmas, the resolution of which requires the exercise of sophisticated problem-solving skills. A paradigmatic example of a *practical ethical problem* is the story told several years ago by Arthur Caplan about how he "solved the oxygen machine crunch" in the emergency room. With the hot summer weather, persons with emphysema and other respiratory ailments were crowding into the emergency room to receive oxygen; unfortunately, there were only two oxygen machines. Instead of solving the allocation problem by developing equitable patient-selection criteria, Caplan sought to address the source of the scarcity. Physicians could prescribe air conditioners to persons suffering from respiratory ailments and the cost would be reimbursed by Medicaid or Medicare.[1] As for the *moral dilemma,* the classic example in contemporary healthcare is the conflict that arises between the commitment to promote the patient's best interest and the commitment to respect patient autonomy when the patient's wishes conflict with what others believe to be in his or her best interest. Moral dilemmas arise when there are obligations to pursue two or more conflicting courses of action and there is no obvious reason to prefer one course of action over the other(s). They can also arise when some evidence suggests that a particular course of action is morally right, other evidence suggests that it is morally wrong, and in each case the evidence is inconclusive.[2]

In the clinical setting, however, framing ethical problems in such narrow terms as either practical problems or moral dilemmas fails to capture what might be called our "experience of the ethical," as this framework does not recognize the experience of moral uncertainty and moral distress. Andrew Jameton describes *moral uncertainty* as follows: "one is unsure what moral principles or values apply, or even what the moral problems is."[3] This aptly describes those situations in which there is an initial sense that something is not quite right, but clarity on this point is lacking. This uncertainty may be nondiscursive and sometimes as basic as a feeling in the pit of one's stomach.

Moral distress, on the other hand, is when there is incoherence between one's beliefs and one's actions, and possibly also outcomes (that is, between what one sincerely believes to be right, what one actually does, and what eventually transpires). For Jameton, moral distress arises "when one knows the right thing to do, but institutional constraints make it nearly impossible to pursue the right course of action."[4] This definition, although appropriately oriented, is too narrow. Moral distress may also arise when one fails to pursue what one believes to be the right course of action (or fails to do so to one's satisfaction) for one or more of the following reasons: an error of judgment, some personal failing (for example, a weakness or crimp in one's character such as a pattern of "systemic avoidance"), or other circumstances truly beyond one's control.

This chapter is about the healthcare ethics consultant's experience of moral distress that can lead to compromised integrity and *moral residue*.[5] Moral residue is that which each of us carries with us from those times in our lives when in the face of moral distress we have seriously compromised ourselves or allowed ourselves to be compromised.[6] These times are usually very painful because they threaten or sometimes betray deeply held and cherished beliefs and values. They are usually also lasting and powerfully concentrated in our thoughts; hence the term moral *residue*.

Interestingly, the experience of moral residue can be the result of error or the cause of error. In the first instance, the experience results from the realization of error, as when one recognizes having chosen a particular course of action for reasons of expediency, laziness, or cowardice; or, one may simply have the perception of error as when, irrespective of any objective evaluation, one believes that one has erred. In the second instance, with moral residue as the cause of error, the critical factor is the incremental loss of commitment to previously held values for reasons of self-interest, such as self-protection or self-promotion.

THE WORKPLACE

The healthcare ethics consultant working in the clinical setting invariably encounters situations where there is pressure or temptation to compromise. This pressure or temptation is particularly acute when there is pervasive uncertainty, or when there is serious disagreement between the ethics consultant and individual practitioners, patients, residents, substitute decision makers, members of the hospital ethics committee, or the employer. Two situations that capture an "acute" experience of moral distress followed by compromise are summarized below.

PROGNOSTIC UNCERTAINTY: "I'M GLAD I FOUGHT
AS HARD AS I DID TO KEEP TREATMENT GOING."

A young woman who broadsided a school bus with her motorcar had been in the neurology intensive care unit for approximately one week when the ethics consultant was consulted by the attending neurosurgeon. A meeting took place with the neurosurgeon, the patient's husband, the patient's father, and the ethics consultant. The husband and father wanted all treatment discontinued immediately, especially the feeding tube that had been inserted earlier in the week. They explained that their wife/daughter would not want to live in these circumstances. The patient had worked with children with disabilities and had previously indicated that she would not want to live if she had to endure what some of the children suffered.

The neurosurgeon was extremely ambivalent about the family's request. He asked the ethics consultant for an opinion. The consultant noted that there was considerable prognostic uncertainty, as the neurosurgeon had indicated in his summary of the patient's situation. The patient had already lived longer than anyone expected and, although her condition was still serious, she was stable and off the ventilator. The ethics consultant thought it might be worthwhile to wait a bit longer to see if the prognosis would become more clear. Among the issues discussed was the recommendation that a "trial period" of feeding by artificial means be attempted given the prognostic uncertainty. The family adamantly refused to consider any alternatives. They wanted all treatment discontinued immediately. The neurosurgeon remained ambivalent. He said that he was not prepared to act on their request at this time but that he was not, in principle, opposed to their request. He wanted more time to think through the situation.

The problem for the ethics consultant in this case was what to do (if anything) if the neurosurgeon reluctantly acquiesced to the family's demands. The consultant was deeply concerned about the haste with which decisions were being made and the apparent failure to attend properly to the interests of the patient, who was voiceless and truly vulnerable. The request to discontinue all treatment and withhold any future interventions would most certainly lead to the patient's death because of the extensive nature of her injuries. If the surgeon acquiesced, would the ethics consultant have an obligation to pursue the matter? If the consultant's role is one of facilitator of moral inquiry, arguably nothing more need be done because such inquiry had been facilitated. Similarly, if the consultant's role is advisory (to assist others in making decisions), again there was nothing more for the consultant to do in this case because advice and assistance had been given. In fact, based on most of the widely accepted job descriptions of the ethics consultant, there was nothing more the consultant could or should do. The question confronting the ethics consultant in this case, however, was whether in these particular circumstances his job should include saving a patient's life.[7] More generally, Laurie Zoloth and Susan B. Rubin ask whether "concern about certain kinds of violations or certain devastating consequences should ever compel [ethics consultants] to do more than merely offer advice upon request. . . . Do we ever have a duty to utterly stop an act we judge as evil from happening?"[8] In our view, the response to this question must be a resounding yes. In the face of perceived serious wrongdoing, the ethics consultant must take a moral stance. Now for some, a question arises as to whether doing so is required because of personal or professional obligations. This question is not explored here because it is not clear that a distinction can be drawn between personal and professional integrity.

"NO PAIN MEDICATION FOR MOTHER, THANK YOU VERY MUCH!"

An elderly woman suffering from shortness of breath was brought to the emergency department by her daughter. She had an elevated temperature and seemed confused and disoriented. Her medical history indicated that she had suffered a cerebrovascular accident (a stroke) approximately a year ago.

On admission, it was noted that the woman had a gangrenous foot and ankle and a mottled leg up to and above her knee. Later, on the ward, the nursing staff noticed that when they moved the patient she appeared to be in considerable pain from the bad leg. They recommended analgesia, and the attending physician concurred. The patient's daughter, however, who was her only child and only living relative, refused to allow any pain medication. The daughter was a retired pharmacist and she said that analgesia would shorten her mother's life. Further, she informed the staff that her mother had an unusually high pain threshold. For example, her mother had never used any freezing at the dentist, and when she had suffered a bad burn on her arm she never took anything for the pain. Caregivers tried to negotiate with the daughter, but to no avail. She emphatically stated: "No pain medication for mother, thank you very much!"

The ethics consultant was called about one week after the patient's admission. The ethicist was not able to communicate with the patient who remained confused and disoriented, and so met with her daughter. The story was similar to that relayed by the staff. In a later team meeting, the attending physician stated that the situation was untenable and it would be unconscionable to continue to not give the patient pain medication. The charge nurse stated that many of her staff were not sleeping at night and found it increasingly difficult to look after the patient because of the daughter's refusal to allow pain medication. At the end of the meeting, the physician noted that the daughter was the legal substitute decision maker and that, although she personally did not agree with the daughter's request, she had "no choice" because she was not prepared to go against the legally recognized substitute decision maker and risk a lawsuit. The nursing staff and chaplain remained silent, and the ethics consultant meekly asked: "But what about the patient?" The physician exploded and said that it was easy for an ethics consultant to raise difficult questions because the ethics consultant had no responsibility for decision making. "No deal. If the daughter says no pain medication—no pain medication." The meeting ended, and nothing more was said.

The ethics consultant later wrote: "I went home and endured (as I recall) one of the most difficult weekends of my life. I felt so morally compromised by the situation, yet I wasn't clear in my own mind what my next step should be. I thought of the patient when I played with my children, when I walked my dog Izabelle, when I dried the dishes, when I put the laundry through the washer and dryer."[9] The ethics consultant went to work early on Monday morning and was called by the charge nurse. Over the weekend, the patient's condition had deteriorated. The daughter had met with the surgeon and had been told that her mother's gangrenous leg was reaching a critical point (sepsis and systemic infection). The only option, if there was to be any hope of saving her life, was amputation. The daughter agreed to the surgery, and the elderly woman's leg was amputated on Sunday; anesthesia was provided in such a way that the patient's lung function was not further compromised. The anesthetic was now wearing off; when the staff approached the daughter about giving the patient postsurgical analgesia, the daughter adamantly refused.

CASE DISCUSSION

In both of these cases, the ethics consultant experienced profound moral distress because of perceived constraints imposed by the institution, the social structures of healthcare, and prevailing role relationships that appeared to preclude the pursuit of right action. Personal moral integrity was compromised as a combination of fear, uncertainty, and doubt led the consultant to remain silent. The ethicist (temporarily) set aside deeply held moral principles and values because there did not appear to be any other option. The ethicist experienced anguish and, on reflection, lasting remorse.

In these types of cases, a critical question for ethics consultants and those who work with them is whether there was also avoidable error. Notably, not all unfortunate outcomes of ethics consultations and not all experiences of moral residue are connected with error. As the second author (FB) noted elsewhere, "Errors can happen because a [person]. . . doesn't know something she should know, doesn't properly execute a requisite . . . skill, or doesn't bring together the facts of the case in a manner that promotes good judgment."[10] The experience of moral residue may arise because of failings in one or more of these areas, but it may also arise when one exercises the requisite knowledge and skills, but circumstances still prevail.

COMPROMISE

Compromise on the part of the ethics consultant may be viewed in positive terms as evidence of desired character traits (such as tolerance and prudence), as well as evidence of a commitment to procedural fairness. Alternatively, compromise may be perceived (and experienced) as an erosion of personal moral integrity and as evidence of a lack of moral courage. As such, compromise is a complex and difficult concept.

In exploring the multiple meanings of compromise, Martin Benjamin suggests at least three different understandings of this concept: (1) compromise as outcome and process, (2) compromise as betrayal, and (3) compromise as prudence.[11] Compromise in the standard sense refers to both outcome and process. Compromise as outcome describes a situation where two or more parties to a dispute accept a position different from the one they originally held—typically a position that more or less "splits the difference" between the contending parties. The compromise position is the fruit of a conciliatory process, also called a compromise, whereby parties in conflict adjust their conflicting claims by making mutual concessions in the hope of finding some middle ground acceptable to all. This might include consideration of one or more options not previously identified. When all parties to the dispute are able to modify their positions and achieve agreement, without compromising on basic principles or values, it can be said that a principled or integrity-preserving compromise has been achieved. In sharp contrast, when the compromise is not predicated on mutually accepted basic principles, but instead requires a shift in fundamental values or commitments simply for the sake of agreement and not as a result of considered judgment, there is compromise as betrayal.[12] Finally, there is compromise as prudence, where external constraints and conditions impose a measured or prudential approach to the pursuit of one's ultimate goals.

In ethics consultation, compromise as process and compromise as prudence are *de rigueur*. Compromise as betrayal, on the other hand, takes us beyond negotiating or finding an acceptable or tolerable middle ground, or a means to a desired end, and focuses our attention on the moral agent. Compromise as betrayal is invariably evidence of a moral failing in that it involves a "retreat on matters of ethical principle."[13] When there is a moral failing, and it is perceived as such, there is likely to be moral distress and moral residue. In Benjamin's terms, "To compromise fundamental principles is to compromise not simply a contingent or readily interchangeable interest, but rather what we regard as an essential aspect of the self. It is to alter one's fundamental convictions and perhaps to weaken or betray one's wholeness or integrity as a particular self—as a person with a determinate identity who stands for some things rather than others."[14] With compromise as betrayal, identity-conferring commitments—"commitments that make us who we are"[15]—are sacrificed. One's moral identity—who one is (or wants to be), and what one stands for—is called into question. The experience of "being compromised" thus overshadows the goal of "reaching a compromise."

INTEGRITY

While many agree that good character, particularly integrity, is important for ethics consultation, individual moral integrity remains one of the more controversial characteristics of working as an ethicist.[16] In part this is because of the significant theoretical problems associated with this characteristic. As Benjamin Freedman notes: "What counts as integrity? Integrity to what? Who decides?"[17] Like compromise, integrity is a complex and difficult concept.

A key element of integrity is coherence. According to Lynne McFall, there are three kinds of coherence: simple consistency, coherence between principle and action, and coherence between principle and motivation. She writes the following: "The requirement of coherence is fairly complicated. In addition to simple consistency, it puts constraints on the way in which one's principles may be held (the 'first-person' requirement), on how one may act given one's principles (coherence between principle and action), and how one may be motivated in acting on them (coherence between principle and motivation)."[18]

For the purpose of our discussion, we focus on the second kind of coherence—namely, coherence between behaviors and beliefs. Here, McFall says: "Integrity requires 'sticking to one's principles,' moral or otherwise, in the face of temptation, including the temptation to re-description."[19] More generally, in the face of either temptation or coercion, a person of integrity acts in a manner that is consistent with his or her avowed principles and commitments, even when there may be serious personal consequences. "Weakness of the will" or "lacking the courage of one's convictions" are among integrity's opposites.

Like McFall, Benjamin also believes that individual integrity is about wholeness or completeness and a certain "fit" between one's beliefs and actions. It consists of "(1) a reasonably coherent and relatively stable set of highly cherished values and principles, (2) verbal behavior expressing these values and principles, and (3) conduct embodying one's values and principles and consistent with what one says."[20] For Benjamin, personal integrity is ineluctably linked with personal identity. Taken together, the elements of integrity "constitute the formal structure of one's identity as a person."[21] And so it is that the experience of compromise as betrayal links directly with compromised personal moral integrity.

Integrity in ethics consultation requires that one speak and act in a manner consistent with one's deeply held values, beliefs, and principles and that, as the need arises, one acts with courage.

THE EXPERIENCE OF MORAL RESIDUE

The experience of compromised integrity that involves the setting aside or violation of deeply held (and publicly professed) beliefs, values, and principles can sear the heart. The passage of time may blunt the acute distress, the profound uncertainty and fear, the guilt, and the remorse, but our experience suggests that people who have lived through serious moral compromise carry the remnants of the experience for many years, if not a lifetime. As Jerome Miller writes: "When the very centre of the self is deeply affected . . . one's whole way of thinking about the world, as well as one's whole way of feeling about it, is profoundly and permanently altered. No part of the self is exempt from such an experience. One is touched in depths one did not know one had but whose reality one cannot possibly doubt."[22]

A poignant remark by a young medical student makes this point very forcefully. The student was told to repeat a pelvic exam on a patient who was anesthetized in the operating room (she was one of five students so instructed). Fearful of the consequences of refusing to perform the pelvic exam, she did what she was told to do. When asked to elaborate on her feelings regarding this experience of compromise, she paused and then said: "It must feel something like a woman who has been sexually violated. You can't get rid of the feeling that you are now somehow dirty or unclean. In the deepest part of yourself, you feel you will never be the same and you carry this with you for the rest of your life." Serious moral compromise (that is, compromised integrity) irreversibly alters the self. One does not experience serious moral compromise and survive as the person one was.

Persons who recognize that their integrity has been compromised typically experience moral residue. For some, this experience leads to the erosion and fragmentation of their sense of meaning and purpose in the world. For others, the experience is not as devastating, but it does create a fissure in the self that may color future actions and decisions; for good or ill, moral residue is incorporated into their lived experience. In very general terms, the change is for the better when the person comes to know with greater clarity what he or she will or will not tolerate or cooperate with in the future. The change is for the worse when the person adapts by constantly shifting his or her values. With the passage of time, that person's values become so changeable that it is nearly impossible for the person to articulate what he or she sincerely believes in. The person—a moral chameleon[23]—becomes desensitized to wrongdoing, willing to tolerate morally questionable or morally impermissible actions.

MORAL RESIDUE "FOR GOOD"

An acute experience of compromised integrity and subsequent moral residue (whether as a consequence of an error of judgment, some personal failing, or institutional or other constraints) can be a positive instructive experience, as when it helps one to become clearer about one's identity-conferring moral, religious, and philosophical commitments. This is important if one accepts the description of the ethics consultant as, among other things, a person with "a strong sense of personal and professional integrity . . . [able to] distinguish outcomes that one will not, on moral grounds, endorse/sanction (e.g., an outcome that violates an important moral principle, but is chosen to avoid confrontation) from outcomes that one disagrees with, but will endorse/sanction (e.g., an outcome within communal and institutional norms)."[24]

The experience of moral residue may help the consultant hone the ability to distinguish between: (1) situations where a proposed course of action appears to contravene deeply held, universalizable principles and so an appropriate response on the part of the ethics consultant would be to intervene; and (2) situations where the course of action appears to contravene personal moral convictions but coheres with communal and institutional norms, so that an appropriate response might be withdrawal or tolerance depending upon the circumstances.

In the first instance, the ethics consultant's considered response would be: "I don't agree with the decision or action taken, and I can't cooperate with this because to do so would profoundly compromise my personal moral integrity." In the second instance, the consultant might say: "I don't personally agree with the decision or action taken, but I accept that I must live with it."

The personal struggle to clarify one's personal moral boundaries and thresholds or to discover what "tips the scale" goes to the very heart of the moral life. Exploring this terrain requires humility and no little moral courage. It also demands an almost unrelenting intellectual honesty. These requirements are, in human terms, often difficult to realize. It is here that one perhaps feels most vulnerable, and it is here that one might choose a route of least resistance because other options appear to be too arduous, contrary to one's interests, or excruciatingly painful. Moral residue may help one to stay the course and sharpen the demarcation line between integrity-preserving compromise and compromise as betrayal.

MORAL RESIDUE "FOR ILL"

Just as the experience of moral residue may yield greater clarity and insight and strengthen one's resolve to do better the next time, the weight of moral residue may lead one to error. Commonly the error will take one of three forms— denial of the incoherence between beliefs and actions, trivialization of the incoherence between beliefs and actions, or unreflective acceptance of the incoherence between beliefs and actions.

In the first instance—denial of the inconsistencies between beliefs and actions—the compromised individual engages in elaborate self-deception that relies on "distorted reasoning, deliberate ignorance, and self-directed lies."[25] Believing his or her integrity to be intact, the individual comes to ignore or overlook wrongdoing. Typically, the individual uses one or both of the following strategies to evade or redescribe the truth about inconsistencies between personal beliefs and actions (that is, inconsistencies between what the person thinks should be done and what the person actually does). The first strategy glosses over certain truths by insisting on a distinction between personal and professional roles. The self is compartmentalized and, further, is persuaded that compromise in the workplace does not threaten personal integrity; the professional self is somehow not a crucial part of the rest of the self. The second strategy typically builds upon the first strategy that bifurcates the self and involves narrowing the description of one's professional role and responsibilities in such a way as to absolve oneself of moral responsibility for one's actions in the workplace. So long as one does one's (limited) job, professional integrity is not compromised.[26]

In the second instance—trivialization of the inconsistencies between beliefs and actions—the compromised individual and others may discount the relevance of any dissonance between beliefs and actions by suggesting that, under the circumstances, the incoherence is unimportant and inconsequential. Over time, the individual becomes less and less clear about the difference between trivial and serious transgressions. From this perspective, no transgression is ever so serious that it cannot be trivialized.

In the third instance—unreflective acceptance—the compromised individual attempts to redress any inconsistencies between beliefs and actions by changing or abandoning his or her principles. That is, for pragmatic (as contrasted with principled) reasons, the individual alters or revises personal beliefs, values, and principles such that actions previously judged morally wrong are no longer perceived as such. Now, this is not to suggest that moral beliefs and values are static and that any change in one's previously avowed principles is indicative of error. Individuals do autonomously shift, modify, or qualify their moral principles and commitments. But, clearly, there is a significant difference between a change occasioned by life experience and critical reflection, and a change motivated by fear, expedience, or self-preservation.

MORAL RESIDUE: FINDING ONE'S WAY

A good healthcare ethics consultant expects to compromise—to participate in a process where mutual concessions are made in an effort to resolve disagreement and to exercise prudence in the pursuit of long-term goals. At all costs, however, most ethics consultants (like other parties to the conflict) want to avoid being compromised—that is, conceding basic principles or commitments as happens with compromise as betrayal. Personal moral integrity is not to be traded upon lightly. What then of the heavy burdens and sometimes very rigid constraints imposed on ethics consultants in the clinical setting that incline the consultant to compromise integrity, most frequently by remaining silent?

One of the many constraining factors in healthcare ethics consultation is the structure and culture of the clinical setting. For example, it is not uncommon for an ethics consultant to be told: "There is no ethical issue here, this is a clinical issue, an operational issue, a management issue, a medical decision," and so on. In this way, the ethical issue is camouflaged in the ordinariness of things, as familiar nonmoral language and categories are used to describe normative issues. In addition to difficulties associated with identifying and naming ethical issues is the apparent willingness of some healthcare providers and institutions to dismiss or trivialize certain ethical concerns and overlook or sidestep others. In some institutions, for example, ethics consultants (and healthcare professionals) have been disciplined or reprimanded for raising challenging ethical questions at team meetings or rounds. There is tremendous pressure to "get along by going along."[27] In refusing to do, one risks isolation and marginalization, loss of employment, or other personal loss. Taken together, these factors foster an environment where the pressure to compromise is tremendous, as is the risk of being compromised.

How should ethics consultants and healthcare facilities attend to this? What kind of "fit" should there be between the ethics consultant's personal and professional values and the values of the wider community in which the consultant works? Should the ethics consultant be free to express deeply held convictions and beliefs? If so, to whom? In what context? And to what end? How should an ethics consultant conscientiously object to institutional practices or ethics consultations deemed morally objectionable? How should the institution respond to the conscientious objections of ethics consultants and others? What if the ethics consultant's moral views are suspect or gravely erroneous? How might this be determined?

PERSONAL AND
COMMUNAL DISCERNMENT

Ethics consultants need to explore more fully questions that go beyond what some have called "quandary ethics." In framing ethical questions only as puzzles to be solved, it is easy to overlook issues having to do with the kind of people we are as we struggle for clarity, insight, and wisdom in the midst of difficult and sometimes almost impossible situations often fraught with uncertainty. Going back to the two experiences of moral residue summarized earlier, the ethics consultant was concerned not only about the quality and clarity of his thinking (or lack thereof) in terms of knowledge and analytical skills, but also about who he was in each of these situations. He was also concerned about his relationship with colleagues and the wider hospital community. What to do? We believe that the experiences of moral distress, moral compromise, and moral residue must be addressed at both the personal and communal level.

At the personal level, one response would be truthfulness with oneself and with others. The ethics consultant would critically review his or her intentions, as well as his or her beliefs and actions in an effort to be clear about what has happened and eventually to share personal insights with others. But this presumes (sometimes erroneously) that ethics consultants are capable of honestly questioning themselves and the quality of their work and that the institution employing them would promote this type of response.

As regards the first of these issues, not everyone is able or willing to expose, even to themselves let alone others, their uncertainties, fears, and failings. For some, honest reflection following an experience of moral residue opens new horizons that can lead to greater clarity about the events that contributed to compromised integrity. For others, however, an attempt at honest self-appraisal in search of personal insight only serves to preclude any further consideration of the issue at hand; the naked truth is too threatening and so better that it remain cloaked in ambiguity and uncertainty. Coming to know oneself (in some coherent and intelligible fashion) is imperative, however. A healthy response to the experience of moral residue has the ethics consultant engage in what Charles Taylor calls "strong evaluation."[28] In an effort to redress wholeness and integrity, the ethics consultant engages in critical self-reflection, where the goal is to evaluate and then either embolden or restructure one's identity-conferring commitments.

In addition to personal reflection about the self, the ethics consultant must engage in informed, honest, critical self-reflection with the support and constructive criticism of well-meaning colleagues. However, taking personal concerns forward in the clinical setting is no easy task. Much depends on the extent to which the work environment is seen to be a moral community. Healthcare institutions must develop and implement mechanisms for understanding and evaluating institutional and institutionalized patterns of behaviors that may contribute to moral distress and all that ensues. This is absolutely necessary if the institution is to meet one of the basic working conditions for ethics consultants—namely, "the ability to do [one's] job without compromising conscience."[29] Following Freedman, we suggest that institutions commit "to protect the ethics consultant from intrainstitutional pressures and . . . [to maintain] the job security of one who acts conscientiously in the course of employment."[30]

In closing, it is perhaps instructive to revisit the first case summarized in this chapter. The day after the consultation, the patient's husband asked the attending physician to "forget" everything that had been discussed because his wife had said hello to him. Some weeks later, the ethics consultant met the husband in the hallway of the hospital. He was pushing his wife in a wheelchair, returning from physiotherapy. He stopped and introduced his wife. She shook hands and said hello. In the course of the conversation, the husband told the consultant that he was pleased he had pushed so hard to continue treatment, because his wife was now doing so well.[31]

One could say, "All is well that ends well," but it is important to recognize that things might just as easily have ended otherwise. Treatment could have been discontinued and the patient could have died with no one ever knowing of the potential for recovery. This highlights the need for healthcare facilities to encourage ethics consultants and others to bring ethical concerns to light and deal with these in a thorough manner that promotes shared understanding and mutual respect—prerequisites for integrity-preserving moral compromise. For, as Zoloth and Rubin note: "While each of our consciences can appropriately be a source of deep inner moral knowledge about the right path in the face of challenge, neither we nor our consciences exist in a vacuum. . . . [An] 'act taken in good conscience' is a social act that has a structural and institutional impact in the workplace and the wider community."[32]

To this they add, " 'Conscientious objections' to, for example a draft policy, or to a medical practice, make no sense unless they are witnessed and honored by the community, and no point unless they are taken as an act of resistance to a given collective normative expectation."[33] These claims underscore the importance of viewing the workplace as a moral community where there is coherence between what healthcare institutions publicly profess to be—namely, helping, healing, caring environments that embrace the virtues intrinsic to the practice of healthcare and what employees, patients, and others both witness and participate in.

The experience of moral compromise and moral residue can be difficult, even painful. However, it can also be a profound teaching moment; one can live through the experience and find it instructive, perhaps even healing. As members of the bioethics community (and other communities), we must address questions about moral compromise and integrity in our healthcare institutions, universities, and ethics centers. While this is not without peril (and may require considerable strength of character and moral courage), choosing not to address these issues is all the more perilous because we risk legitimizing and perpetuating practices and behaviors that ultimately will erode the very fabric of our personal lives and the life we share as a moral community.

ACKNOWLEDGMENT

We would like to thank Pat Murphy, a Clinical Ethicist at St. Boniface General Hospital in Winnipeg, Manitoba, Canada, for helpful comments on an earlier draft of this chapter.

NOTES

1. A.L. Caplan, "Can Applied Ethics Be Effective in Health Care and Should It Strive to Be?" *Ethics* 93 (1983): 311-9.

2. For a brief discussion of moral dilemmas, see T.L. Beauchamp and J.F. Childress, *Principles of Biomedical Ethics* (New York: Oxford University Press, 1994), 11-3.

3. A. Jameton, *Nursing Practice: The Ethical Issues* (Englewood Cliffs, N.J.: Prentice-Hall, 1984), 6.

4. Ibid.

5. The experience of moral residue is not unique to healthcare ethics consultants. For example, nurses frequently experience moral residue because of institutional constraints, and increasingly physicians experience it because of fiscal constraints. For a chilling account of moral residue experienced by nurses, see B. Sibbald, "A Right to Be Heard," *The Canadian Nurse/L'infirmiere canadienne* (November 1997): 23-30.

6. G. Webster, "Moral Residue: The Problem of Moral Compromise," (Paper presented at the Annual Meeting of the Canadian Bioethics Society, Vancouver, B.C., 24 November 1995).

7. B. Freedman, "Should an Ethics Consultant Save a Patient's Life? The Limits of Justice of Neighbours," (Paper presented at the Annual Meeting of the Society for Bioethics Consultation, Toronto, Ontario, 5 September 1991). See also B. Freedman, "From Avocation to Vocation: Working Conditions for Clinical Health Care Ethics Consultants," in *The Health Care Ethics Consultant,* ed. F. Baylis (Totowa, N.J.: Humana, 1994), 113.

8. L. Zoloth-Dorfman and S.B. Rubin, "Insider Trading: Conscience and Critique in Bioethics," *HEC Forum* 10 (1998): 28.

9. From a written account by George C. Webster.

10. F. Baylis, "Errors in Medicine: Nurturing Truthfulness," *The Journal of Clinical Ethics* 8, no. 4 (Winter 1997): 337.

11. M. Benjamin, *Splitting the Difference: Compromise and Integrity in Ethics and Politics* (Lawrence, Kans.: University Press of Kansas, 1990), 4-23.

12. A. Rand, *The Virtue of Selfishness* (New York: Signet, 1964), 79-81.

13. See note 11 above, p. 12.

14. Ibid., 13-4.

15. L. McFall, "Integrity," *Ethics* 98 (1987): 13.

16. Society for Health and Human Values/Society for Bioethics Consultation Task Force on Standards for Bioethics Consultation, *Core Competencies for Health Care Ethics Consultation* (Glenview, Ill.: American Society for Bioethics and Humanities, 1998), 25-6.

17. See note 7 above, p. 123.

18. See note 15 above, p. 8.

19. Ibid., 7.

20. See note 11 above, p. 51.

21. Ibid., 51.

22. J. Miller, "The Way of Suffering: A Reasoning of the Heart," *Second Opinion* 17 (1992): 21.

23. See note 11 above, p. 8.

24. F. Baylis, "A Profile of the Health Care Ethics Consultant," in *The Health Care Ethics Consultant,* ed. F. Baylis (Totowa, N.J.: Humana, 1994), 35.

25. M. Martin, *Self-Deception and Morality* (Lawrence, Kans.: University Press of Kansas, 1986),

1. This is an excellent, thought-provoking discussion of self-deception and morality.

26. C. Mitchell, "Integrity in Interprofessional Relationships," in *Responsibility in Health Care,* ed. G.J. Agich (Dordrecht, The Netherlands: D. Reidel, 1982), 163-84.

27. B. Freedman, "Where Are the Heroes of Bioethics?" *The Journal of Clinical Ethics* 7, no. 4 (Winter 1996): 298.

28. C. Taylor, "Responsibility for Self," in *The Identities of Persons,* ed. A.O. Rorty (Berkeley: University of California Press, 1976), 281-99.

29. See note 7 above, p. 123.

30. Ibid., 127. We recognize, as does Freedman, that while this offers needed protection for persons of conscience, unscrupulous persons may abuse their job security "to cover deficiencies in other areas of performance" (p. 128).

31. This account of things is an interesting example of redescription and self-deception. While the ethics consultant experienced moral residue, it seems clear that this patient's husband had re-described things to accommodate a new reality that he had not anticipated in his earlier conversation with the medical team about her treatment and care.

32. See note 8 above, p. 30.

33. Ibid., 31.

15

Quality and Error in Bioethics Consultation: A Puzzle in Pieces

Paul J. Reitemeier

INTRODUCTION

Philosophy traditionally seats ethical authority not in its ability to levy sanctions or rewards (as is possible with legal authority) but solely in its ability to persuade the rational inquirer. Rational persuasion requires recognized starting points of shared assumptions about the nature of the world and the nature and value of human ethical reasoning in it. Numerous attempts to establish ethical authority have been made within various metaethical theories, indicating that disagreement and diversity of thought occur at the most fundamentally abstract levels of rational inquiry. For example, following David Hume, emotivists deny that authority exists in ethics but allow that veracity does exist, at least in terms of the distinction between authentic and inauthentic approval by moral agents. Kantian rationalists claim that ethical expertise and its associated authority are limited to the ability to draw logically valid inferences and form conclusions from within the conceptual constraints of a particular ethical theory itself. They leave to others the difficult pragmatic application of such conclusions in the empirical world of human experience. In contrast, pragmatists following Dewey require ethical theory to enable one to draw true conclusions about true and false moral beliefs, but also admit that this requires competency in the relevant empirical subject areas.[1]

Despite these metatheoretic disagreements, philosophers nevertheless argue that truth and error are possible in moral judgments. What are the relevant capacities needed in making moral judgments, and how is individual competency assessed in each of them? Competency is most often described as a rational faculty operating within specified ranges of decision making and according to which an individual is judged to be capable or incapable of making rationally coherent decisions concerning his life, person, and property. It is characterized as a psychological condition involving sufficiently well-functioning cognitive processes and memory to enable the competent person to reach rational conclusions, to use them to make decisions, and to explain how he did so. Occupational competency assumes that, in addition to this rational faculty, one possesses a specific set of definable skills and uses them appropriately according to predetermined standards.

Thus, a *descriptive definition* of competence in bioethics specifies the intellectual, communicative, and other capacities needed to perform a minimum set of identifiable and role-specific functions, while a *threshold definition* focuses on the relationship between having these minimum capacities and the legal authority to perform the necessary functions.[2] Bioethicists have a roughly approximate descriptive definition for their own functions,[3] but thus far there is no basis for establishing a threshold definition of competence. Nonetheless, error in bioethics is certainly possible insofar as bioethics is a rationally constrained discussion of ethical matters in healthcare. Patterns of repeated error in bioethics, as in other intellectual fields, would constitute incompetence in the field. Yet if philosophers diverge so much in their identification of the competency skills needed for reasoning in ethical theory, how can bioethical competency ever be defined and individual abilities assessed?

CERTAINTY, AUTHORITY, AND EXPERTISE

Absolute certainty in ethics, as in clinical science, has never been attained. The currently received view about the nature of truth in either science or ethics is that of provisional commitments to certain facts and propositions that are probably true, but that are not known to be logically or necessarily true. Authority in science and ethics is related to expertise, which is defined in terms of demonstrated mastery of specific knowledge bases that are relevantly applied to the problem-solving tasks at hand. According to Howard Brody, the nature and operation of authority are best understood as socially legitimated power.[4] Power relies for its own legitimacy upon a system of beliefs concerning competency and expertise that is widely shared by those seeking assistance from the presumed authority. Identification of such authority is accomplished in part by the authority's own persuasiveness (claims of competency) and in part by effective manipulation of the physical world for purposes that are valued by those seeking assistance in problem solving. Bioethicists have been much more successful at persuading others of the values of their work than in demonstrating measurable effectiveness in improving the quality of healthcare services through enhanced ethical reflection.[5] Thus, the degree of socially legitimated power in bioethics lags considerably behind that of licensed clinical practitioners.

There is no formal training requirement, evaluative process, or licensure mechanism for persons who seek to function as bioethicists. Moreover, there is no standard intellectual or disciplinary approach such that all bioethicists can be said to share a common base of subject-specific knowledge, however modest.

Similarly, with respect to the methodologies of bioethics, practitioners use a wide variety of methods and agendas and aim at a plethora of goals. As a consequence of this wide diversity in intellectual process and purpose, there is no standardized or authoritative procedure or office through which a bioethicist who commits a professional error can be recognized, his or her professional activities reviewed, and corrective or disciplinary action taken. At the same time, aside from self-identified peer recognition, there is no process or office authorized to formally recognize significant accomplishments in bioethics by individuals or groups. Numerous self-selected, voluntary associations in bioethics have formed, grown, ebbed, and evolved, with some groups merging and others disappearing, but none instituting selective criteria for membership beyond a willingness to self-affiliate and pay the required (and comparatively modest) financial dues.[6] Indeed, the largest bioethics organization in the United States is actively seeking ways to enlarge its own membership, including the consideration of awarding incentives to current members for identifying potential new members as targets for organized recruitment efforts.[7]

Despite the absence of any socially legitimated authority for bioethics, scores of conferences have been held, thousands of articles and books have been published (including an impressive, five-volume *Encyclopedia of Bioethics*),[8] the U.S. Congress and several presidential administrations have sought consultation, and many courts have heard expert testimony from bioethicists during civil and criminal trials. Hundreds of self-described bioethicists have been interviewed by the media on breaking news involving ethical issues. Even the most prestigious awards for significant accomplishment in the field of bioethics are presented to recipients by the elected leadership of a voluntary and self-selected membership. Bioethics is perhaps best described as a kind of friendly club of intellectual inquisitors that virtually anyone can join. How then can one discern whether the advice and counsel received from a randomly selected bioethicist is of high quality, is only minimally competent, or is filled with errors that other bioethicists are more likely to avoid making?

It is tempting to consider the intellectual field of bioethics to be the creatively reflective application of conceptual precision and logical rigor to evaluations of morally good and bad human agency in the context of organizing, delivering, and financing healthcare, and to assume that bioethics includes a penetrating examination of medical care's relative social value. If that were true, error in bioethics might well be identifiable through an assessment of its reasoning processes and evaluation of bioethicists' behaviors as more or less consistent with some ideal intellectual standard. Yet the long-standing intellectual and methodological diversity of bioethics precludes such a simple analysis. The field of bioethics perhaps can be understood most accurately as a wide-ranging intellectual practice of reasoning and judgment about how well or poorly medical care experiences, in all varieties of expression, consistently and comprehensively cohere with those values and principles of right action and morally good ends that are claimed by the larger social community in which they occur. The major methodological approaches to bioethics include principalism, casuistry, virtue theory, and narrative ethics. What these approaches share is a deep concern with ethical reflection as a central component in socially worthy interpersonal (and for some, interspecies) relationships concerning welfare and, in particular, healthcare.

COMPETENCY AND ERROR
IN BIOETHICS

In general, erroneous statements have two components: they are contrary to established fact (that is, they are false), and they reflect the speaker's true or actual belief about that fact.[9] All bioethicists recognize that they make unintentionally erroneous statements, although they do not know they do so at the time they make them. Moreover, not all misstatements are errors, nor are all errors morally blameworthy. It is presumed that competent bioethicists keep current with relevant literature in bioethics and related fields, sincerely express their beliefs and uncertainties, and genuinely respect the dissenting opinions of others. When bioethicists discover on retrospection that they have erred, it is presumed that they will make a reasonable effort to share that discovery with those persons who may have been materially affected by it. However, because there is a paucity of general agreement concerning many components of bioethics consultation methodology and content, established facts in consultation are few and distinguishing errors from mere disagreements is difficult and complex.

TYPES OF ERROR

To make an error, one must make a mistake that is practically avoidable by either refraining from doing something or acting differently (that is, choosing a different discernible path[10] that leads to a measurably different process or outcome). Errors in bioethics are of two distinct but related types: outcome errors and procedural errors.

OUTCOME ERRORS
Outcome errors are judged (prospectively or retrospectively) to be undesirable because (1) they consist of negatively valued effects on identifiable persons, and (2) they are avoidable outcomes. Examples of outcome errors include loss or diminishment of the trust relationship or feelings of confidence and well-being among two or more of the principals (patient, family, health professionals); and significant diminishment of a patient's physical well-being. In any case, the outcome must have been avoidable through alternative decisions or different methods of reaching those decisions. Because the moral life partially consists in tragedy, not all negatively valued outcomes result from errors.

PROCEDURAL ERRORS
Procedural errors include the following: errors in identifying, gathering, and using relevant information including medical and legal facts; cognitive-pro-

cessing errors, especially logic, critical thinking, and moral imagining; use of an inappropriate perspective; an underappreciation of the importance of others' emotional vulnerability and the role emotion plays in rational deliberation; inadequate understanding or integration of theological and spiritual commitments, beliefs, and obligations in healthcare contexts; failure to recognize personal incompetence in a given circumstance; and failure to seek assistance when personal incompetence is recognized. Procedural errors may or may not result in outcome errors. In rare cases, procedural errors can result in good outcomes. Even if no procedural errors of reasoning are involved, the results of that reasoning may be applied in a given instance in inappropriate ways or in pursuit of unworthy social ends. Several types of procedural errors are discussed below.

Information-based errors. Because bioethics is a new field, it is often difficult to know when one is adequately detached from the issue at hand to be capable of providing a constructively critical analysis of its ethical dimensions both as perceived and unperceived by the principal players. The empirical, speculative, and interpersonal features that an ethics consultant decides to believe to be true about a particular case arise from at least three distinct sources of information and their associated claims for accuracy and completeness.

First are the oral reports, beginning with the case overview information that is communicated when the bioethicist initially receives a request for a consultation; these initial oral reports are later augmented with comments from different members of the healthcare team. Second are the written notes and factual records in the patient's medical chart that concern the ethical issues directly or indirectly. These may or may not include an explanation of why an ethics consultation is deemed appropriate. Third are the verbal comments, physical behaviors, and other types of input received from the patient, the patient's family, various health professionals, and other concerned parties whom the bioethicist interviews during the consultation process. Harvesting relevant information from these three sources is a difficult and complex task that requires well-developed moral imagination and broadly inquisitive searching techniques.

Cognitive-processing errors. It is tempting but wrong to conceive of the bioethics consultant as merely an intellectual receptacle for factual data and emotive and spiritual inputs. On such a view, the consultant analyzes the collected input within a selected ethical framework and uses the processed output to facilitate a consensus of opinion among the principals. Group consensus is grounded in the shared ethical findings as articulated by the bioethics consultant, and these findings are used to develop specific agreements and recommendations for decision making. The bioethics consultant never personally enters into the mix. Such a detached, impersonal role of positional objectivity suggests a comprehensive and carefully considered view of the case, but would actually be held by no one in particular. In practice, positional objectivity is an idealized state that, however deeply desired, can never be fully realized.[11]

Failure to recognize and to own one's personally influential role in the ethics consultation process is perhaps the most easily committed error, especially by inexperienced consultants. The very sequence of one's questions to others and the tonal influences with which they are posed can influence the respondents' choices and characterization of answers. The other involved parties often fail to appreciate this effect. Because positional objectivity is practically unachievable, the consultant's positional subjectivity must be acknowledged and self-critically assessed for its potential to influence the process of ethical reflection by others.

One of the bioethicist's most difficult tasks in case consultation and teaching is to ensure that one's efforts both accept and nurture the sovereignty of the persons with whom one is working. Sovereignty is the ability to be completely one's full self in an external world.[12] Ethical nurturing of others must be done in their own regard and not into the form, behavior, practice, or idea that the institution or bioethicist thinks is best for them. But sovereignty is not simply allowing the other person to do whatever he or she desires. Educational shepherding is required. The bioethicist provides his or her own self in guiding and shaping others to become more fully themselves.

In ethics case analysis, it is not uncommon for different observational claims and assessments to be both dependent upon health professionals and person-invariant. For example, nurses may view an ethical issue in the same way, and so too might respiratory therapists and physicians, but each group may disagree with the others' observational claims as the most accurate account of the relevant ethical features and how the tensions should be characterized and their importance prioritized. The bioethics consultant must hear and incorporate those diverse opinions within his or her own analysis, but then go beyond the shared beliefs and individual disagreements to facilitate a consensus for decision making. Under ideal circumstances, and with much supervised practice, an ethics consultant may be able to approximate a trans-positional scrutiny of ethical reasoning—but adopting the perspective of no one in particular is never fully achievable. No matter how personally disengaged bioethics consultants attempt to become, their reasoning and understanding of ethical matters depend in part on the knowledge and skills they learned in training as ethics consultants (and before) and on the type(s) of reasoning they are able to use under the circumstances. All of these influences contain the potential for contributing to procedural errors if they are not sensitively appreciated by the ethics consultant.

It is presumed that a properly trained and skilled ethics consultant will be well informed on the full range of ethical and other matters relevant to the case as a result of reading the bioethics literature and participating in professional conferences. The ethics consultant's expansive awareness and appreciation of the moral, legal, emotional, spiritual, interpersonal, communicative, and other complexities is thereby potentially greater than that of any other single participant in a case consultation. As a consequence, the competent ethics consultant may find more avenues of ethical agreement and consolidation among disputing or indecisive participants than the participants see themselves, and may use that understanding to facilitate a consensus among them. Alternatively, the consultant may find that there is actually more serious ethical disagreement among the participants than at first appears to them; the consultant may elect to illuminate gently that disagreement before the participants rush to judgment in apparent agreement concerning a particular decision that they may view retrospectively as ill advised or wrong.

In ethics consultation a facilitated discussion among the principals often identifies incomplete or inefficient prior communication or even miscommunication that, when uncovered and corrected, suggests a natural pathway out of the current conflict to well-grounded consensus. By illuminating these similarities and differences in beliefs, the bioethics consultant may be able to defuse conflict and find a pattern of shared beliefs that point toward resolution.[13] The consultant can show that more focused and exploratory discussion among the principals is critical and that a cooperatively developed care plan incorporating all relevant considerations would be helpful.

The chief danger for consultants in this role is mistaking their own ethical perceptions and judgments about what should be done and why as being somehow closer to the "truth" of the matter than are the ethical perceptions and judgments of others. Because their training in bioethics is itself the product of selective information and focused emphasis for analysis, ethics consultants cannot project their own perspectives as if they were a view from no place in particular. The consultant's perspective, like that of all the others, is itself position-dependent. Moreover, although the bioethics consultant should have diminished expectations of others' skills in ethical analysis, that is only because bioethics operates in an abnormal moral context, and not because the consultant is somehow ethically or intellectually superior to the other involved parties.[14] The position-dependence of the consultant's perspective suggests a third type of procedural error—perspective-based error.

Perspective-based error. In analyzing the various functions in bioethics consultation we might ask to what degree the gathering of data, methodological reasoning, formation of judgments, and drawing of conclusions should be expected to approximate positional invariance among different bioethics consultants. However, because ethics consultants are quite varied in their formal disciplinary training (philosophy, nursing, medicine, social work, religious studies, and so forth), agreement with a wide consensus among other consultants may be an unreasonable measurement in evaluating an individual's competency. An outlier's opinion may or may not be outright wrong. Three possible explanations for diversity in approaches to ethics consultation must be considered. First, it may be that the intellectual influences acquired during the consultant's prior disciplinary education and training were effectively neutralized through the process of ethics consultation training or experience itself, in whatever form it may have occurred. This seems unlikely, given the divergence between the subject matter of ethics and that of the other intellectual disciplines from which ethics consultants typically come (other than moral philosophy). A second possibility is that, although training in bioethics consultation may not neutralize one's existing intellectual habits and dominant perspective, it nonetheless may produce quite similar perspectives and attitudes among consultants with similar disciplinary backgrounds (such as philosophy, nursing, and so forth). If that is true, then philosophers trained as bioethics consultants will gather facts, reason, and formulate conclusions in roughly similar manners to one another, and so will nurses, although the two groups will do so in measurably different ways from each other. This too seems unlikely, although perhaps slightly more probable than the first possibility.

The third possibility is that formal ethics consultation training may have no discernible effect on trainees' existing reasoning methods and, thus, no reliable predictions can be made as to how a particular ethicist will address, consider, or draw conclusions about a particular case. Given the wide diversity in ethics consultation training and the absence of any clear standards for objectively measuring the content of case consultations, this last possibility seems more likely than the other two, but still far short of a general tendency. Evidence of thoroughgoing diversity in consultation opinions can be found in the wide variety of case commentaries that appear regularly in bioethics journals such as the *Hastings Center Report* and *HEC Forum*. On the other hand, as Ken Kipnis has pointed out, the diversity of consultants' opinions may be much more common in unusual or cutting-edge cases than in those more commonly occurring.[15]

These three possible explanations for diversity in bioethicists' perspectives and procedural approaches may or may not be ethically important. Whether variations in analytic methodologies contain errors of ethical significance depends more on how those methods contribute to empirically distinct outcomes than on whether some methods are better than others, independent of the outcomes they produce. The identification of error in ethics consultation is initially generated from an outcome that is perceived to be bad (one that is negatively valued), which catalyzes a review of the procedure that is used to attempt to explain how the undesired outcome came about. To argue, as some clinicians do, that philosophers, attorneys, religiously trained individuals, or nurses are not qualified to do clinical ethics consultation, because they cannot approximate the physician's perspective within the physician-patient relationship, requires more than equating perspective-based variation with error. It requires pointing to an empirically bad outcome that would not have occurred had the ethics consultant been a physician. But identifying a bad outcome as arising from a poor consultation process presupposes that there exists a gold standard of evaluative perspective from which such judgments can unerringly be made. The richly diverse disciplinary mix of bioethics provides evidence that such a singularly accurate perspective simply does not exist.

Underappreciation of the role of emotion. Virtually every bioethics case consultation involves significant emotional energy on the part of one or more of the principals involved. Emotional energy can both skew and enhance rationality, although having both effects simultaneously is rare. Emotional energy can be exacerbated or dulled by fatigue, nutritional imbalance, sleep deprivation, and other factors common in critical care, where the majority of bioethics consultations occur. Emotionality and rationality are not discreet psychological capacities, processes, or states, and the competent bioethics consultant needs to understand how the rationality of emotion and the emotionality of reason are interrelated.[16] Failure to do so can precipitate the error of dismissing the voice or sovereignty of emotionally charged principals. Equally erroneous perhaps is paying too much attention to the voice of nonemotional principals, mistaking their calculated logical voice for proper ethical orientation.

Inadequate understanding or integration of spiritual commitments. Just as bioethics consultants need to develop sensitivity to and proper integration of emotional rationality, they also need to understand and incorporate the importance of the spiritual dimensions of patient care. These dimensions are generally manifest through the claimed commitments of various participants. Spiritual beliefs and commitments partially define individual persons as moral agents. Offending, disregarding, misunderstanding, or showing other insensitivity to the importance of spiritual beliefs can hamper or distort proper ethical analysis through failing to respect the persons involved as the persons they are.

Consultants who practice in religiously supported institutions understand the theological values and principles that guide and motivate the institution's ministry of healthcare. Consultants who practice exclusively in public or secular institutions have no less of a need to appreciate the ethical importance of the religious commitments held by the case participants. Comprehensive understanding of comparative religious beliefs pertaining to healthcare decisions cannot reasonably be required, but understanding their relevance and importance can be required. For example, a non-Roman Catholic bioethics consultant may not be familiar with the U.S. Council of Catholic Bishops' Ethical and Religious Directives on medical care or what implications they hold for a Catholic physician managing the care of a pregnant, Roman Catholic patient with severe head trauma. But a competent consultant should recognize the importance of the patient's and the physician's theological commitments and seek additional ethical consultation with more knowledgeable colleagues, especially if a local priest is also unfamiliar with the directives, as often is the case. Failure to recognize the need to seek such help is another type of procedural error, that of experiential immaturity.

Experiential immaturity. Because bioethics consultation is an evolving intellectual enterprise, it is by nature a moving target. The consensus opinions of bioethicists generally and the professional maturity of individual bioethicists increase over time as a consequence of experiential and reflective maturation. Moreover, each bioethicist functions within a self-constructed and ever-maturing inner frame of reference within which he or she makes individual discernments, judgments, and decisions. As bioethicists mature and evolve in understanding, their abilities to discern and comprehend more complex ethical tensions and to respond to increasingly sophisticated clients also grow. Similar to what happens with health professionals, the experientially mature bioethicist develops a professional humbleness and self-critical awareness.

Just as skills and knowledge increase with experience, so too do one's personally established standards of performance. Teaching the same topic in bioethics to different groups such as medical students, residents, nursing students, nurses in the intensive care unit, administrators, and others requires different communication and pedagogic skills, not all of which can develop at the same time. A particular pedagogic approach that is well received by members of one group may not work equally well with other learners with different histories of experience in clinical contexts. Finding personal connections to experiences in different learners' memories usually requires drawing from a range of illustrative examples that are specific to particular work environments and professional roles. This diversity among learners' backgrounds often requires bioethics educators to employ widely differing pedagogic approaches in making the same moral point. Moreover, the bioethicist's own interpretation of which laws, institutional policies, professional ethical principles, and obligations are familiar to different learners will vary in proportion to their clinical experience, role within the institution, and personal interests. All of these factors must be assimilated by the bioethicist and used in various ways according to the manner and objectives of ethics educational presentations, including case consultations.

Bioethicists with limited experience will predictably make errors that more experienced bioethicists will anticipate and avoid. But this is no more true in bioethics than in any other profession that encompasses a range of human needs, attitudes, vulnerabilities, and goals. Key to avoiding error in this regard is the ability to recognize one's personal limitations and to seek appropriate assistance before participating further in the consultation. When an institution employs only one ethics consultant, that individual may find it difficult to admit to experiential shortcomings and to withdraw from a case for that reason; however, doing so would both reflect and enhance the consultant's occupational integrity.

Finally, the field of bioethics itself is rapidly maturing. Today bioethicists routinely discuss topics that previously did not garner attention. They have changed the way that they approach certain issues, recognizing that their earlier methods may have been simplistic or simply wrong (for example, pervasive clinical paternalism or insensitivity to different cultural and ethnic ethical perspectives). Judgments of error in bioethics always require a clear grasp of what was known and understood at the time the particular judgment was made. Retrospective identification of personal error, therefore, does not always require or justify retroactive blaming of the person who erred.

DISCOVERY OF ERROR

Occasional error in bioethics—as in any intellectual, emotional, and spiritual human enterprise—is ubiquitous and unavoidable. Human reasoning is not simple calculation and computation, and proper analytic reasoning in bioethics is richly emotive and spiritually sensitive. It is not merely a clinical-ethical subspecies of logical reasoning. Discovery of personal error by bioethicists may arise from a number of sources. These include attending conferences and reading relevant literature for new insights and deeper understanding of important relationships; uncovering new medical interventions; and applying new legal regulations, judicial rulings, and legislative precedents. New insights also can arise from learning new ways of perceiving ethical issues and their tensions as contained in the emotional or spiritual reactions to specific features of an ethics case or problem.

Each bioethicist functions with irreducible psychological influences on his or her perception and judgment of facts and events. Differences in perception and judgment create the potential for significant separation between (1) the contents of one's private consciousness and awareness; (2) the clinical, interrelational, and other features that are empirically present in the facts of the case; and (3) the perceptions and evaluations of those same features by other observers. These differences may account to a large extent for the reason that many disagreements in bioethics are factual or heuristic, rather than ethical.[17] Like all other participants, the bioethics consultant lacks thoroughgoing objectivity. On retrospection, a bioethicist may come to recognize an error as arising from a preconscious enhancement or diminishment of certain features of a case that reflects personally biased background beliefs, attitudes and sensitivities, agendas, mental imagery, thought processes, or priorities.

Communal perspective. The most consistently reliable reference frame from which judgments of error in bioethics can responsibly be drawn is the collective opinion of other bioethicists. Substantively divergent opinions about a particular case or issue in terms of the appropriate conceptual analysis or decision must rationally be justified to the satisfaction of other bioethicists. Failure to do so risks others' collective judgment that the outlier's opinions are not merely divergent but the result of one or more types of procedural error discussed above. Those with sustained patterns of opinion that diverge from the collective opinion of other bioethicists risk being labeled incompetent by the wider community. However, a general consensus may well be difficult to attain on deeply controversial issues; in regard to cases involving such controversial issues, widely held judgments of individual error—as opposed to respectful disagreements—are rare.[18]

EVALUATING ERROR IN BIOETHICS CONSULTATION

Error in case consultation, like error in any field, can be evaluated a number of ways. From an analytic standpoint, procedural errors may be the result of mistakes involving the aforementioned six components of information gathering, cognitive processing, perspective, emotional rationality, spiritual understanding, or experiential immaturity. Outcome errors may result from procedural errors, or they may be motivated by willfully intending to cause embarrassment or other harm to some identifiable person or institutional entity. Specific errors may be evaluated as morally blameworthy, even if the error was unintended, if it resulted from impaired or incompetent actions by the error maker. An important but separate question is whether ethics consultants can make errors of an unprofessional nature.

BIOETHICS CONSULTANTS AS PROFESSIONALS

Bioethics is an emerging intellectual field aimed at developing and perfecting specific forms of moral reflection on matters involving clinical skills and health policy. However, it lacks the internal authority and external recognition that fully established professions enjoy and the social expectations and obligations they serve. According to David Ozar, the key to a legitimate profession's authority is the relationship between the professional and client, which aims at bringing about certain values that the client desires or needs and are otherwise unavailable without the assistance of the professional's expertise. Moreover, professionals are expected to undertake certain personal sacrifices in service to their clients that other persons are not expected to undertake, such as health or financial risks by healthcare professionals, and social loss or criticism by legal professionals.[19] These values and risks are not part of the practice of bioethics in either its educational or clinical consultative roles. More importantly, there is no formally recognized set of professional norms or practices to which all ethics consultants agree. Indeed, there is not even an appropriately selective mechanism for identifying ethics consultants as distinctly skilled persons.[20]

If bioethics consultation is not a profession, it seems unlikely that practitioners can properly be accused of unprofessional conduct. At worst some may be described as acting in incompetent or unethical ways in reference to one or more of the methodological approaches currently in use. But such behaviors cannot be deemed unprofessional; there is no standard of performance unique to bioethics consultation by virtue of which any particular behavior can be externally judged to be competent or ethical, and therefore incompetent or unethical, except insofar as grossly incompetent and unethical behaviors can be readily identified by anyone, even nonconsultants. In this regard, the current practice of bioethics consultation services includes a risk of unknown magnitude of contributing to bad outcomes for innocent, trusting persons, under the guise of providing a service to enhance ethically reflective patient care by licensed health professionals.

EVALUATING THE ETHICS CONSULTANT

In what sense can the bioethics consultant be said to have gotten the consultation "right" in some minimally objective sense of right? That is, what counts as error in ethics case consultation, and by reference to what standard does it count as error? There are several ways to approach this question.

Beliefs. One evaluative standard is to examine how similar or different are various consultants' comments concerning the same case. This type of evaluation is comparable to the medical model in which clinical trainees' diagnoses and treatment plans are judged by attending physicians for clinical appropriateness. For instance, we might ask whether ethics consultants are like other healthcare professionals in that—although their training covers different times, methods, and instructors—their functional output upon completion of training is comparable. Do different ethics consultants' actions (that is, process, outcome, and reflective assessment) resemble one another in ways that are similar enough that a well-educated and experienced ethics consultant can provide "expert testimony" regarding a standard of care and whether that standard has been breached in a given case? Although this sounds like a reasonable empirical question, it has never been systematically tested on any basis involving large numbers of practicing consultants in different contexts, and therefore cannot serve as a reference standard for identifying error.

Setting aside normative questions concerning bioethics education,[21] is it possible to find a reasonable grounding for retrospective judgments of error in ethics consultations?[22] That is, given the diversity of background training and experiences among practicing ethics consultants and the absence of anything resembling a common content and training standard, from what perspective might one venture to say: "Consultant A made a mistake in case X"? Appeal to a consensus opinion of a cross-section of ethics consultation reviewers may not result in an internally consistent conclusion[23] or a consistent method of arriving at that conclusion. Indeed, given the variability in backgrounds and training of consultants, finding general agreement on the appropriateness of consultant A's actions might be even surprising. Moreover, there is a notable lack of consensus on the important aspects of consultation itself; some argue that substantive capability such as solid grounding in ethical theory is *de rigueur,* while others insist that communication skills and experience in mediation, arbitration, and conflict resolution are equally important as familiarity with ethical theory.[24]

Practices. If case consultation is not suited to statistical methods of evaluating appropriateness, perhaps a characterization of the roles or behaviors of clinical bioethicists would receive general agreement as either grievously objectionable or laudably exemplary, based on a widely shared understanding of the consultant's professional responsibility. In general, bioethics consultants seek to enhance ethical reflection in patient care and institutional policies. Building and advancing consensus of decision making among the principals is the most common activity.

Special duties. Are there additional responsibilities that befall bioethics consultants that are not generally assumed by other health professionals? Acting ethically is every professional's equal responsibility, but what about reporting unethical behavior by others? Is whistle-blowing a special moral requirement for bioethicists or an example of a courageously heroic act? Susan Sherwin argues as follows: "Silence in the face of [institutional or behavioral] moral wrongs is a serious breach of ethics for any profession, but it seems especially objectionable on the part of people whose profession is centered on questions of ethics."[25]

Whistle-blowing. A quick inventory of published reports concerning whistle-blowing in healthcare turns up precious few instances of ethics consultants' reporting of errors committed by their colleagues, despite a presumed expectation that ethics consultants would be more willing than other professionals to do so. This hesitancy to whistle-blow may be for practical reasons more than lack of courage.[26] To understand error in this regard, we must be clear about the relationship between legal and moral obligations so we can make sense of the moral concept of supererogation. Supererogation, which is defined as exceeding one's duty beyond what is minimally required, often serves as the identifying characteristic of moral heroes. When healthcare ethics is subsumed under healthcare law, the possibility of moral behavior becomes difficult to distinguish from lawful behavior. Supererogatory acts may even become rationally precluded, for if supererogation exists, it must be achievable by ordinary people. At the same time, failing to act in supererogatory ways can in no way be morally blameworthy, and this includes ethics consultants. The result of this complexity concerning whether bioethics consultants have special duties is that, as Sherwin states, "It is unclear how "success" [or failure] in the practice of ethics consultation is to be evaluated . . . [and there is] no obvious basis on which to resolve many of the difficult ethical disputes that exist among practitioners; there is not even any agreed on methodology available for discussing such issues."[27]

Policy development and revision. Bioethicists involved in patient care consultation sometimes uncover ethical issues with organizational parameters that may not be widely perceived as present. It is incumbent on the bioethicist not to mistake absence of open conflict for moral harmony in terms of the interpersonal relationships within a hospital unit. For example, even in well-functioning hospital units, there sometimes occur systematic but undetected deprivations of the rights and privileges of some participants, especially as they pertain to decision making. Concomitantly, bioethics consultants must be vigilantly cognizant of the type and degree of assistance they have been explicitly requested to provide, and acutely aware that they operate within a confounded, structured moral space that may itself reflect the hierarchical power structure of the employing institution.[28]

A bioethicist involved in a case consultation must be aware of the conceptual and operational distinctions between medical and organizational ethics and the consultant's role with respect to each. Rather than immediately addressing all of the ethically problematic issues he or she may perceive in a particular case, the ethics consultant needs to discern the range of his or her responsibilities and obligations owed to different participants in different regards. Thus, bioethicists who determine that conflict about patient care arises from a particular institutional policy may need to pursue a two-step resolution. Initially, a negotiated settlement may be pursued by seeking a one-time exception to an established but presently problematic policy. Later, a long-term resolution may be pursued at the level of administrative and organizational ethics. To illustrate, gay partners of patients may be excluded from overnight stays in some hospitals ostensibly because they are not related family members. Such a policy may warrant its own ethical review following a case in which the policy precipitates a conflict between a patient and the healthcare team. Often ethically problematic organizational issues are not readily apparent and require focused investigation to uncover. Upon review, the institution may elect to modify a particular policy or to encourage physicians to explicitly notify affected patients of a policy's existence prior to admission to the institution.

It has been suggested that one of the roles of an ethics consultant is to speak truth to those in power,[29] so perhaps engaging the institution's administration on organizational ethical issues (such as institutional pollution of the environment, justice in employment relations and practices, or obligations to serve the poor) also falls within the range of the healthcare ethics consultant's role.[30] On the other hand, if organizational ethics is outside the responsibility of particular ethics consultants, then those who choose to so engage their institutions on these matters are in error relative to the range of their proscribed duties and responsibilities. They are guilty of overstepping the boundaries of authority in which they are employed to work. Self-imposed limitation on one's work requires the exercise of discernment and judgment in carving out a domain of professional activity and then maintaining a moral stance within that domain. It becomes challenging to the ethicist's personal and occupational integrity, however, when obvious ethical wrongs exist within the institution and he or she is told to ignore them because they are not occupationally related concerns.[31]

These observations support the view that an internal morality of bioethics has not yet been developed and is not likely to appear soon. Before any profession's internal morality can be delineated, general agreement as to its overall goals and outcomes must be specified. This consensus is necessary so that evaluative measures can be developed to establish a standard of care for the profession and the range of reasonable and appropriate employer expectations.[32] An important determination in this latter regard is whether the role of the ethics consultant is understood to be strictly limited to the context of medical care or to encompass a broader scope of institutional and organizational issues. The final determination is likely to vary among institutions and individual consultants.

TOWARD A GENERAL STANDARD OF PRACTICE FOR BIOETHICS CONSULTATION

ERRORS IN JUDGMENT

Bioethics consultation begins but does not end with an ability to identify and consider the relevant ethical dimensions of a case, consult the appropriate resources, determine whether consensus exists on particular points, provide a referenced account of that consideration, and then facilitate consensus building among the principal decision makers involved in the case. Discernment and judgment tempered by practical wisdom are needed in each of these activities. The relevant bioethics and other literature is only rarely directly applicable to the details of an actual case consultation. This is because the range of published views by commentators is too wide, the issues and cases commonly discussed are rarely directly aligned with the one immediately at hand, and local interpersonal disagreements often abound, usually for unstated or unclear reasons.[33] Moreover, bioethics authors sometimes strive to make their position clear by overstating its cogency or overemphasizing its logical structure. Such philosophical rigor risks underappreciating the psychological-emotional, intellectual-spiritual, and other personal nuances wherein empirical (rather than theoretical) ethical tensions germinate and take shape. To take a commentator's opinion on a hypothetical case from the literature and dump it wholesale on an actual case would be an error in judgment; it would treat the contextually rich actual case as if it were ethically as thin as the published case description, which cases rarely exceed a couple of paragraphs.

Error in judgment itself must be further examined. How detailed must the competent consultant's judgment be? Must a consultant be able to address every aspect of a particular case in ethical detail? Logical perfection, exhaustive comprehensiveness of relevant considerations, and heuristic infallibility are unreasonable minimum standards in ethics consultation, just as they are in any intellectual activity. For a reasonable standard of care in bioethics consultation to exist, it must be widely applicable in different institutional contexts and sufficiently sensitive to personal differences that it avoids rigidly mechanical procedures. Before bioethicists rush to develop a standard of care, they should cautiously consider its advisability.

DEVELOPING BIOETHICS CONSULTATION GUIDELINES

In medicine, the standard of care is based on the considered opinions of recognized authorities with expertise in particular fields of medicine. Clinical practice guidelines have been developed to augment practitioners' interpretations of appropriate medical care and to provide an additional degree of stability to their understanding of the standard of care as articulated by the authorities. The Institute of Medicine defines clinical practice guidelines as "systematically developed statements to assist practitioner and patient decisions about appropriate health care for specific clinical circumstances."[34]

Bioethics has nothing resembling clinical practice guidelines at present. Before bioethicists consider developing and implementing such guidelines, they should carefully examine the motivations supporting this activity. Several important points can be gleaned from experience with clinical practice guidelines in medicine. When these guidelines are combined with considerations of financial costs of care, they can lead to questions of quality improvement imperatives versus stewardship responsibilities. Daniel Callahan has warned that as clinical practice guidelines increase in number, institutions can be tempted to pursue cost containment under the cloak of quality improvement and to implement guidelines without adequate empirical justification.[35] For all their supporting arguments, clinical practice guidelines raise problems related to quality control, methods used to develop them, and interrater reliability.[36]

Practice guidelines in ethics consultation are likely to face even more pronounced difficulties than their clinical counterparts. While guidelines aimed at improving clinical practice admit of certain ethical advantages, practice guidelines in ethics consultation likely will not be able to draw on the same expert panel consensus on substantive matters, resulting in a dearth of guidance precisely where it is most needed. For example, one of the reported ethical advantages of practice guidelines is clarification of individual ethical goals of medical care through improved communication between practitioners and patients. But there is no cause-and-effect relationship between clarifying ethical differences and resolving them that ethics consultation can effect, as some might hope. Indeed, clarifying disagreements may serve to accentuate them in stark contrast, thereby risking the deepening of disagreement into open conflict. In such cases, the bioethics consultation could have the unhappy effect of making matters worse. Whereas clinical guidelines may help delineate certain factors pertaining to triage under the parameters of managed care, ethics guidelines may instead question the very triage method that clinicians are expected to use. Here, again, the line separating clinical ethics and organizational ethics becomes seriously blurred.

Practice guidelines also carry several inherent risks related to expert judgment. In the early years of clinical practice guidelines, a shortage of appropriately focused, well-designed empirical studies required an over-reliance on the expert judgment of panels of selected authorities. Typically the authorities were specialist clinicians known anecdotally for their standards of excellence in the delivery of healthcare or by impressive published records using statistical techniques to analyze treatment outcomes.[37] In ethics consultation the problem is exacerbated, for there are precious few consultants specializing in sub-areas of clinical ethics, such as neonatal intensive care, geriatric medicine, or mental health. Most ethics consultants function as generalists. Moreover, the absence of well-designed empirical studies in clinical ethics literature has been a comparatively long-standing deficiency.[38]

If ethics practice guidelines eventually are developed, however imperfectly, ethics consultation may risk becoming rigidly defined in terms of those guidelines, both in substance and process. If that occurs, variation in consultation methods and objectives may significantly diminish or even cease, especially among consultants who are cautious about litigation. The opportunity to learn from nonstandard consultation techniques would, concomitantly, disappear. This last point was a key reason the Society for Health and Human Values-Society for Bioethics Consultation Task Force on Standards for Bioethics Consultation (SHHV-SBC Task Force) rejected the credentialing of bioethics consultants as a model for developing increased professionalism and socially legitimated power.[39] The current variation in consultation techniques and rich mixture of disciplinary backgrounds is a catalyst for keeping bioethics consultation, scholarship, and conferences vitally alive and thoroughly engaged in a wide range of issues.

The greatest challenge may be to design ethics consultation practice guidelines in a controlled but flexible way so that the emerging standard of care can grow and mature. New analytic and investigative techniques and ways of understanding religious faith traditions, feminist concerns and methods, and the special ethical needs of cognitively and physically challenged patients must be carefully studied. Sensitivity to detecting, synthesizing, and analyzing rapid development in these regards requires careful follow-up collection and analysis of outcomes data from standard as well as innovative interventions.[40] Currently, outcomes data in ethics consultation are almost nonexistent beyond simple satisfaction surveys sent, after the fact, to selected subgroups of consultation "consumers," and analysis of even those data has been frustratingly inconclusive. A further question is whether the development of practice guidelines can safeguard patients' values rather than becoming a tool for institutional or organizational imperialism.[41] Finally, there is some reason to believe that the values of laypersons may differ from those of professional bioethicists, even if they were to agree on the same medical facts of particular cases.[42]

THE BIG PICTURE IN BIOETHICS CONSULTATION: A PUZZLE IN PIECES

The initial goals of ethics case consultation were to develop modes of ethical inquiry within the clinical context and to focus on particular patients' circumstances. Middle-level ethical principles and time-tested moral rules were identified as appropriate guides for analysis of ethical issues and conflicts, with the intent of resolving ethical uncertainty, confusion, and conflict. However, critics of those principles argued that they were too narrow or too abstract to be useful in responding to the range of issues arising in acute-care settings, and these critics called for a theoretical augmentation to principalism.[43] Proponents of casuistry, virtue ethics, and narrative ethics each spoke up in response to this call, and the end result was that no single methodological approach was widely judged to be adequate to the task as globally conceived. As these theoretic and metatheoretic matters were being developed and debated, several practical matters also emerged that suggested that a widespread confusion existed over the proper role of the ethics consultant as distinct from other roles that were already well established in the clinical setting. Some argued that the function of ethics consultation was embedded in everyone's responsibility, and therefore a new, explicit role was not required. The functions were performed piecemeal by clinicians, utilization review, quality assurance, pastoral care, and patient advocates in the admissions or business offices. The proper role of clinical ethicist *qua* ethicist is still a matter of debate, but general agreement has been reached on four illegitimate roles: ethics social worker, ethics police officer, secular clergy, and patient advocate.[44]

The current state of affairs in bioethics consultation is decidedly undecided. There are troubling pragmatic questions regarding the goals, roles, methods, and training of clinical ethicists. There is lack of agreement as to the proper relationship of clinical ethics to moral philosophy, law, medicine, religion, and organizational ethics. This lack of agreement is more the result of widespread uncertainty than of disagreement among those with strongly held positions. Still, some areas with broad consensus do exist and can be used to identify potential areas for marking identifiable errors in clinical ethics consultation.

The most common reasons for requesting ethics consultations include reassurance that adequate and appropriate consideration of ethically relevant matters has been accomplished; mediation of interpersonal conflict involving participants; emotional support in care of the dying; identification or clarification of ethical issues in complex cases; minimization of exposure to legal liability; and interpretation and explanation of institutional policies, or law, or both. Proper goals of ethics consultations include responding directly to the reasons for requesting consultations mentioned above with the exception of reducing legal liability (and, for some commentators, conflict mediation). A range of specific objectives for reaching these goals include the following: avoiding ethically poor outcomes by focusing on enforcement of legal requirements, institutional policies, and established hierarchy of decision making; ensuring ethically appropriate process by focusing on patients' autonomy through assessment of competency, advance directives, and shared decision making with the patient, a proxy, or families, as appropriate; achieving the best possible ethical outcomes through proper use of integrity-preserving compromise;[45] enhancing self-awareness and increased knowledge of relevant ethical principles, methodology, and justification; and balancing the ethical primacy of individual autonomy with responsible stewardship of resources.[46]

ENFORCING ETHICS

One reason clinical ethics remains adrift methodologically is that it feels, even to itself, like a round peg in a square hole. The medical model of consultation is most familiar to health professionals and emphasizes a hierarchy of authority with the attending physician at the summit. Ethics consultation, in contrast, relies much more on shared participation among multiple participants and a balance of authority, with the competent patient or proxy nominally at the summit. This is not a small difference in the perception of appropriate authority. Many health professionals feel their authority to be at risk by engaging in deliberations so differently structured. Some ethics consultants may seek a widely participatory deliberative process and argue that whatever results from a good process is, by definition, the best possible ethical outcome. But many health professionals believe that an evaluation focused solely or even principally on a patient-centered deliberative process—rather than on achievement of the best possible outcomes from medically appropriate interventions—risks suboptimal medical-ethical outcomes. In addition, health professionals note that patients' or proxies' authoritative decision-making power is often encumbered by medical ignorance, overemphasis on fear of pain, impairment of mobility, disfigurement, or other considerations that health professionals deem peripheral to good decision making. The relative clinical authority of an ethics consultant and that of a medical consultant are not directly analogous, and the patient's authority is of a third kind—a negotiated power that exists within a specific professional-client relationship. It is important that bioethicists not allow themselves to come between the two parties simply because their points of discussion have ethically rich content.[47] Ethics is not law, and bioethics consultation is not a club to be used to force health professionals, patients, or family members to behave as others want them to behave.

One basic difference between ethics and law turns on the ability of their respective conclusions to effect change in the world. Law has the power of enforceable sanctions behind its rulings, whereas ethical arguments, however persuasively concluded, end with the hope that the listener will act in accord with the conclusion. The ethicist recognizes that there generally is no recourse if the listener opts for the ethically inferior, even morally blameworthy, act. This is one frustration occasionally voiced by ethics consultants. They may offer well-considered insights and occasionally even advice, only to have them disregarded;

at the same time, they are told that they are still valued because "ethics had its moment." Sometimes the ethics consultant feels marginalized and ineffective because his or her contribution never became operational. The consultant has only persuasive power with which to effect change, and simply being well heard feels personally inadequate.

Moral philosophers and theologians have long recognized a distinction between legal and ethical rights and duties. However, the evolving corporatization of healthcare organizations and the subsequent need to standardize relationships across increasingly large employee and patient groups enhances the effects of institutionalization on interpersonal relations. This often leads to the creation of rules and policies powered by legal rather than ethical concerns. Some organizations attempt to protectively enforce morally obligatory behaviors by subsuming them under legal requirements and subjecting affected participants to regulatory oversight. These combined legal-ethical duties apply to all combinations of relations among patients, health professionals, and their associated corporate healthcare entities. The nesting together of ethical rights and duties under legal rights and duties changes the essentially personal ethics context into an impersonal and legal one, and thereby risks the depersonalization of interpersonal relations. Concern with this trend may partially explain why attorneys are the fastest-growing subgroup among bioethicists.[48]

Although conceptual philosophic distinctions between ethics and law can still be made, distinguishing their empirical contents in modern healthcare contexts is more difficult. Law is a social value aimed at establishing and maintaining the social order through settled opinions and normative judgments. Ethics is a cultural value aimed at clarification of issues pertaining to personal identity and integrity, and interpersonal or intergroup relationships, rights, and obligations. When bioethicists seek a pathway to enable others to achieve their own moral sovereignty, perfection is not possible, and making mistakes in bioethics is an inevitable component of its educational as well as consultative activities. The bioethicist's objective cannot be to avoid mistakes completely, so that if he or she fails to avoid all mistakes he or she somehow has failed globally. Rather, the goal is to avoid obvious, easy mistakes, to recognize one's own mistakes when they occur, and to learn from them. One especially important caution to bioethicists when doing ethics education or consultation is to avoid having preconceived expectations of the outcome. When that happens, those expectations get in the way of one's own efforts at freeing the others to seek their own pathways to improved well-being. The bioethicist ends up striving for some predetermined end point rather than receiving what is there as the raw, autonomous material with which to work.

CONCLUSION

Ethical authority is grounded in rational persuasion using shared assumptions as starting points. Descriptively, competency in bioethics consultation is a rational faculty of investigation, discovery, processing, decision making, and critical reflection concerning ethical issues in healthcare. Normatively, a minimum threshold standard of competency has never been established and, therefore, evaluating an individual's competence for quality and error is difficult and complex. It is difficult because the field of bioethics does not have an identifiable body of knowledge that all competent consultants are known to have mastered according to standardized measurements, and it does not use methodologies that are widely recognized as consistently producing desired results. The goals of bioethics consultation vary significantly in particular circumstances, and the social legitimation of authority in bioethics is not formally recognized by any credentialing body or office. Judgments of error in bioethics consultation are not made using standardized review mechanisms or accepted standards of professional performance. Finally, bioethics consultation, by nature, is principally educational and advisory, which limits the effective power of consultations to persuading clinicians and other principals of the need and value of self-critical ethical reflection. Attributing error to an ethics consultant therefore requires consideration of the responsibility of the consultation "consumer" to be a prudent purchaser of ethical insight and advice.

Errors in bioethics consultation can be distinguished according to whether they are or are not morally blameworthy. Some errors result from personal inexperience and must be considered part of the normal risk of using otherwise competent consultants who have not fully matured, just as is the case with competent clinicians of varying experience and expertise. Morally blameworthy errors occur when the consultant personally contributes to an avoidable event or outcome that should have been anticipated. Identifying an error requires also identifying the alternative pathway that should have been recognized as superior and that could reasonably be known to avoid the bad outcome that occurred. Error in bioethics consultation can be either well or poorly motivated and reflect either good or bad character in the bioethicist. Character considerations notwithstanding, error in bioethics consultation can be distinguished along two basic lines—outcome errors and procedural errors.

Outcome errors are negatively valued effects on one or more of the principals and include a diminishment or loss of trust, confidence, or well-being. Procedural errors include avoidable mistakes involving information gathering, cognitive processing, perspective, emotional rationality, spiritual understanding, and experiential immaturity. Self-discovery of procedural errors proceeds from one's own maturing insight into psychological influences on discernment and judgment and as measured against the collective opinions of respected consultant colleagues.

NOTES

1. B. Gert, C.M. Culver, and K.D. Clouser, *Bioethics: A Return to Fundamentals* (New York: Oxford University Press, 1997).

2. R.M. Wettstein, "Competence," in *Encyclopedia of Bioethics*, ed. W.T. Reich (New York: Simon & Schuster Macmillan, 1995), 1: 445-51.

3. See F.E. Baylis, "A Profile of the Health Care Ethics Consultant," in *The Health Care Ethics*

Consultant, ed. F.E. Baylis (Totowa, N.J.: Humana, 1994), 25-44; Society for Health and Human Values-Society for Bioethics Consultation Task Force on Standards for Bioethics Consultation, *Core Competencies for Health Care Ethics Consultation* (Glenview, Ill.: American Society for Bioethics and Humanities, 1998).

4. H. Brody, *The Healer's Power* (New Haven, Conn.: Yale University Press, 1992).

5. See S.M. Wolf, "Quality Assessment of Ethics in Health Care: The Accountability Revolution," *American Journal of Law & Medicine* 20, no. 1 & 2 (1994): 105-28; S. Fry-Revere, "Some Suggestions for Holding Bioethics Committees and Consultants Accountable," *Cambridge Quarterly of Healthcare Ethics* 2 (1993): 449-55; and L.S. Schierton, "Measuring Hospital Ethics Committee Success," *Cambridge Quarterly of Healthcare Ethics* 2 (1993): 495-504.

6. In the mid-1980s the original requirements for membership to the Society for Bioethics Consultation included a nomination and review process. That requirement was withdrawn as the society's financial solvency became threatened from low numbers of eligible dues-paying members.

7. American Society for Bioethics and Humanities Membership Committee, personal communication, February 1999.

8. W.T. Reich, ed., *Encyclopedia of Bioethics,* 2nd ed. (New York: Simon & Schuster Macmillan, 1995).

9. I. Thalberg, "Error," in *Encyclopedia of Philosophy,* ed. P. Edwards (New York: Macmillan, 1967), 45-8.

10. I owe this notion of a "discernibly path" in this context to T.A. Cavanaugh's remarks at the International Association of Bioethicists Annual Meeting, Tokyo, Japan, November 1998.

11. A. Sen, "Positional Objectivity," *Philosophy and Public Affairs* 22, no. 2 (1993): 126-45.

12. M. Kabat-Zinn and J. Kabat-Zinn, *Everyday Blessings: The Art of Mindful Parenting* (New York: Hyperion, 1997).

13. B.J. Spielman, "Conflict in Medical Ethics Cases: Seeking Patterns of Resolution," *The Journal of Clinical Ethics* 4, no. 3 (Fall 1993): 212-8.

14. For a discussion of diminished expectations of others in abnormal moral context, see C. Calhoun, "Responsibility and Reproach," *Ethics* 99 (1989): 389-406; T. Isaacs, "Cultural Context and Moral Responsibility," *Ethics* 107 (1997): 670-84.

15. K. Kipnis, Internet-based MCW bioethics discussion forum, 1998. The MCW Bioethics discussion forum is a restricted access site on the worldwide web and is administered through the Medical College of Wisconsin, Milwaukee. For more information about the discussion forum, please contact the author at < paulj@kvi.net >.

16. R. DeSousa, *The Rationality of Emotion* (Boston: MIT Press, 1987).

17. See note 1 above, p. 45.

18. The assisted suicide of more than 130 persons by Jack Kevorkian is an example of behavior receiving virtually universal disapproval by bioethicists, including those who strongly advocate for the legalization of assisted suicide. More controversial, however, is the proposal for recognizing a "care ethic" in bioethics as only a concept and not a complete theory or ethical framework. Those supporting recognizing a care ethic include C. Gilligan, *In a Different Voice: Psychological Theory and Women's Development* (Cambridge, Mass.: Harvard University Press, 1982); N. Noddings, *Caring: A Feminist Approach to Ethics and Moral Education* (Berkeley, Calif.: University of California Press, 1984); P. Benner and J. Wrubel, *The Primacy of Caring: Stress and Coping in Health and Illness* (Menlo Park, Calif.: Addison-Wesley, 1989).

Published criticisms of this approach as less than a full theoretic foundation and methodology include H.L. Nelson, "Against Caring," *The Journal of Clinical Ethics* 3, no. 1 (Spring 1992): 8-15; E.H. Loewy, "Care Ethics: A Concept in Search of a Framework," *Cambridge Quarterly of Healthcare Ethics* 4, no. 1 (1995): 56-83, and E. Loewy, "Of Sentiment, Caring and Anecephalics: A Response to Sytsma," *Theoretical Medicine and Bioethics: Philosophy of Medical Research and Practice* 19, no. 12 (1998): 21-34.

19. See D. Ozar, "Profession and Professional Ethics," in *Encyclopedia of Bioethics,* ed. W.T. Reich (New York: Simon & Schuster Macmillan, 1995), 2103-11.

20. The American Society for Bioethics and Humanities guidelines, *Core Competencies for Health Care Ethics Consultation,* is a new and promising effort to address this problem of ethics consultants' skills. See note 3 above.

21. S. Sherwin, "Certification of Health Care Ethics Consultants: Advantages and Disadvantages," in *The Health Care Ethics Consultant,* ed. F.E. Baylis (Totowa, N.J.: Humana, 1994), 11.

22. I am not considering here situations in which an ethics consultant makes patently obvious errors of fact or logic. Such errors are readily identifiable by nonconsultants as well, and errors of this type are common in all professional activities. Thus, they are not controversial as errors specific to the practice of ethics consultation.

23. See E. Fox's discussion of a case study showing wide variation on remarks by bioethics consultants, in J.A. Tulsky and E. Fox, "Evaluating Ethics Consultation: Framing the Question," *The Journal of Clinical Ethics* 7, no. 2 (Summer 1996): 109-15.

24. A. Lynch, ". . . Has Knowledge of [Interpersonal] Facilitation Techniques and Theory: Has the Ability to Facilitate [Interpersonally] . . . " in *The Health Care Ethics Consultant,* ed. F.E. Baylis, (Totowa, N.J.: Humana, 1994), 45-62. See also the interim report of the SHHV-SBC Task Force on Standards for Bioethics Consultation. The final version appears as the *Core Competencies for Health Care Ethics Consultation,* see note 3 above.

25. See note 21 above, p. 14.

26. B. Freedman, "From Avocation to Vocation: Working Conditions for Health Care Ethics Consultants," in *The Health Care Ethics Consultant,* ed. F.E. Baylis (Totowa, N.J.: Humana, 1994), 109-32 at 128; B. Freedman, "Where Are the Heroes of Bioethics?" *The Journal of Clinical Ethics* 7, no. 4 (Winter 1996): 297-300. See also P.J. Reitemeier, "Perhaps We All Be Heroes," *The Journal of Clinical Ethics* 7, no. 4 (Winter 1996): 307-9.

27. See note 21 above, p. 48.

28. S.E. Kelly et al., "Understanding the Practice of Ethics Consultation: Results of an Ethnographic Multi-Site Study," *The Journal of Clinical Ethics* 8, no. 2 (Summer 1997): 136-49.

29. This interpretation of the healthcare ethics professional was suggested by Judith Andre at an Ethics Grand Rounds, Medical College of Wisconsin, Milwaukee, May 1997.

30. D. Schiedermayer and J. LaPuma, "The Ethics Consultant and Ethics Committees, and their Acronyms: IRBs, HECs, RM, QA, UM, PROs, ICPs, and HREAPs," *Cambridge Quarterly of Healthcare Ethics* 2 (1993): 469-75.

31. P.J. Reitemeier, "Integrity and the Role of the Pharmacist," in *Ethical Dimensions of Pharmaceutical Care,* ed. A.M. Haddad and R.A. Buerki (New York: Haworth, 1996), 125-36.

32. Freedman, "From Avocation to Vocation," see note 26 above, 116.

33. Freedman makes a similar point in "From Avocation to Vocation," ibid.

34. Quoted in K.N. Lohr, "Guidelines for Clinical Practice: What They Are and Why They Count," *Journal of Law, Medicine and Ethics* 23, no. 1 (1995): 49-56.

35. D. Callahan, *Setting Limits: Medical Goals in an Aging Society* (New York: Simon & Schuster, 1987).

36. See note 34 above.

37. R.L. Kane, "Creating Practice Guidelines: The Dangers of Overreliance on Expert Judgment," *Journal of Law, Medicine and Ethics* 23, no. 1 (1995): 62-4.

38. B. Brody, "Assessing Empirical Research in Bioethics," *Theoretical Medicine* 14, no. 3 (September 1993): 211-9; J. Sugarman, "Should Hospital Ethics Committees Do Research?" *The Journal of Clinical Ethics* 5, no. 2 (Summer 1994): 121-5; E. Pellegrino, "The Limitation of Empirical Research in Ethics," *The Journal of Clinical Ethics* 6, no. 2 (Summer 1995): 161-2.

39. SHHV-SBC Task Force on Standards for Bioethics Consultation, "Discussion Draft," 14 October 1997, see note 24 above.

40. See note 37 above.

41. J. Halpern, "Can the Development of Practice Guidelines Safeguard Patient Values?" *Journal of Law, Medicine and Ethics* 23, no. 1 (Spring 1995): 75-81.

42. R.M. Veatch, "Consensus of Expertise: The Role of Consensus of Experts in Formulating Public Policy and Estimating Facts," *Journal of Medicine and Philosophy* 16 (1991): 427-45.

43. See, for instance, "Theories and Methods in Bioethics: Principlism and its Critics," a special issue of the *Kennedy Institute of Ethics Journal* 5, no. 3 (September 1995); R.B. Davis, "The Principlism Debate: A Critical Overview," *Journal of Medicine and Philosophy* 20 (1995): 85-105.

44. T.F. Ackerman, "Medical Ethics in the Clinical Setting: A Critical Review of Its Consultive, Pedagogical and Investigative Methods," in *Clinical Medical Ethics: Exploration and Assessment,* ed. T.F. Ackerman et al. (Lanham, Md.: University Press of America, 1987): 145-73.

45. The best discussion of integrity-preserving compromise is in M. Benjamin, *Splitting the Difference: Compromise and Integrity in Ethics and Politics* (Lawrence, Kans.: University Press of Kansas, 1990).

46. G. Kanoti and S. Youngner, "Ethics Consultation," in *Encyclopedia of Bioethics*, ed. W.T. Reich (New York: Simon & Schuster Macmillan, 1995): 404.

47. B.J. Crigger, "Negotiating the Moral Order: Paradoxes of Ethics Consultation," *Kennedy Institute of Ethics Journal* 5, no. 2 (1995): 89-112.

48. Unpublished demographic data from my 1996 survey of registered members of three leading bioethics organizations in the United States (American Association of Bioethics, Society for Bioethics Consultation, and Society for Health and Human Values). In 1998 these three organizations merged to form the American Society for Bioethics and Humanities (ASBH), which is now the leading organization of its kind. Presented in poster form at the annual meeting of ASBH in Houston, Texas, November 1998, and as an invited paper presented at the 4th World Congress, International Association of Bioethics, Tokyo, Japan, November 1998.

16

Errors in Ethics Consultation

Ellen W. Bernal

INTRODUCTION: SKILLS AND COMPETENCIES
IN ETHICS CONSULTATION

There has been a perplexing lack of conversation about errors in ethics consultation. The relative silence may result from personal and professional concerns about the profession's early stage of development. Even though ethics consultation has considerable historical background in medical consultation, religious traditions, and research ethics, the first "ethics consultants" only began practice in the 1960s and 1970s.[1] For those who now wish to establish and maintain an ethics consultation practice, talking about errors can raise sensitive concerns about the legitimacy of the profession and even of one's own expertise. If there is lack of consensus about the goals and standards of ethics consultation, identifying mistakes will also be an uncertain enterprise.

The recently published report of the American Society for Bioethics and Humanities (ASBH Report), *Core Competencies for Health Care Ethics Consultation,* is a significant step forward. The document describes the skills, competencies, and habits that ethics consultants should use as they seek to help patients and others directly involved in patient care with difficult questions that may arise in clinical settings. The *Core Competencies* state that the general goal of ethics consultation is to "improve the provision of health care and its outcome through the identification, analysis, and resolution of ethical issues as they emerge in consultation regarding particular clinical cases in health care institutions."[2] Intermediary goals include identifying and analyzing the nature of the value uncertainty or conflict that underlies a consultation, facilitating resolution of conflicts, developing policies and quality improvement activities, and providing ethics education. The *Core Competencies* then describes the skills in ethical assessment, skills in process, and interpersonal skills that the ethics consultant, consulting team, or full ethics committee requires to be effective.

Many organizations and professionals have joined and contributed to the effort of defining ethics consultation. One noteworthy example is the Sparrow Hospital Task Force in East Lansing, Michigan. The task force spent a year evaluating ethics consultations at Sparrow Hospital. They agreed that "the purpose of an ethics consultation is to promote ethical resolution of 'uncertainties and disagreements' in health care settings." Because the Sparrow Hospital report was developed for a particular institution, it is more specific and detailed than the *Core Competencies*. The hospital task force created operational statements of all the identified goals, a form for evaluating consultations, a guide for doing ethics consultation in the future, and useful examples for case reports that would be helpful for someone "learning the trade" and to the hospital specifically.[3] In contrast to the *Core Competencies*, the Sparrow Hospital report emphasizes the importance of using respectful communication to help those involved to work through ethical issues on their own.

The *Core Competencies* document and the Sparrow Hospital document offer descriptions of current practice, according to its development over the past 30 years. When the modern bioethics movement first began, even such foundational terms as *ethical principles, bioethicist,* and *ethics consultation* needed definition. The general meaning of these terms is now routine for bioethicists, and the current expanse of literature, professional societies, and educational organizations speaks to the field's development. In effect, the documents provide shorthand descriptions of the accumulated skills and competencies of experienced ethics consultants. But the fact that at times we still need to define our role to patients and surrogates is a reminder that this taken-for-granted knowledge does rest on construction of meaning.

The *Core Competencies* and the Sparrow Hospital description open rich opportunities for dialogue with others about ethics consultation. They may eventually lead to specific curricula, rules of conduct, and quality standards. But even with these documents or later versions, we will never be able to specify fully, in advance, the correct actions that an ethics consultant should take in a particular situation, or show how to avoid all errors. Despite advances in detailed description, ethics consultation remains a complex, skilled performance that unfolds over time. Even routine ethics cases require skilled judgment. An especially difficult, complex, or unusual case requires greater innovation on the part of the ethics consultant, and it involves a greater risk of error.

This chapter distinguishes between mistakes and errors, and outlines their relation to routine and innovative action; describes ethics consultation as a skilled achievement that cannot be fully specified in rules; describes and comments on four personal accounts of error provided by ethics consultant colleagues; and draws out implications and suggestions for ways to support ethics consultants and committees so that practice can continue to develop and improve.

THE RELATION OF MISTAKES AND ERRORS
TO ROUTINE AND INNOVATIVE PERFORMANCE

A number of modern social theorists have claimed that mistakes are a product of ordinarily hidden, self-serving motivations.[4] Freud claimed that mistakes reveal "drives,"[5] and Goffman asserts that "unmeant gestures" spoil the public impression a group is trying to "stage, in order to maintain social control and power."[6] Both of these perspectives overlook the creative, responsible features of human activity, particularly in the professions. Although it is certainly important to examine critically the foundations of ethics consultation and the motivations and character of those who provide it, the present discussion assumes that ethics consultation is a professional service activity, provided by persons of good character and will.

As persons, we live and act in a temporal context—Merleau-Ponty's "being in the world."[7] On a daily and lifetime basis, we accomplish any number of projects in collaboration with many other people. Through learning and experience, we develop skills and interpretive frameworks so that many of our achievements are accomplished routinely, and seemingly without effort. In routine performance, intellectual effort is dormant but not absent. In innovative, complex, or difficult performance, the person's struggle to comprehend and influence a situation becomes more apparent.[8]

Mistakes and errors are signs of situations in which a person's actions, taken to accomplish a particular task, prove to be ineffective. The origins of the words *mistake* and *error* each call attention to construction of meaning in time.[9] A mistake is a relatively isolated incident in a relatively short time frame. Here we say, "I made a mistake" or "I was wrong about that." We do not ordinarily say that one has "persisted in a mistake." A mistake can be based on a misapprehension of the significance of a particular situation or event, or a misunderstanding of our own obligations in the situation. It seems to refer to an overreach of skills in perception and identification. As an example, an ethics consultant is speaking with the adult son of an acutely ill trauma patient. The nursing staff has described the son, who is demanding to see the attending physician immediately, as "difficult" and "suspicious," and at first the ethics consultant had this same impression. But, with further discussion, the ethics consultant recognizes the basis for the son's demands: his father's sudden, devastating injury; ongoing problems in meeting with the physician; the son's lack of sleep; and the strangeness of the hospital setting. Once the ethics consultant's perception shifts, reorientation and redirection can follow, along with enhanced effectiveness in helping the family member. We often redirect our actions before a potential mistake or, after the fact, recognize that we have made a mistake and seek ways to adjust the situation to a better course.

An error is more persistent and extended than a mistake. The term *error* means "wandering" or "straying from a path" and requires greater reinterpretation and reorientation of the situation.[10] An error also seems to strike more deeply at one's own sense of person. We are more likely to identify with an error by saying "I was wrong." An error in ethics consultation may also have more serious consequences for the patient or others involved.

We are more likely to make both mistakes and errors in situations that are out of the ordinary, complex, or novel, because the requirement of greater innovation carries with it the possibility of greater risk. In these situations, we are "pioneering" rather than taking a familiar path.[11] But even in routine ethics consultations, the consultant is continually shaping meaning and understanding, changing actions according to the situation at hand. A typical, composite ethics consultation often goes something like this:

> The unit coordinator of the cardiac stepdown unit calls to say that the family of Mr. A. would like to speak to the ethicist. The patient's nurse has suggested the ethics consultation. In speaking with her briefly, I learn that the patient is a 68-year-old, married gentleman recently retired from teaching chemistry at the university. He and his wife have three adult children. He was admitted for cardiac surgery after experiencing increased pain and difficulty with activity. After the surgery, he had a series of unexpected complications, including a stroke, infection, and problems with breathing. He is currently receiving ventilator support. His wife and adult children are struggling with decisions about life-sustaining treatment. Upon arriving on the unit, I learn that a meeting between the family and attending physician is about to take place, and I ask if I can join. When everyone agrees, I participate in the meeting. I help the family speak with the physician about Mr. A.'s diagnosis and prognosis, and help them explore what the patient's goals might be in light of his current circumstances. I outline the ethical basis for decisions that may need to be made and provide appropriate levels of ethical, spiritual, and emotional support. By inquiring about religious background, I learn that the family has a strong religious faith, and I offer to call the hospital chaplain for additional support. The family and physician reach an agreement that they will try a few more days of intensive support, and then reconsider options.
>
> During follow-up, I speak with the physician and learn that there was little additional improvement in Mr. A.'s condition, and as a result of further discussion the family and physician have decided to discontinue ventilator support and provide full comfort measures to Mr. A. The physician indicates that the family expressed appreciation for the support and respect they received from everyone involved.

This ethics consultation went well. There was consensus, spiritual and emotional support, an appropriate decision, and later appreciation expressed by the family. The ethics consultant used skills of ethical assessment, process, and interpersonal skills without severe difficulty, mistakes, or error. There was no great need for innovation, and the consultant's skills were relatively invisible. Nevertheless, the consultant did attend to, evaluate, and tailor her own actions to the situation at hand, depending on the course of events and how people were responding at the time. Someone without experience in the field of ethics consultation would not even know how to begin. "What is a bioethicist, and what is an ethics consultation? Where is the cardiac stepdown unit? What is a value decision, and what is an ethical principle? Why is this patient on a ventilator? Have there ever been any similar cases, nationally and locally, in which a ventilator has been stopped when a person is still living? Should I write anything in the medical record?" And so on. Ethics consultation is much more complex than simply applying bioethical principles—although there is no question that beginning to name principles and theories, in the early days of bioethics, did begin to create a common language for the profession. The consultant actively makes sense and seeks to influence each novel situation, even those that present no great difficulty, by using the vocabulary of bioethics, interpretive frameworks, skills, and goals, as first outlined approximately 30 years ago and further elaborated over time. The active shaping of each consultation through the use of skills in assessment, process, and working with others is the reason why there is a greater likelihood of mistakes and errors in complex, unusual, or difficult cases. However, these pioneering experiences also offer significant opportunities for enhanced understanding and professional skills.

ETHICS CONSULTATION
AS A SKILLED ACHIEVEMENT

The work of the scientist and philosopher Michael Polanyi provides further understanding of knowledge as personal achievement. This in turn leads to a further understanding of the meaning of mistakes and errors, and how we can seek to avoid them by enhancing skills in ethics consultation.

Polanyi was defending intellectual freedom in science when he noticed that an attempt to specify fully the rules for the conduct of science—for example, by stipulating that it must only focus on those inquiries that will result in predetermined benefits for society—will fail, because specifiable rules cannot, in and of themselves, account for the way that scientific inquiry proceeds. "No rules can account for the way a good idea is produced for starting an enquiry; and there are no rules either for the verification or the refutation of a proposed solution of a problem. Rules widely current may be plausible enough, but scientific enquiry often proceeds and triumphs by contradicting them."[12] Scientists accept scientific traditions and knowledge, yet on this basis make new discoveries. Scientific progress was regarded as the result of strictly objective processes at the time Polanyi was writing, but he identified its actual source as the innovations of skilled scientists. An incorrect understanding of the conduct of science has little direct effect on that discipline, but to the extent that we attempt to apply a similar understanding to pursuits in the humanities and professions, we risk assuming that skills and knowledge are fully specifiable. As a result, we might overlook the ways that we can develop ethics consultants' skills with teaching, support, and appropriate organizational structures.

Polanyi documents the modern tendency to overlook the creative, personal achievement underlying all knowledge, even scientific knowledge. In the process of achieving knowledge (or "knowing"), the "knower actively creates an interpretive framework, or Gestalt, by subordinating a set of particulars, as clues or tools, to the shaping of a skillful achievement, whether practical or theoretical."[13] In all intellectual performances (scientific discovery, diagnosing illness using x-rays, or reading a text) there are at least two forms of awareness. The knower has a "subsidiary awareness" of particulars within a "focal awareness" of the coherent entity that he or she achieves.[14] In a similar fashion, the ethics consultant subsumes the core skills of ethical assessment, process direction, and interpersonal communication in the service of the goals of ethics consultation.

The ethics consultant actively shapes meaning by alternately observing the reactions of others, testing the worthiness of principles and theories, listening, and speaking. As the consultant observes others in conversation, he or she can at one time be focally aware of this impression, and at other times shift attention to other matters.[15] The complexity of ethics consultation can be traced to the consultant's exercise of attention in this fashion, while always keeping the goals of bioethics in mind.

When an ethics consultation case is more routine, we are better able to specify the rules and principles underlying the consultant's activity. The interpretive framework in this instance is more fixed, and can be summarized in documents such as the *Core Competencies*. When a consultation is more novel, complex, or difficult, the ethics consultant must adapt an existing framework to comprise the lessons of a new experience. Following Polanyi, we would identify that:

> The first is a routine performance, the second a heuristic act. A paradigm of the first is counting, which leaves its interpretative framework—the numbers used in counting—quite unchanged; the ideal of the second is found in the originality of poetic phrasing or of new mathematical notations covering new conceptions. Ideally, the first is strictly reversible, while the second is essentially irreversible. For to modify our idiom is to modify the frame of reference within which we shall henceforth interpret our experience; it is to modify ourselves. In contrast to a formal procedure which we can recapitulate at will and trace back to its premises, it entails a conversion to new premises not accessible by any strict argument from those previously held. It is a decision, originating in our own personal judgment, to modify the premises of our judgment.[16]

In this sophisticated domain, the ethics consultant may experience mental uneasiness due to the feeling that his or her previous interpretation of the situation does not accord with reality. This leads to a correction of the way we define, interpret, and address the situation or, alternatively, a revision in the underlying premises of the profession.

The ethics consultant begins by identifying the ethical problem. Hunter states: "Is this a case of physician-assisted suicide? Or is it rather a withdrawal of treatment at the patient's request? The circular, hermeneutic procedure that ensues is equally familiar to lawyers, physicians, and moral reasoners, all of whom are required to fit the overarching laws of their disciplinary world view to the particular circumstances."[17]

AN ETHNOGRAPHIC STUDY OF ETHICS CONSULTANTS' PERCEPTIONS OF MISTAKES AND ERRORS

In an attempt to understand how ethics consultants perceive and define mistakes, I invited approximately 20 bioethics colleagues to write a first-person account of a mistake or error that occurred when they were providing an ethics consultation as an individual consultant, consultation team member, or member of an ethics committee. I requested that participants answer the following questions:

1. How long ago did this perceived mistake occur?
2. Were you acting as an individual consultant, member of a consulting team, or committee member?

3. How many consultations had you been involved in at the time? At present, approximately how many consultations have you been involved in?
4. How did you first become aware of the perceived mistake?
5. Why do you think the mistake occurred?
6. Have you given any thought as to how you might "classify" this mistake?
7. Did the perceived mistake change the outcome of the consultation?
8. Any personal responses?
9. Any professional responses or follow-up?
10. Have you identified anything that might help minimize, avoid, or deal with mistakes in the future?
11. Other comments or observations.

The four responses that follow offer a beginning description of errors in ethics consultation. While it is not the intent of this chapter to determine whether the consultant's actions were right or wrong, the discussion will classify the situations as "mistake" or "error," identify the relative skill domains, compare the consultants' personal and professional responses, and make suggestions for ways to provide ongoing education for ethics consultants to minimize future errors.

A NEUROSURGERY PATIENT

The ethics consultant in this situation is a clinician who provided consultation along with a chaplain who was also a member of the ethics committee.

We had a case of a young or middle-aged man who was chronically depressed and had therefore shot himself through the temple. He had left a phone suicide message for his boss, who received the message sooner than expected and found the patient injured but not dead. The patient was brought by helicopter to our tertiary-care center, where he underwent surgery and was aggressively treated for several days. Surprisingly, he survived, but it was clear that he would have neurologic impairments. At this point the family—parents and sister (an emergency room nurse)—decided they wanted to discontinue the ventilator and let him die. The neurosurgeons were reluctant to do so, and the family requested an ethics consultation. The neurosurgeons argued that the patient was not clearly ventilator dependent at the time, but he needed a ventilator partly to hyperventilate him to ensure the best possible neurological outcome. They were concerned that if the ventilator were discontinued, the patient might survive with a worse outcome than otherwise. However, they were willing to consider discontinuing the ventilator if we felt strongly that they should do so. We told the family that we agreed with the neurosurgeons and that it might not be legal to discontinue the ventilator in that situation (which I think is not really true). The worst part is that he then developed pneumonia and would certainly have died if we had stopped the ventilator. But at that point, the parents were resigned and the sister was furious, so there was no further discussion after the first meeting. Part of the trouble was that the sister wanted a decision "now." This was difficult for the neurosurgeon, but in retrospect we should have discontinued the ventilator. Eventually the patient went to rehabilitation and then to a nursing home. Last I heard, he was aware, but minimally communicative. Whether he was still depressed or aware of his situation, I don't know. That was about one and a half years ago—I don't know if he is still alive.

The ethics consultant and chaplain had been concerned about how they handled the case from the beginning; they became more convinced that they had erred over time, partly based on the patient's poor neurological outcome. The experience has been a source of regret and stress for the consultant; he feels that he wronged the patient and the family and that he failed in his duty as an ethics consultant. He believes that the mistake occurred because of "feeling we had to make a decision right away; overemphasizing legal concerns, thereby boxing ourselves into a corner; not keeping lines of communication open; not insisting that a delayed decision was preferable to a wrong decision; overreliance on the hopeful prognosis and concerns of the neurosurgeon."

The consultant classifies this perceived mistake as an error of judgment and an error of process. The perceived mistake changed the outcome of the consultation, in that the patient survived with minimal quality of life instead of dying. As a result of this experience, the consultant now tries to ensure adequate time, open communication, and enough emphasis on ethical concerns along with reasonable legal concerns. He also notes that this is the only case he can remember that was handled badly.

A DIALYSIS PATIENT

The person who wrote about the following situation was providing ethics services as an individual consultant. This situation was early in his career.

It was one of my first five consultations. In reading the chart and talking to nurses and residents, I "determined" that the patient was being irreversibly dialyzed (that is, he would not recover kidney function sufficient to stop dialysis). I factored this into the recommendation that we could respect his family's preference to withhold and withdraw medical treatments.

The nephrologist called me at home at about 10 o'clock on a Friday night. He read my note. He liked the note, but he asked why I had said that this patient could not survive withdrawal of dialysis. The nephrologist said that in perhaps a few weeks, the patient might very well survive withdrawal of dialysis. My stomach dropped. I was speechless. I felt like I had made a big mistake. Indeed, several. I felt that I had not consulted sufficiently, and that someone might inappropriately die because of my mistake.

I said these things to the nephrologist. He replied, in effect, that there was no problem because he thought the patient's overall condition and prognosis warranted respecting the family's preferences. Immediately, I agreed with him, but I realized that I had dodged the bullet this time. I have not underconsulted since. Today, I cannot remember thinking or feeling I made any other mistakes. I realize how either prideful or unaware that sounds. The thing is, I took ethics case consultation very seriously and very conscientiously. So, that might be why I made few conscious mistakes.

The consultant in this situation received a surprising weekend phone call that suddenly brought the mistake to his attention, leading to a strong personal reaction. He states that he "underconsulted" in this situation, meaning that he failed to get enough information. This would fall under "gathering relevant data" of the "qualified facilitation model" in the *Core Competencies*. The perceived error led to increased thoroughness on the part of this consultant. He states that he cannot recall any later errors like this.

A SERIOUSLY ILL NEWBORN

The ethics consultant in this case acted first as an individual consultant, then with the involvement of the infant bioethics committee. This was the consultant's 50th ethics consultation. He had been providing ethics services for two years at the time, but primarily for cases involving adult patients.

> The head nurse of labor and delivery called me to talk with Mrs. A., who had given birth to a baby with hydrocephalus and a neural tube defect. The parents had been expecting a normal infant, because prenatal testing had not revealed any abnormalities. Mrs. A. wanted more information on the infant's long-term quality of life and prognosis, what resources would be available for short- and long-term care, and whether it would be possible to limit life-sustaining treatment while continuing to provide comfort measures. I described the role of the bioethics committee and said that, in general, parents were the decision makers for their children, but that if the hospital believed that the parents' choices were not in an infant's best interest, the hospital might step in to limit parents' choices. I offered a bioethics committee meeting in her hospital room, but Mrs. A. declined because she was gathering information from physicians. I felt a connection to Mrs. A., and I wanted to help her as she worked her way through the difficult choices ahead of her and her husband.
>
> Different physicians gave the parents different information. A geneticist indicated to the parents that the infant might have serious mental deficits. One neonatologist recommended a nonaggressive approach and another believed that it was necessary to wait a period of time to see how the baby was going to do. After surgery to place a shunt for drainage of excess cerebrospinal fluid from the infant's head, the infant could not be weaned from the ventilator, and the healthcare team found that he had a diaphragmatic hernia. The consulting surgeon recommended against surgery, but stated that he would perform the surgery if the parents insisted.
>
> I spoke with the chair of the infant bioethics committee (IBC) and we agreed that, even though the parents did not specifically request a meeting, one should be held to try to work out the issues among the caregivers and the family. The committee reviewed medical and ethical perspectives. They reached consensus to "support the parents as decision makers, along with the attending physician," but at the same time many committee members believed that the surgery was advisable.
>
> One month after the IBC meeting, the surgical repair still had not been done and the infant remained on the ventilator. The infant was showing some neurological improvement, and more of the physicians and consultants were becoming convinced that surgery was in the infant's best interest. The parents were offered consultation from outside physicians. A second meeting of the IBC was scheduled, and then it was postponed when it appeared that the parents were about to agree to surgery. A few days later, the infant unexpectedly died. I experienced remorse and guilt over this outcome, and I spoke to a hospital chaplain and many colleagues about it.

The consultant became aware of the perceived error in the course of the consultation. He believes that he should have been more clear about his role as ethics consultant at the initial meeting with the parents, by explaining that he cannot be an advocate for parents if their choices do not appear to be in the best interest of the infant. The first IBC meeting was unclear in its recommendations. The statement that the committee "supported the parents as decision makers" left a major issue unresolved: would the committee abide by the parents' decision under any circumstances, even if the parents continued to refuse surgical intervention that might be in the infant's best interest? In addition, more information about current standards of care for seriously ill newborns would have been useful. The IBC made process errors and an error in information gathering.

The ethics consultant states that he now moves cases more quickly to the IBC. The committee has carefully reviewed its policies and procedures and improved the way it reviews cases and makes recommendations.

LUCIENDA'S STORY

This description is taken from a short story written by an ethics consultant who was troubled by the case at the time. The "I" in the story, Dr. Everson, represents the ethics consultant-author. At the time, he had done approximately 20 ethics consultations; at present, he has provided more than 350.

Lucienda Peak was the kind of woman whose views of life and death brought a smile to your face. Immensely practical and immensely wise. She came to the hospital after a visit to her family doctor. During her examination, Dr. Thomas had noticed a large growth in Lucienda's stomach the size of a grapefruit. Dr. Thomas assumed it was cancer and wanted to work it up. Even if it were benign, it was growing fast enough that it would probably need to be removed.

Lucienda, herself, had been noticing an increase in stomach problems but wasn't attributing it to any growth. Instead she would insist that this was "the piles." Seeing a growth this size, Dr. Thomas knew that the surgeons would want to cut it out. But he also knew Lucienda and he knew that Lucienda would not want the surgery. So when he sent Lucienda to the hospital, he also called me in to talk to her. I was supposed to evaluate Lucienda's ability to understand her situation and see if she could understand enough to refuse consent for surgery.

I am always amazed at the way doctors can sum up the life of a person in such a brief statement. "Lucienda is an 86-year-old black female with a history of dementia who was admitted to rule out cancer in her stomach." As I entered her room, I saw an elderly black woman with blue tinted hair sitting up in a chair in the corner of the room reading the *Reader's Digest*. She looked up at me and set her book in her lap.

"Mrs. Peak? My name is Dr. Everson. How are you today?"

"Ahm doin' jist fine, Docta," she said with a southern drawl that was pleasantly conspicuous in our Midwestern surroundings. " 'Cept I got the piles. My momma had the same probl'm. It's gettin' bett'r tho. I jist gotta keep eatin' mah greens."

[Dr. Everson tries to determine whether Mrs. Peak has decisional capacity to refuse surgery. He notices that she has difficulty keeping her facts straight and forgets what she has already said. He tries to assess her understanding of her condition, the nature and effect of the proposed treatment, and the risks of pursuing or not pursuing the treatment. He repeatedly attempts to help Mrs. Peak understand the medical interpretation of her condition and why the doctors say she needs surgery, but to no avail.]

Mrs. Peak insists, "Ah don't need no one cuttin' on me. Don't you docta's know no bettern' ta cut on an 86-year-old woman? Ah been cut on befo' and I don't wanna be cut on again. Besides, like I told ya, I ain't got no growth. I got da piles. My momma had da same thang."

Later, Dr. Everson speaks with Wilmalou Jefferson, Mrs. Peak's daughter, who feels that her mother is "just a confused old lady who doesn't know what's good for her."

In tears, Wilmalou says that she has to take good care of her mother, because "I got family in Tennessee who keep calling me, asking me what it is . . . I've got to tell them something. What if she dies and I have to say I don't know what caused it? They'll say I wasn't taking care of her and that's all I have been doing."

[Dr. Everson understands that Wilmalou would choose surgery for her mother, but he also knows that the risks and pain are Lucienda's. He wants to avoid sending her to surgery, but he isn't sure how to justify it.]

Dr. Everson: I was convinced of two things. I was convinced that this was not a case of so-called informed refusal. Mrs. Peak was not convinced she had a growth, so how could she be aware of the risks of having surgery? But I was also convinced that she was opposed to surgery. She had been through surgery before, so she was aware of the risks.

Trying to find a compromise, I went in to see her. "Let me ask you a question, Mrs. Peak. I know you think you just have the piles, but if you thought you did have a growth in your stomach, if you knew you had cancer, would you want the doctor to remove it?"

"By cuttin' on me? All I got is da piles and I don't need no one cuttin' on me for that."

"But if you did . . .," I tried.

"But ah don't!" she stated emphatically.

After a few more minutes, I went to speak with Dr. Thomas. "I can't help feeling that the refusal of surgery is fundamental—she wouldn't want surgery in any case. It seems we have three choices. First, we could give Wilmalou permission to decide, which we know will be for surgery. Second, we could argue that Lucienda has knowingly refused surgery—probably the hardest to justify, at least to others. Three, we stall. She is pain free now. Maybe we could send her home with pain medications and get her to promise to come back in when her pain gets worse."

[Dr. Everson and Dr. Thomas agree on the third option and explain the plan to Wilmalou. The daughter has strong doubts about whether she can get her mother to come back to the hospital but agrees to the plan. Mrs. Peak promises to come back in and goes home the next morning. Dr. Everson finishes the story.]

Lucienda died almost two years later of an obstruction in her stomach. I saw her occasionally when she came in for her checkups. When she walked I could see her pain. She would stand all bent over, slowly moving one foot at a time and not able to do even this without the help of her daughter. Her daughter was the physical support that allowed her to walk, the financial support that kept her on her feet, and the emotional support that allowed her to survive two years of increasing pain and discomfort.

After the decision was made to avoid surgery, I felt good for Lucienda but I pitied her daughter. Now the pain has ended for them both. As for me, I wanted to write this story as a memorial to Lucienda. But I couldn't write it until I knew how it ended. I would ask Dr. Thomas how she was and I would follow the obituaries looking for her name. We knew she would die but we didn't know when or how. We didn't know if it would be painful or if she would go quickly. As I watched for her name I would wonder how the story might have ended if she had gone to surgery to have that mass removed. I wondered whether the ending would have been easier for Lucienda and for her daughter, whether they would have both been happier. But I knew in my heart that if she had gone to surgery, this would no longer have been Lucienda's story.[18]

The ethics consultant states that he was troubled at the time about how to address this case. He was balancing two values "but knew the balance I chose was less than defensible." He thinks that the mistake occurred because he was acting on what "felt like the right thing to do." He wrote the story as personal catharsis to try to address the situation in his mind. Professionally, he has spent a lot of time addressing the issue of capacity to consent or refuse treatment.

ANALYSIS OF THE CASES

Exhibits 16-1 through 16-4 compare information from the four case descriptions. The case of the dialysis patient and Lucienda's case were both addressed by individual ethics consultants. The neurosurgery case was addressed by a small consultant team, and the seriously ill newborn situation began as an individual consultation and then moved to the full infant bioethics committee.

The consultants remembered these cases clearly, even though they had occurred from one and one-half to 10 years ago. The consultants considered themselves to be relatively inexperienced at the time of these cases, but, at present, three of the consultants have provided more than 300 consultations each. The fourth ethics consultant has provided approximately 30 consultations at the present time (see Exhibit 16-1).

The ethics consultants described how the mistake or error became apparent (see Exhibit 16-2). Only in the dialysis case did the consultant become immediately aware of misinformation, through a nighttime telephone call from the nephrologist. The other consultants were uneasy early on, but over time became more concerned. The duration of the problem suggests that the consultant's action in the dialysis case more resembles an isolated "mistake," while the actions in the other cases more resemble "errors." Each consultant felt responsibility for the patient's poor outcome. All four consultants experienced personal responses such as regret, stress, grief, feelings of failure, and concern about the patient's later suffering. It is worth remembering that ethics consultants are not solely responsible for the suffering and outcomes that patients may experience. The bioethicist does not cause the unfortunate or tragic circumstances of the patient's illness and suffering, and the consultant is not the primary decision maker in any case. Nevertheless, these ethics consultants all experienced regret and sympathy when they witnessed their patients' suffering.

All four ethics consultants questioned their professional role as a result of these experiences. They took specific actions to improve their practice and to avoid similar mistakes in the future. The consultant for the neurosurgery patient noted particular attention to allowing time, keeping communication open, and avoiding excessive emphasis on legal concerns or an overly optimistic prognosis. The consultant in the dialysis case has redoubled efforts to take consultation very seriously and gather information very carefully. The consultant in the case of the seriously ill newborn is careful to explain the role of the consultant and the IBC, has reviewed and revised IBC policies, and keeps current on standards of practice for seriously ill newborns. The consultant in Lucienda's story has studied capacity to consent, refers difficult cases to the full committee, and uses difficult or troubling cases in teaching. All four commented that the cases they submitted were rare.

The four ethics consultants were asked to "classify" their mistakes (see Exhibit 16-3). The neurosurgery case consultant saw the problem as an error of judgment and error of process, which could be prevented by keeping lines of communication open and maintaining an appropriate emphasis on legal and medical issues. The *Core Competencies* analyze value uncertainty(2) and building moral consensus(4). The corresponding Sparrow Hospital operationalized goals are promoting ethical resolution, ensuring respect for the wishes of the patient (IA), and ensuring respectful communication among parties involved (IIB). These interpretations are not inconsistent, but there is a difference in their level of generalization.

In the dialysis case, the consultant identified the problem as insufficient information gathering. The corresponding skill area in the *Core Competencies* would be identifying the nature of value uncertainty (1). The Sparrow Hospital Task Force views gathering information as the "preparation" phase of consultation.

The consultant in the case of the seriously ill newborn identified a lack of clarity about the roles and responsibilities of the ethics consultant and the infant bioethics committee. The corresponding skills listed in the *Core Competencies* are analyzing value uncertainty (2) and facilitating informal and formal meetings(3). The Sparrow Hospital goal statements, evaluation forms, or guides do not appear to address specific role issues.[19]

Exhibit 16-1
Ethics Consultants' Experiences

Case	Consultation Style	How Long Ago Mistake Occurred (Years)	Number of Consults Provided at Time of Mistake	Number of Consults Provided at Present Time
Neurosurgery patient	Small consulting team	1.5	20	30
Dialysis patient	Individual consultant	10.0	5	400
Seriously ill newborn	Individual consultant, then full infant bioethics committee	2.0	50	300
Lucienda's story	Individual consultant	2.0	20	350

Exhibit 16-2
Ethics Consultants' Appraisals of Mistakes

Facts about the Mistake	Neurosurgery Patient	Dialysis Patient	Seriously Ill Newborn	Lucienda's Story
First awareness of mistake	From beginning, more over time, partly based on poor neurological outcome	Upon receiving call from nephrologist	One month after first infant bioethics committee meeting, delay in surgery, then death of patient	When developing possible courses of action
Perceived responsibility for patient's outcome	Life-sustaining treatment continued; patient survived with poor quality of life	Sense of narrowly avoiding inappropriate death of patient	Possible influence on delay of surgical treatment death of patient	Patient did not have surgery, survived 2 more years with discomfort and suffering
Personal response	Source of regret and stress, feeling of wronging the family	Stomach dropped, speechless at nephrologist's telephone call	Feelings of guilt, grief	Troubled by decision and Lucienda's suffering; wrote story as a catharsis
Professional response	Feeling of failure in duty as ethics consultant	Felt I had made a big mistake, had "underconsulted"	Spoke with clergy and colleagues	Wrote the story as personal catharsis
Attempts to minimize or avoid similar mistakes in the future	Give enough time, keep lines of communication open, do not overemphasize legal concerns or rely too heavily on the attending physician's hopeful prognosis	Takes ethics consultation very seriously, very conscientious in gathering information	Explains role of ethics consultant and committee very carefully, further study of ethical and medical practice related to seriously ill newborns, review of committee policies and procedures, sends infant cases to committee more readily	Has studied capacity to consent, refers difficult cases to the full committee, uses difficult or troubling cases in teaching
Comment on frequency of errors	Only recalls one case like this one	Is not aware of other mistakes in later practice	Case that elicited the strongest personal response and regret	Mistakes are rare because the ethics consultant only recommends options; others are available to review

In Lucienda's case, the consultant identified the problem as an incongruity between the ethical requirements for informed refusal and an awareness that, even if the patient had understood, she most likely would not have chosen surgery. Another tension was that fact that all parties involved in selecting the third option—delay—strongly suspected that the patient would not return to the hospital even if her pain did get worse. It was a difficult case of the type that the consultant now more readily refers to the full ethics committee. The ASBH skill area would be building moral consensus, but this does not truly capture the nature of the uncertainty. The consultant seemed to meet the Sparrow Hospital goals of promoting ethical resolution, ensuring respect for the patient's wishes (IA), recommending treatment that would most benefit the patient (IB), and identifying the appropriate decision maker (IC). It seems that, in this case, it may be necessary to define a subcategory of skills: knowing when agreed-upon moral rules do not seem to promote the patient's wishes or best interest. Lucienda's case is one that causes us to review and possibly revise the interpretive framework used by ethics consultants.

CONCLUSIONS AND RECOMMENDATIONS

Errors and mistakes are most likely to occur when the ethics consultant is entering the unfamiliar territory of cases that are difficult, complex, or unusual. When confronted with such cases, the consultant must extend the reach of routine practice to accommodate a different set of circumstances. We should not expect that all mistakes and errors can be prevented; at the same time, however, there should be ways for ethics consultants to enhance their skills through ongoing education. There are many formal opportunities for professional growth, including publications, professional meetings, ethics committee meetings, case discussions for interdisciplinary groups, and rounds. As noted in the *Core Competencies* document, organizations have an obligation to ensure that these and other educational resources are available to the ethics consultants they employ.[20]

However, informal case discussions and peer review and support are also advisable. Ethics consultants remember situations in which they have made mistakes and errors, and can use these mistakes to modify and improve their practice. We can best help one another learn and develop expert practice if we allow conversation about mistakes and errors, as well as the "midcourse corrections" that occur on a daily basis. Case narratives are excellent learning devices, as noted previously with respect to medical error.[21] I encourage ethics consultants and committees to develop informal peer review of their consultations.

The *Core Competencies* document is an excellent description of bioethics goals and competencies, with a high degree of generalization. The report will meet its intended use in developing curricula, educational opportunities, and practice standards. While the Sparrow Hospital goals are not inconsistent with the *Core Competencies*, one significant different is the attempt to "operationalize" goals by moving to a level that, at times, verges on the conversational.

Exhibit 16-3
Consultants' Classifications of Mistakes/Errors Compared to *Core Competencies* and Sparrow Hospital Goals

Case	Consultant's Classification	Consultant's Recommendation to Avoid Similar Mistakes, Errors	*Core Competencies*	Sparrow Hospital Operationalized Goals
Neurosurgery patient	Error of judgment and error of process, incorrect view of law	Give enough time, keep communication open, proper emphasis on legal concerns and attending physician's prognosis	Analyzing value uncertainty (2) Building moral consensus (4)	Promoting ethical resolution, trying to ensure respect wishes of the patient (IA) Respectful communication among parties involved (IIB)
Dialysis patient	"Underconsultation," not getting enough information	Serious, conscientious approach to ethics consultation	Identifying nature of value uncertainty (1)	Preparation phase: gathering information
Seriously Ill newborn	Lack of clarity about role responsibilities of the ethics consultant and the infant bioethics committee	Careful explanation of consultant's and committee's role, ongoing review of ethical and medical practice related to infants	Analyzing value uncertainty (2) Facilitating informal and formal meetings (3)	Promoting ethical resolution recommending treatment that would most benefit the patient (IB)
Lucienda's case	Requirement for informed refusal not met, awareness that patient would not follow through on plan to return to the hospital	Refers difficult cases to the full ethics committee, uses difficult or troubling cases in teaching	Building moral consensus (4) but not a good fit Balancing competing demands of bioethics analysis and the patient's wishes	Promoting ethical resolution trying to ensure respect for the patient's wishes (IA) Recommending treatment that would most benefit patient (IB) Identifying appropriate decision maker (IC)

Exhibit 16-4
Recommendations and Comments on Perceived Errors

	Neurosurgery Patient	Dialysis Patient	Seriously Ill Newborn	Lucienda's Case
Recommendations to minimize or avoid similar mistakes in the future	Give enough time, keep communication open, proper emphasis on legal concerns and attending's prognosis	Serious, conscientious approach to ethics consultation	Careful explanation of consultant and committee's role, ongoing review of ethical and medical practice related to infants	Refers difficult cases to the full ethics committee, uses difficult or troubling cases in teaching
Time frame	Course of consultation	Brief	Course of consultation	Course of consultation
What I would want to say to this consultant in conversation:	You attempted to safeguard the best interest of the patient. It is not always possible to keep family members from feeling frustration. Even when we do all the right things, the results may not be ideal. It might be helpful to explore process, communication, and the limits of our ability to influence others	No additional harm came to the patient from your temporary misunderstanding of his renal prognosis. Because of the chart note, the physician caught the misunderstanding.	The situation was complex. The infant had multiple nomalies and many consultants, each with a separate opinion. The parents kept a strong stance against aggressive treatment, and you made sure that their voices were heard. Clarity about your professional role still might not have changed the outcome.	Even though the exact requirements for informed refusal were not met, you tried diligently to identify and act upon Lucienda's wishes. Lucienda did experience suffering, but this might not have been avoidable. The case did remain "Lucienda's story."

Operationalized goals would more readily lend themselves to informal case reviews and the face to face conversation about errors that would help all of us to improve practice.

ACKNOWLEDGMENT

I would like to express sincere thanks to the ethics consultant colleagues who allowed me to use their descriptions of errors in this chapter.

NOTES

1. J.C. Fletcher, N. Quist, and A. Jonson; "Ethics Consultation in Health Care: Rationale and History," *Ethics Consultation in Health Care* (Ann Arbor, Mich.: Health Administration Press, 1989), 1-15.

2. Society for Health and Human Values-Society for Bioethics Consultation Task Force on Standards for Bioethics Consultation, *Core Competencies for Health Care Ethics Consultation* (Glenview, Ill.: American Society for Bioethics and Humanities, 1998), 8.

3. J. Andre, "Goals of Ethics Consultation: Toward Clarity, Utility and Fidelity," *The Journal of Clinical Ethics* 8, no. 2 (Summer 1997), 193-8 at 193.

4. See S. MacIntyre, *After Virtue: A Study in Moral Theory* (Notre Dame, Ind.: University of Notre Dame Press, 1981).

5. S. Freud, *The Psychopathology of Everyday Life,* trans. A. Tyson (New York: W.W. Norton, 1960).

6. E. Goffman, *The Presentation of Self in Everyday Life* (New York: Doubleday Anchor, 1959), 208.

7. M. Merleau-Ponty, *Phenomenology of Perception,* trans. C. Smith (New York: Humanities, 1962).

8. M. Polanyi, *Personal Knowledge: Towards a Post-Critical Philosophy* (New York: Harper Torchbooks, 1962).

9. E. Partridge, *Origins: A Short Etymological Dictionary of Modern English* (New York: Macmillan, 1966).

10. K. Hunter, "Narrative, Literature, and the Clinical Exercise of Practical Reason," *Journal of Medicine and Philosophy* 21 (1966): 303-20, at 305.

11. See note 8 above, pp. 89.

12. Ibid., ix.

13. Ibid., xiii.

14. Ibid., 55-65.

15. Ibid.

16. Ibid., 105.

17. See note 10 above, p. 305.

18. N. Edinger, "Lucienda's Story," (unpublished manuscript), used with permission.

19. J. Andre et al., *Evaluating Ethics Consultations* (Lansing, Mich.: Sparrow Hospital and Michigan State University, 1997).

20. "Institutional Obligations to Patients, Providers and Consultants," Section 5.2. of SHHV-SBC *Core Competencies,* see note 2 above.

21. See D. Hilfiker, "Facing Our Mistakes," *New England Journal of Medicine* 310, no. 2 (12 January 1984): 118-22 [Hilfiker's article is reprinted as chapter 6 of this volume—ED.]; J. Christensen et al., "The Heart of Darkness: The Impact of Perceived Mistakes on Physicians," *Journal of General Internal Medicine* 7 (July-August 1992): 424-31; J. Rachels, "Responsibility to Monitor and Remedy Quality-of-Care Mistakes," in *Ethics in Emergency Medicine* 2nd ed., ed. K. Iserson, A. Sanders, and D. Mathieu (Tucson, Ariz.: Galen, 346-350); C.L. Bosk, *Forgive and Remember: Managing Medical Failure* (Chicago: University of Chicago Press, 1979).

17

Margin of Error: The Sociology of Ethics Consultation

Charles L. Bosk

INTRODUCTION

The title of this volume is divided by a colon. The first three words of that title, "Margin of Error," appear to the left of the colon and are an implied question, a world of interpretive possibilities suggested by a phrase evocative in its ambiguity. This world is erased by the more exacting semantic construction that appears to the right of the colon in the original working title: "The Nature, Inevitability, and Ethics of Mistakes in Medicine and Bioethics Consultation." The title is a binary opposition. The left is the raw; the wild; the animal; the sacred; the dark; and, of course the left. The right is the cooked; the tamed; the human; the profane; the light; and, of course, the right.

The right, being both the side that it is and the part of the opposition that it expresses is capable of much further subdivision. The disciplined and disciplinary half of the colonic divide, it represents our scientific, theological, and philosophic understanding. It is the side in which the terms *margin* and *error* come to have operational definitions both for those such as ethics consultants or clinical ethicists who need to act in situations of risky choice where help is needed and for those who are trying to make sense out of these newly specialized and socially visible activities that we call clinical ethics consultation.

The tension of this volume is that the right side of the title seeks to make sense of the left, but the left always has an incalculable element of terrifying mystery and awesome power. When we cross the divide of the colon—when we transform error into mistake—we perform an important collective ritual affirming, denying, and thereby neutralizing that mystery and power that resides leftwards of the colon. In this ritual, whatever form it takes, we press for and provide a social accounting for the error. This social accounting assigns to each error a cause, identifies warning signals to prevent such errors in the future, provides ground rules for understanding and action the next time, and reaffirms first principles for pressing on with the enterprise now that we have addressed the problem.

Untamed error exists as the Kennedy assassination; the launch of the Challenger and its subsequent explosion; the fiery crash of TWA Flight 800; the immolation of the Branch Davidian compound; the assault of Rodney King by Los Angeles police officers; and, closer to my home, the bombing by the Philadelphia police of the MOVE headquarters or the explosive collision of U.S. Senator John Heinz's private jet and a helicopter over a schoolyard during lunch recess. All of these are examples of errors in their pure state. Errors are, above all, a breakdown in the normal organization of social life as a practical accomplishment, an ongoing natural order within a meaningful world. Many of the above errors were all the more threatening to our sense of how the world works by the fact of their being captured on film or tape for endless playing and replaying. Each new viewing raises again the fundamental question: How could this happen? At the same time, each reviewing deadens our collective horror and wonder of the world gone awry. Public disaster and the implications it carries of human failing so ruptures our taken-for-granted sense of how the world works—our normal expectations—that a collective search for the explanation of error is necessary.

These public errors have their shocking properties removed through a public process that turns the incomprehensible mishap into a mistake that had its reasons. These reasons allow blame to be assigned to individuals and the more structural, global implications of error to be evaded. With serious error—undeniable breaches to the normal order—there is something like a ritual order for the restoration of the everyday: an impartial blue-ribbon panel is set up to investigate the rending of normal expectations, the error. Panels are comprised of members selected for disciplinary or technical expertise, demographic diversity, and political centrality. Panels then find a set of specific reasons to explain this error in the natural order; they tame error by labeling and categorizing the mistakes that allowed it to occur, reducing the intrinsic tragedy of error to a set of mere miscalculations avoidable in the future. Panels sometimes find that their pronouncements are met with profound skepticism in some quarters. Error is not so easily tamed as the right side of its existence likes to pretend; those who read left-sided meanings into error's inevitable existence resist official normalizing accounts. The political dexterity needed to turn errors into mistakes is seen as a sinister plot by those who find in errors other, more primordial meanings.

But, error in medicine and bioethics consultation is surely different from the kind of error that results in socially visible catastrophe. The Challenger, TWA Flight 800, Pan Am Flight 104, Bhopal, Chernobyl, Three Mile Island—their occurrence and the subsequent need to account for that existential fact—these surely share few characteristics with the errors of medicine and bioethics consultation. At the surface, the denial of any commonalities seems sensible. Socially visible errors are accounted for in and with very public processes; public hearings, testimonials, and reports provide the democratic transparency of a public inquiry, the social openness of a visible collective grappling with human failure, and the public judgment of a final report.

Error in medicine and bioethics consultation occurs in a different social space entirely. Social accounts for error are certainly, on occasion, necessary. But errors, for the most part, are internalized by the provider organization, however this is defined, or the appropriate operating unit of the organization identified as responsible for that error. In the socially visible error of the public catastrophe, the fact of error is inescapable. An analysis of decision making will lead back to causes and the identification of responsible parties. In the arena of medicine, the process of identifying and accounting for mistakes is very different. Whether error, in fact, occurred is often hotly contested. Who is the responsible agent is also a source of debate without resolution. Even when errors are acknowledged, there is still very rarely public reporting of specific incidents. Rarer still is the public linking of individuals with particular mistakes. This is to say the social accounting system in medicine is much more private. The difference in the type of event that sparks an inquiry and the processes then used to account for that error suggests that there is little to learn by comparing publicly visible catastrophe to the more quiet disaster of medicine and bioethics consultation. Practically speaking, the margin of error in medicine and bioethics is so wide that we can live happily on the right side of the colon of this volume's title. This essay questions that assumption by surveying what we know of medical error in the context of what we know about public catastrophe. What we learn from supplementing one perspective on error and mistakes with the other is then applied to discuss error and mistakes in bioethics consultations.

TWO SOCIOLOGIES OF ERROR

Error and the social accounts offered to explain it are relatively underdeveloped domains within sociology. Sociological theory has more often concentrated on explaining success. In many ways our theories echo a public ideology or American civil religion; the accent is on progress, development, and programmatic action to overcome obstacles and barriers to social achievement. Despite the minimal emphasis on how errors are identified, categorized, understood, and managed, two disparate, albeit complementary perspectives have emerged for viewing error. One perspective concentrates on organizational features of error; the other focuses on emergent understandings in the everyday life of the work group.

THE ORGANIZATION OF NORMAL ERROR

Charles Perrow is a leading proponent of the organizational approach to error.[1] He contends that modern technological systems are error-prone and that we should think of certain catastrophes, such as mishaps at nuclear power plants, as "normal accidents." For Perrow, certain accidents are not produced by individual human failings—what he call the "ubiquitous operator error." Rather, certain catastrophes are an inevitable result of features embedded in many enterprises of the modern world. The two features most important to the production of normal accidents are interactive complexity and tight coupling; that is, each system component is itself intrinsically complicated at the same time that each component part's performance affects the functioning of other system components. As a result, errors ramify through systems, creating large catastrophes. This is simply a fact of life for many of our complex technological undertakings. Or, as Perrow says: "If interactive complexity and tight coupling—system characteristics—inevitably will produce an accident, I believe we are justified in calling it a *normal accident* or *system accident*. The odd term *normal accident* is meant to signal that, given the system characteristics, multiple and unexpected interactions of failure are inevitable. This is an expression of an integral part of the system, not a statement of frequency."[2]

We cannot, says Perrow, prevent normal accidents by simply building more elaborate warning and backup safety systems. These systems add to the complexity and tight coupling of the organization of the original enterprise. They become as likely to malfunction as any other part of the system. Safety devices then multiply the possibilities for normal error. Any reduction in the probability of error is more than offset by the new component with its own unique possibility for failing and sending mistaken signals to other components of the system. Perrow's survey of normal accidents in high-risk systems is a mind-numbing catalogue of all the ways a concern for safety creates complacency, misperception, or misjudgment in the face of alarming dangers. For Perrow, what is needed is not merely better safety systems or more diligence, for the marginal gain from these is just too unpredictable. What is needed is better wisdom about which high-risk technologies to encourage and which to abandon.

The most extensive empirical treatment of a normal accident is Diane Vaughan's *The Challenger Launch Decision*.[3] To watch, as a nation of schoolchildren did, the technological pomp and ceremony surrounding this launch (which featured Christa McAuliffe, the nation's first teacher-astronaut-shuttle passenger), then witness the explosion of the spacecraft in real time, watch the visible, smoke-flumed pieces of wreckage drop into the ocean, and listen to startled newscasters search for adequate words to describe and explain what happened, was to experience firsthand the power, horror, and mystery of error on the left side of our volume's title. Vaughan's historical ethnography accomplishes two separate explanatory tasks.

First Vaughan shows the social and organizational work needed to remove the horror, mystery, and power of the visual images of original error—to normalize the explosion as a "deviant outcome," one not rooted in the organizational culture of the National Aeronautics and Space Administration (NASA) and private aerospace contractors like Morton-Thiokol. To do this, Vaughan analyzes how the official "Rogers Commission" report constructed an explanation that emphasized the decision to launch as a mistake that ignored previous warnings that something was amiss with the O-rings. The official understanding of the event lays the blame at a few reckless individuals who foolishly overrode the evidence of past performance and the expertise of fearful engineers. This scripting of the final report satisfies certain cultural requirements for adequate social accounting for error by locating the source of the disaster, demonstrating how far that source was from our normal expectations, and underlining how what was learned in analyzing this disaster will prevent its recurrence in the future.

Second, and more importantly, Vaughan demonstrates that the official account of the decision to launch the Challenger is a "just-so" song we whistle to ourselves as we walk alone through the graveyards of high-risk technologies at night. The problem with the official account is that it is inaccurate. In Vaughan's judgment, the decision to launch the Challenger was not the result of deviant behavior by NASA personnel. On the contrary, the decision was the result of sets of interacting workers following work group norms that had developed over time. The most important of these were the normalization of deviant performance of the O-rings over several flights; a production culture that had made accommodations to the built-in budgetary constraints of the shuttle program; and patterns of communication between operating units of the launch team that created a structure of secrecy as an artifact of bureaucratic reporting requirements. Information was passed up the organization but not necessarily shared between parallel subunits. This pattern of communication brought into being what David Matza, in the far different context of explaining juvenile delinquency, identified as zones of "pluralistic ignorance."[4] Those with doubts and misgivings were not in a position where they could share their thoughts and misgivings with anyone but their organizational superiors. The opportunities for "private troubles" to escalate into "public issues" were constricted as a result.

If it does nothing else, this abbreviated account of normal accidents underscores that the workplace of the tertiary-care hospital shares features with workplaces said to be most typical of those where normal accidents occur. There is interactive complexity and tight coupling. Clinical emergencies that demand action before information is complete are commonplace. There are laboratory tests and bedside monitoring units that perform just as erratically as O-rings. Work groups develop a production culture where economic constraint is a brutal fact of any calculation of what to do. Patterns of everyday interaction create zones of pluralistic ignorance between operating units of the organization. As a raw fact of organizational life, there is an irreducible structure of secrecy in tertiary care that is a contributing factor to much of the normal error that occurs. Although normal errors have tragic consequences, although they are all too costly and frequent, and although efforts to reduce such errors are necessary, once a basic investment in safety is made, further investment is likely to provide disappointing marginal gains. Some activities such as space travel or healthcare, activities premised on highly sophisticated technological processes, are "error-ridden."

THE CULTURE AND PRODUCTION OF ERROR ON THE SHOP FLOOR

The organizational approach sees error as one of the normal products of task organization. The second approach in the sociology of error begins where the organizational approach leaves off. Starting with the assumption that work is "error-ridden," this second perspective revolves around the culture and production of error on the shop floor. Some of the first studies of error are literally of shop floors: production crews in the aircraft industry,[5] workers in a machine shop,[6] street-level bureaucrats,[7] or managers in an industrial plant.[8] However, the most sustained treatment of workplace error concentrates on the shop floor of the academic hospital.

The classic orienting statement for understanding medical error is Everett C. Hughes's essay "Mistakes at Work."[9] For Hughes, all work can be categorized as either routines or emergencies. Routines, when routinely attended to with success, reinforce a sense of mastery. Routines that do not yield success create emergencies. Emergencies, when handled with aplomb, create routines and thereby reestablish a sense of competence and mastery. Emergencies that spiral out of control create the sense that a culpable error or mistake was made, and that sense is a threat to the integrity of the work activity. Mistakes and errors create the impression that those involved do not know what they are doing. Hughes suggests that we can create a calculus for mistakes and errors out of the experience of the worker and the routineness of the task.

Because academic hospitals often involve front-line workers (students and residents) who may have little experience, and because the clinical problems encountered there are often very far from routine on any standard index, we might expect to find a fair number of mistakes and errors. But, says Hughes, hospital work is organized in such a way as both to control and limit the actual occurrence of mistakes and to filter out any recognition of individual responsibility or accountability for mistakes. Hughes describes the organization of hospital work as a set of "risk-sharing" and "guilt-shifting" devices that make it difficult to say if or exactly where in the chain of events the error or mistake occurred. These work practices include supervision, consultation, cross-coverage, and case conferences. All of these devices make it harder to see individual mistakes. A course of action is not any one individual's property or agency, but rather it is shared within a community of fellow workers who second decisions all along the way. For Hughes errors are normal, and there is an elaborated social division of labor that keeps errors and mistakes from coming plainly into view. In his recent discussions of training for certainty, Paul Atkinson has clearly restated this position and given it greater empirical specificity.[10] Paget[11] and West[12] have provided two leading accounts detailing how mistakes are embedded in the everyday order and language of the group. The old folk adage, "Doctors bury their mistakes," describes better the social process that surrounds mistakes and errors than it does the literal fate of patients. Not all mistakes are so meaningful, so fateful.

Even so, not all medical mistakes can be buried. Some outcomes of care raise a strong, if rebuttable, presumption that a serious error has occurred. These outcomes are public and visible, as are the social accounting practices and collective rituals employed to rebut the more serious implications of fateful error. Light extends Hughes's discussion of mistakes at work by looking at the type of negative outcome that is not so easily folded into the life of the group, not so easily hidden from view.[13] The error that Light examines is suicide from the perspective of the treating physician (a resident) and the work group (the ward and the training program). His account of a suicide review sounds a number of important points for our understanding of mistakes at work and recognizes suicide review as a workplace ritual that serves a number of group needs. First, the artful discussion of the case models professional standards at precisely the moment the event being reviewed makes a mockery of claims to competent practice. Second, the faults of the individual therapist in handling the case are pointed out in such a gentle way as to suggest that these misjudgments could (indeed, would) have been made by anyone—that the errors involved were inevitable and unavoidable; hence, the errors need not weigh too heavily on the head of the therapist or the supervisor. And third, the lessons of the case taken away from the review, in Light's words, provide "a reaffirmation of how fine psychiatry is; for in its darkest hour, a clear lesson can be drawn by a model of the profession (the reviewer)."[14] Errors are inevitable and unfortunate. But they also serve as an occasion for reviewing behavior and for correcting faulty practice. However, as Light points out, the perforce *ad hoc* and episodic nature of suicide review prevents us from making broad generalizations about the lessons from suicides.

It is on the generalizable dimensions of the social accounting for error that I concentrate in *Forgive and Remember: Managing Medical Failure.*[15] This ethnographic study examines how surgical residents learn to separate blameless error from blameworthy mistakes in the course of their training. Errors appear blameless, by and large, if they are seen as part of the normal learning process. Inexperienced residents are expected to make some technical or judgmental mistakes. These errors are considered a normal consequence of providing opportunities to the unpracticed. Such difficulties have the following characteristics: the resident quickly recognizes the problem; the resident seeks appropriate help for it; the resident learns a "lesson" from the entire incident; and the resident does not repeat that mistake during the rotation. These are normal errors; like Perrow's normal accidents that are built into the system of technology, these are built into the system of training. These normal errors allow the attending physician and resident to take the role of teacher and student, respectively. Attending physicians say they "forgive and remember" the normal errors of their residents. They forgive because such errors are inevitable in a field like surgery. They remember just in case such errors are repeated, become part of a pattern, and thereby indicate that something in addition to the normal fallibility of a diligent and scrupulous resident is causing these errors.

If error that can be seen as part of the educational process is seen as both normal and blameless, then errors are blameworthy when the reading of events makes it difficult to sustain a claim that the resident acted in good faith. Errors are blameworthy when they involve normative breaches—that is, when they break universal rules about how a responsible doctor acts. Also blameworthy are quasi-normative breaches or the failure to abide by an attending physician's cherished but often unannounced way of doing things. A source of great confusion to residents is the fact that attending physicians treat breaches of their personal rules as seriously as they do breaches of universal rules. Hence residents' views of egregious errors are often at odds with these of attending physicians, especially if the attending physicians have confused their personal preferences with the moral order. Difficulties likely to be coded as normative have the following characteristics: the resident failed to recognize problems sufficiently early or attempted to cover them up; the resident failed to seek appropriate help; the resident failed to improve his or her performance over successive trials; and the resident made the same mistake on repeated occasions. These errors are not seen as a normal part of the educational process, but rather they signal that a resident lacks the skills or fails to honor the commitments that surgery as a profession requires. When such mistakes occur, attending physicians approach residents as wrathful and righteous judges eager to root out heresy. All those errors that are seen as blameworthy indicate that a resident is either in need of serious remediation or in need of dismissal from the training program.

One striking feature of categorizing residents' errors into the blameless and blameworthy is how easily the process may turn into a self-fulfilling prophecy. That is, a resident's good reputation exerts a protective or deviance-reducing effect while a bad one generates a destructive or deviance-amplifying effect. If a resident is considered trustworthy, monitoring by attending physicians is decreased. Therefore, deficiencies are less likely to be discovered. Conversely, if a resident is suspect, monitoring increases. Convinced that the resident's deficiencies are there for the finding, an attending physician is more likely to look for and find evidence of sloppy work. When the attending physician finds deficiencies, he or she increases surveillance, which again increases the probability of finding other mistakes. Clearly suspicion alone does not create residents who are judged unfit; after all, something creates the suspicion. Nonetheless, being suspect is for a resident a very vulnerable and demoralizing position. Not only that, being above suspicion gives a fair amount of protection, especially when mistakes need not be seen as innocent error. Given these dynamics, it is not surprising that those who fall short when evaluated (or their attorneys) often characterize the process as arbitrary and capricious.

This sense of unfairness is symbolized for residents by what I called quasi-normative errors. These are breaches of the attending physician's personal preferences, which are read as if they were absolute, universal rules. Residents who make such mistakes often find themselves locked into personality conflicts with attending physicians. Invariably, when these conflicts occur, residents are losers. There are two problems here. First, the seriousness with which these breaches of personal preference are punished undermines the seriousness of the more universal norms attending physicians seek to enforce when they react to normative error. The confusion introduced by treating personal preferences as if they were universal rules allows residents to confuse their profound and trivial lapses and to excuse too easily the serious ones. Second, this confusion is only multiplied when the quasi-normative errors of residents are simply thought of as the personal style or signature of the attending surgeon. To be sanctioned severely on one service for what is acceptable practice on another only reinforces the sense that the coding of mistakes and error is arbitrary and capricious.

ERRORS IN ETHICS CONSULTATION

What is and is not an error, how errors occur, who is culpable, and what needs to be done to prevent their occurrence are never simply matters of defining ever more rigorously and objectively a discrete empirical event—something capable of being captured by a very sophisticated outcome measure. Rather, culpable error and its control are a matter of occupational morals, of situations defined this way rather than that, of administrative classifications about how causality works here, and of implicit social rules that make clear to all but the most obtuse when further questions are not welcome. The social constructedness of error matters, very fatefully in fact, for system participants. This is as true for pilots and airline passengers as it is for doctors and patients.

How then is error socially constructed in the world of ethics consultation? Or, to put the matter more pointedly, is it possible for a clinical ethicist to make a blameworthy error? Although it might seem nonsensical to claim that clinical ethicists do not and, in fact, cannot make blameworthy errors, this does seem to be the case. To avoid unnecessary debate, the bald assertion—the clinical bioethicist or the ethics committee is incapable of making a mistake—needs sharpening, qualifying, and clarifying. It is, possible—even likely—that for any given case the individual clinical ethicist or committee may feel that things could have been handled more smoothly, that critical opportunities were missed, or that a better outcome could have been obtained. But an *ad hoc,* individual sense of regret is not the same thing as an acknowledgment of error, a concrete identification of a specific mistake, and a precise mode of redress to avoid that mistake in the future. The individual clinical ethicist or ethics committee cannot make a mistake, because the structural and cognitive features that make for a shared, collective understanding of mistake are absent. The features that allow for public identification of mistakes in other occupational segments simply do not exist in the world of clinical bioethics. To those who might argue that a public, collective understanding of mistakes and errors is nothing more than a sociological rendering of these events, I would agree. And I would add that, without such a collective or sociological version of mistake and error, the community lacks the resources necessary to assess performance, redress blameworthy mistakes, and exercise the self-regulatory functions said to distinguish the professions from other occupations.

Of those missing structural and cognitive features necessary for a community's possession of an understanding of mistake and error and the capacity to act on that collective understanding when necessary—and here it is important to remember that both forgiveness and negative sanctions are actions—three are most critical. First, without any form of systematic review of problematic cases, there is no public forum in which to develop collective understanding of what counts as adequate or inadequate case management. As Light points out, psychiatry has suicide review, which allows the community to develop standards, pinpoint errors, assess blame, forgive mistakes, and define the limits of individual clinical responsibility. Surgical morbidity and mortality conferences accomplish much of the same work in surgical departments. In these meetings, attending surgeons model and residents learn the standards of professional responsibility, the rhetoric for acceptable accounts of errors, and the boundary between acceptable and unacceptable behavior. One striking similarity between suicide review among psychiatrists and mortality and morbidity conferences among surgeons is that both meetings reassert professional claims to competence at just that moment when events most mock such claims, reassert professional standards when outcomes suggest that they have been breached, and reestablish commitment to professional norms of behavior when they seem to be most in doubt. Whatever other tasks these meetings accomplish, they are a public reaffirmation of what does and what does not count as acceptable practice and of how seriously this professional community takes those standards.

So far as I know, neither ethics consultants nor ethics committees conduct regular case reviews. There are any number of reasons for this. First, there is no outcome from ethics consultation comparable to suicide in psychiatry or mortality and morbidity in surgery. In some sense, psychiatric services are organized to prevent suicide and surgical services to avoid mortality and morbidity. When such events occur, as they inevitably will, an accounting is necessary lest it seem that the professional community is tolerant of such outcomes But, in ethics consultation, this is not the case. There is no outcome that so challenges the professional conscience of the community that it triggers the demand for a collective, public accounting. As a consequence, there are no occupational rituals that serve to articulate, make explicit, and reinforce professional standards.[16] Without such rituals, there is no public space for an understanding of what causes a mistake or error to develop.

The absence of such occupational rituals may itself index nothing so much as how different action within the occupational community of bioethicists is from action within the community of psychiatrists and surgeons. Suicide review in psychiatry and mortality and morbidity conferences in surgery both move forward under a convenient sociological fiction—namely, outcomes are interpreted, until proven differently, as if they were determined exclusively by the actions of psychiatrist and surgeon. Certainly, the review of bioethics consultation can never proceed under this fiction. In fact, if this were true, it is not immediately clear how the consultation could subserve the value of autonomy (assuming that autonomy is one value that the consultants have an interest in preserving). Indeed, it is not even clear how fateful consultation should be in decision making. In good consultations do those whom one has consulted follow recommendations? In good consultations are recommendations given in the alternative (a set of options) with likely costs and benefits attached? Or in good consultations are no recommendations given at all? Rather, instead of concrete suggestions, are the parties to the consultation empowered to frame and assess the options themselves? So, without a clear idea of what role the consultation is supposed to play in unfolding action, it is very difficult to say that a mistake was made in consultation. Beyond that, whatever is ultimately decided in the case is not decided by the bioethicist. Typically to make a mistake or error, one must exercise some exclusive decision-making authority. Bioethicists rarely do this *qua* bioethicists. As a rule, it is hard to assess which streams of their clinical talk in a case are mistaken and which are correct, if only because it is so hard to connect those streams of talk to actions taken and, ultimately, to outcomes.

Finally, there is one last reason that inhibits regular case review in bioethics consultation. Both the psychiatry departments that conduct suicide review conferences and the surgery departments that hold mortality and morbidity conferences are densely peopled. From these conferences, there are impersonal lessons that can be communicated to a broader collegium. This is much less so for those units responsible for bioethics consultation. Most commonly, ethics consultation is managed through a committee. Alternatively, a hospital may have a few individuals who provide consultation services. When committees provide consultation services, it is always the case that members have other, more primary clinical responsibilities. Committee work is an additional service provided to the institution for a wide, if unspecified, range of motives. When individuals provide consulting services, it is also rarely the case that ethics consultations are their primary clinical responsibility. Under these conditions, a regular review of performance is inhibited for two reasons. First, however valuable such a review is, whatever lessons are learned from it, close case review is often stressful, time-consuming, and interpersonally difficult. Because committees need to enlist volunteers and then to motivate their continued involvement, regular case reviews with a focus on what was done wrong may seem to volunteers an undue burden, a heavy price to provide what is often a thankless, extra administrative duty. Additionally, with the ethics committee and also where a few individuals provide consultation services, there is no audience to inform beyond those who already know the details of the case for a review. In short, the community of professionals involved in ethics consultation is very rarely dense enough to support the kind of public review of outcomes found in suicide review and mortality and morbidity conferences. In such small communities of workers, it would be most difficult not to personalize criticism and to focus on impersonal lessons learned.

But even if there were formal case reviews in bioethics to dissect mistakes and to delineate measures to prevent their reoccurrence, it seems highly unlikely that these sessions would be of much value. First, there is too little consensus on what the goals of ethical consultation are. Part of what makes suicide review or mortality and morbidity conference important is that suicide and mortality and morbidity are just those events that psychiatric treatment or surgery are instituted to prevent. The comparable event for ethics consultation, the one that signals that consultation itself has been error-ridden, is hard to specify. There has been an explosive growth in ethics committees and individual ethics consultants in the last decade. This growth has been fueled, in part, by the requirement of the Joint Commission on Accreditation of Healthcare Organizations (JCAHO) that institutions need to have in place a mechanism to resolve the ethical dilemmas arising in the course of care. What the JCAHO is silent about is how these mechanisms are to be organized, how they are to operate, and how institutions are to assess the efficiency of these mechanisms.

This silence presents many difficulties to anyone who wishes to assess whether ethics consultation, however it is organized, properly serves the goals it is intended to serve. The JCAHO's standard suggests that all mechanisms and all resolutions are equally acceptable. This plainly cannot be the case. An ethical dispute can be resolved by the patient's death, by a physician overriding the patient's or family's wish, or by a physician simply acceding to the patient's or family's wishes even if these wishes are morally problematic and beyond the bounds of community standards. Some of these resolutions are clearly preferable to others from the point of view of norms, social process, or both. But, ultimately, in order to assess whether mistakes or errors occurred in an ethics consultation, we would need a more certain sense of how ethics consultations are to resolve ethical conflict. Is the purpose of consultation to provide a forum for protecting the patient's autonomy? Or is ethics consultation a procedure to ensure that some specific overarching cultural values are respected? Or is ethics consultation a process designed to avoid litigation and adverse public relations for hospitals? Without a consensus on questions such as these, the judgment of an action as reasonable and responsible or fatally flawed in conception and execution is difficult, if not impossible, to make.

Knowing the goal of ethics consultation is a necessary but not a sufficient condition for determining if a mistake or error has been made in any particular case consultation. What is also needed, and in this case missing, are some data that suggest that one way of doing consultation provides better outcomes than some other way. Here our knowledge of consultation is flawed on two counts. First, at a theoretical level, there are multiple approaches to doing consultations. Consultants approach their tasks from a variety of paradigms. There are bioethics consultants deeply committed to a principalist, a narrative, a phenomenological, a dialogical, or a virtue-based approach to their work. But this in itself is not a flaw. After all, multiple paradigms exist in psychiatry where the arguments among those who favor behavioral, cognitive, pharmacological, psychodynamic, or family-system approaches to various problems are ceaseless and no less passionate on that account. Likewise, in surgery, there is no lack of debate on the proper approach to specific illnesses or procedures. What these fields possess that bioethics lacks is agreement on outcome measures and controlled clinical trials that compare different approaches. This is the second failing of bioethics consultation, that makes errors and mistakes hard to gauge. Put most simply, there are no data that suggest that any one approach creates different results than another. We do not know what difference the various theoretical operating paradigms make. Beyond that, we do not know what difference the variety of ways these paradigms are implemented makes. Does it make a difference in outcomes whether consultation is by committee or by individuals? Does it matter whether patients and their families are part of the process? Does it matter whether consultants have any specific set of professionally trained competencies? Without this sort of data, it is simply impossible to say that one approach was a mistake or that errors were made.

CONCLUSION

In reviewing the sociology of error and then applying that sociology to bioethics consultation to conclude that consultants cannot make mistakes, I have not meant to imply that consultants are not conscientious individuals who do trying and much-needed work under difficult circumstances in often thankless environments. For it is plainly the case that ethics consultation provides a necessary corrective to many of the least praiseworthy features of modern medical care. It is equally clear that ethics consultants are dedicated, committed, and conscientious workers. Their own writings reveal that they are also self-reflective about the practice of their craft and very far from uncritical about their performance.

What I have tried to do in this essay is not look so much at individual case performance but rather provide a framework for understanding what is necessary in the occupational community of ethics consultants for a collective understanding of mistake and error to emerge—of what work is necessary to move beyond an *ad hoc* assessment of individual consultations. This framework includes three elements: regular case review, agreement on outcomes and a means for assessing them, and systematic data that compare different approaches to ethics consultation. It is most understandable that, in an emerging and often contested domain of professional practice, these elements have not yet developed. But, if ethics consultation is to continue in its institutionalization in healthcare organizations, these three elements demand the attention of the community of practitioners.

NOTES

1. C. Perrow, *Normal Error: Living with High-Risk Technologies* (New York: Basic Books, 1985).

2. Ibid., 5.

3. D. Vaughan, *The Challenger Launch Decision: Risky Technology, Culture and Deviance at NASA* (Chicago: University of Chicago Books, 1996).

4. D. Matza, *Delinquency and Drift* (New York: John Wiley, 1964), 56.

5. J. Bensman and I. Gerver, "Crime and Punishment in the Factory: The Function of Devi-

ance in Maintaining a Social System," *American Sociological Review* 28 (1963): 588-99.

6. D. Roy, "Quota Restriction and Goldbricking in a Machine Shop," *American Journal of Sociology* 57 (1952): 427-42; D. Roy, "Banana Time: Job Satisfaction and Informal Interaction," *Human Organization* 18 (1960): 156-68.

7. M. Lipsky, *Street-Level Bureaucracy* (New York: Russell-Sage, 1980).

8. M. Dalton, *Men Who Manage* (New York: John Wiley, 1959).

9. E.C. Hughes, "Mistakes at Work," in *The Sociological Eye: Selected Papers on Work, Self, and Society* (Chicago: Aldine-Atherton, 1951, 1971), 316-25.

10. P. Atkinson, "Training for Uncertainty," *Social Science & Medicine* 19 (1984): 949-56.

11. M. Paget, *The Unity of Mistakes: The Phenomenological Interpretation of Medical Work* (Philadelphia: Temple University Press, 1988).

12. C. West, *Routine Complications: Troubles with Talk between Doctors and Patients* (Bloomington, Ind.: Indiana University Press, 1984).

13. D. Light, "Psychiatry and Suicide: The Management of a Mistake," *American Sociological Review* 77 (1972): 821-38.

14. Ibid., 835.

15. C.L. Bosk, *Forgive and Remember: Managing Medical Failure* (Chicago: University of Chicago Press, 1979).

16. Ibid.

18

Ethics Consultation and the Law: What Is the Standard of Care?

Robert S. Olick

INTRODUCTION

Recent proliferation of ethics consultants in the halls of hospitals and health systems has engendered a dialogue within the bioethics field about standards for ethics consultation and for the qualifications of ethics consultants. Some have called for a code of ethics for ethicists,[1] while others have called for formal certification.[2] Motivated in large measure by concerns for competence and quality in ethics consultation, the "standards debate" has occasioned scant reflection about the legal implications of the consultant's role and even less about the potential legal significance of the movement toward standards. If consultants (like all of us) make mistakes, do those mistakes have any legal significance? Can the consultant be held legally accountable? In short, can ethics consultants commit malpractice?

The query may at first seem puzzling. After all, while a growing chorus advocates some mechanism for quality assurance, there is no recognized standard of care by which to measure fulfillment of the consultant's responsibilities, or deviation therefrom, either in ethics or in law. Those who hold themselves out as ethics consultants are often professionals, but they are not professional ethicists who can point to generally accepted and publicly legitimated qualifications for engaging in the consultative enterprise. Ethics consultation lacks certain common hallmarks of a "profession," such as systematized, extensive training of members; a defining set of standards generated, embraced, and enforced by members of the profession; and provision of a service widely recognized as important in society.[3] Movement in these directions within the bioethics field suggests that the discipline of ethics consultation might qualify as an emerging profession.[4]

This essay explores the lessons of the medical malpractice model, asking what medical malpractice law instructs us about the possible emergence of a legal standard of care for clinical ethics consultants. Conjointly, the malpractice prism offers a "law's eye" view of recent developments in the field pressing the question of standards, as well as of connected bioethical debates about who the ethicist serves, the goals of ethics consultation, and whether ethicists possess moral expertise. Should a consultant's liability ultimately be adjudicated, a number of signposts of a standard of care could be used by a court called upon to do so. Of particular import is the policy statement produced by the Task Force on Standards for Bioethics Consultation of the Society for Health and Human Values and the Society for Bioethics Consultation (SHHV and SBC, respectively), adapted on 8 May 1998 by American Society for Bioethics and Humanities (ASBH), the national successor organization to the merger of the SHHV and SBC.[5] Neither the fact that ethics consultation is not a publicly legitimated profession complete with licensure or certification requirements, nor the absence of a recognized code of ethics for ethicists, would shield against liability.[6]

This essay does not purport to explicate the full range of issues related to the legal duties of ethics consultants. It has been suggested, for example, that ethics consultants have a number of obligations with legal implications—including confidentiality, truth-telling, even whistle-blowing—that do not fit the malpractice paradigm.[7] Potential legal pitfalls for institutional ethics committees, any number of which might apply to individual consultants (such as aiding and abetting a battery, failure to warn at-risk third parties), have been discussed elsewhere.[8] Fry-Revere's exposition of the accountability of ethics committees and consultants is the most comprehensive account of the nexus between ethical and legal accountability for competence and quality from the standpoint of regulation and self-governance.[9] The inquiry pursued here concerns the more narrow and basic concept of a legal standard of care; whether it makes sense to hold that an ethics consultant has a legal (not solely ethical) obligation to act as a reasonable consultant would under the circumstances, and what it would mean to understand the consultant's role in this way.

To be sure, the risk of legal liability for ethics consultants is quite small. The best known precedent is the *Bouvia* case—still the only reported case naming a hospital ethics committee as a defendant (the claims against the committee were dismissed without opinion).[10] A handful of recent lawsuits have named ethicist-consultants as defendants, but there has been no reported adjudication of these claims.[11] (See chapter 21, "Errors in Healthcare Ethics Consultation"—ED.) If sued, ethicists are likely to be "tag-on" defendants, not the "deep-pocket" targets of the skilled malpractice attorney. Still, the risk is real and increasingly on the minds of those who provide consultation services. One word of counsel: A survey of SHHV members conducted a decade ago found that, of 83 respondents describing themselves as humanist scholars engaged in clinical ethics consultation, approximately 50 percent believed they had professional liability coverage (only slightly more than half of this group had verified their coverage as fact).[12] All would be well advised to procure liability insurance either independently or through the institutions that they serve, or to enter into some form of indemnity agreement with those institutions.

THE MEDICAL MALPRACTICE MODEL: A PRIMER

It is, as the expression goes, "hornbook law" that a patient-plaintiff in a medical malpractice action must prove four elements of the case: (1) duty, (2) breach of duty, (3) causation, and (4) damages. For a duty to exist, a doctor-patient relationship must be established. Three principles emerge from the case law regarding formation of this relationship. Courts have held that a physician-patient relationship exists when (1) the physician exercises independent medical judgment on the patient's behalf, (2) when the patient reasonably relies on the physician's statements (advice), or (3) when the physician's actions create in the patient a reasonable expectation of care. The first formulation holds the status of a majority rule. Once formed, the physician-patient relationship continues until it is intentionally terminated, in a manner clearly understood by the patient and allowing reasonable time for the patient to secure a new physician without placing the patient's well-being in jeopardy. Failure to attend to the patient's needs when a physician-patient relationship exists (and has not been properly terminated) constitutes patient abandonment actionable at law.[13]

Most often the central issue in a malpractice action is what care is due and whether the duty of care has been breached. Here the core inquiry is whether the physician has acted negligently—that is, whether he or she has failed to act with the level of skill, diligence, and judgment as would be exercised by a reasonable physician under the circumstances. The standard of care can be thought of in terms of knowing what one is doing (skill and judgment), and being thorough and careful in the provision of care (diligence).[14] For generalists, the measure of due care is what is reasonably expected of other generalists; for specialists, the relevant skill, knowledge, and diligence is that of others in the same or similar specialty. That the standard of care is one of reasonableness has important implications. The law does not hold physicians to a standard of perfection. Bad outcomes happen, but a physician will not be at fault (legally) for failure to possess or exercise the highest degree of skill possible. Nor is the physician held to be a guarantor of good results (unless perhaps he or she has made an ill-advised promise of this sort).[15]

Even if the physician has failed to act with due care, the patient-plaintiff must also show that the physician's negligence was the cause of the injury or harm and that the bad outcome is compensable in money damages. The common test of causation is one of "but for" causation: the physician is held to be the legal cause of the patient's injury if, "but for" the physician's negligence, the patient would not have suffered the injury. With this established, the court (jury) will go on to assess damages. The most common form of this inquiry is comparison of the patient's condition following the negligence to his or her condition had the negligence not occurred, taking into account such factors as past and future medical expenses, lost wages, impaired earning capacity, and pain and suffering.[16] It follows that a physician may act negligently but not be the cause of the patient's injury—in short, that the physician may commit harmless error. It is also possible for the patient's injury to be caused by the physician's negligence, but not be compensable in monetary terms. Although extremely rare in traditional malpractice cases, this has been the result in wrongful-life cases on behalf of disabled newborns where parents have alleged that, had they been informed of an anomaly *in utero*, they would have chosen to terminate the pregnancy. Although courts have recognized a violation of the mother's right of informed consent (wrongful birth), a clear majority have also declined to assign a monetary value to the difference between a disabled life and nonexistence.[17]

It is often said that a medical malpractice case is a "battle of the experts." The reason is straightforward. The typical manner of proof of deviation or compliance with what the similarly situated reasonable physician would do has for many years been to employ (oftentimes literally) medical experts to attest "customary practice" or (with a modicum of cynicism) to testify to what "I and other reasonable physicians in the defendant's practice area would have done under the circumstances." Expert testimony is also commonly needed to show that the physician's negligence caused the patient's injury. In earlier times expert testimony was to come from the physician's local community (the "locality rule"), but many states now recognize national standards and admit testimony from national experts, especially in suits against specialists. While this characterization of dueling experts for hire remains the reigning paradigm, in recent years a range of other sources have assumed increasing significance in the courtroom. "Generally accepted practice" may be proved by reference to clinical practice guidelines, official statements of professional organizations, institutional policy, pharmaceutical company warnings, recognized texts, and the published literature. In short, a wide variety of sources from within the medical profession itself may be introduced as evidence of the standard of care, each to be weighed and measured for its credibility and authority. In various respects, to define the standard of care is to articulate the consensus or majority rule within the profession and the defendant-physician's practice area.[18]

Although the law's familiar reasonableness standard establishes defining parameters of a standard of care, in critical respects the content of that standard (that is, whether a physician acted reasonably under the circumstances) comes from the medical profession itself. Evidence of consensus about what counts as good medical practice is the crux of the case. Indications of consensus as established by bioethicists themselves would play a similarly essential role in shaping a standard of care for the clinical ethics consultant.

MALPRACTICE IN ETHICS CONSULTATION:
A PARADIGM CASE

It will be helpful to establish a point of reference with an illustrative case.

Consider Mrs. B, a middle-aged woman in a persistent vegetative state (PVS) whose husband is acting as surrogate decision maker without benefit of a proxy directive or living will. The attending physician has obtained the necessary confirmation of the patient's condition from qualified neurologists, but he is uncomfortable with the husband's request to terminate the respirator. Rather, the physician believes life support should be continued, and he has contacted the ethicist employed by the hospital for a consultation. [Assume that the husband's request is based on his understanding of his wife's wishes, which are reasonably clear, and that there is no evidence of malice or ill-motive in his decision.] The consultant's recommendation supports the physician's judgment, not that of the patient and family, and treatment is continued despite Mr. B's persistent protest. Some time later Mrs. B dies, and a lawsuit is brought by her husband and estate; the lawsuit names the ethicist as one of several defendants and alleges that this individual acted negligently and breached a duty of reasonable care to the patient and family. The injury alleged is continuation of life support contrary to the patient's wishes; legal claims are based on wrongful life, battery, and violation of civil and constitutional rights. [Because our concern is with legal accountability *qua* ethicist, imagine that our consultant is a humanist ethicist who does not wear the hat of the physician, nurse, lawyer, or other licensed professional whose obligations in one of these capacities may arguably be implicated when functioning as an ethics consultant.]

Mrs. B's case is familiar, perhaps so much so as to be considered commonplace among bioethicists. Yet there are reasons the scenario is instructive. For one thing, the vast majority of ethics consultations involve decisions regarding care at the end of life.[19] For another, decisions near the end of life for PVS patients have received substantial attention in law, medicine, and society and have been the subject of an extensive literature. It is fair to say that there is ample evidence of consensus that termination of life support for PVS patients is morally licit and legally permissible, without implying that consensus means unanimity. Moreover, the clinical diagnosis of PVS leaves no room for ambiguity or equivocation regarding decision-making capacity or the clinical facts (assuming, of course, proper diagnosis and confirmation). Thus, while there is always an arbitrary quality to selection of hypothetical cases, the case of Mrs. B constructs a useful paradigm for the issue of a standard of care. It also offers a framework for asking whether ethicists can give "wrong" advice for which they can be held to legal account. I suggest that the law's response to this query likely depends on the presence of bioethical consensus translated into the language of reasonableness and due care. To illustrate the point, the discussion later briefly considers a variation of this case—a case in which the spouse insists on continued treatment that the physician considers to be "medically futile." The issue of futility is one of growing significance to the work of ethics consultants, and it continues to generate substantial disagreement at the level of principle.

MALPRACTICE IN ETHICS CONSULTATION: PROVING THE CASE

DOES THE ETHICIST HAVE A DUTY TO THE PATIENT?

There is a lively debate among bioethicists about who the ethics consultant serves, and about the closely connected questions of the functions and goals of case consultation.[20] Whatever position one takes on these matters, there is general agreement that an ethicist cannot conduct a meaningful consultation without at a minimum inquiring of the patient (or, in the case above, the patient's family) as to the patient's wishes and the basis for the family's decision. Assume that this has occurred. This interaction is sufficient to establish a consultant-patient-family relationship. It may be tempting for the ethicist to assert that, when it is the physician who requests the consult, the consultant's duty is to the physician—not the patient. This position finds some support in the literature.[21] But, while the assertion may be true of so-called curbside consultations involving informal and largely educational interactions (if a legally cognizable duty exists here at all), it is not likely to be availing in bona fide (formal) case consultations. Few hold that the ethicist acts for the exclusive benefit of the physician (or the hospital or health system) and has no obligation to serve the interests of the patient. Most of the familiar descriptors of the ethicist's role—facilitator, mediator, problem solver, educator, or some combination of these—defy this narrow characterization.[22] Nor can it be persuasively argued that a competent consultation does not involve the exercise of independent judgment on the patient's behalf (or at least in a way that affects the patient's interests). If, on the peculiar facts of a case, rigorous application of the independent judgment test failed to establish a consultant-patient-family relationship, the alternative formulations that look to the patient's or family's reasonable reliance and expectations would.[23] Note that there may be conflicting duties, since the consultations here also involve, as is often true, judgment and advice for the benefit of the physician and hence a legal duty to the physician.[24] But this in no way negates the consultant's duties to the patient and family. In sum, the family's attorney should be able to establish the first element of a malpractice case against the consultant.

CAN THE ETHICIST BE NEGLIGENT?
IS THERE A STANDARD OF CARE?

Far more interesting questions arise when the family attempts to establish the consultant's failure to meet the standard of care. A decade ago John Robertson wrote that the ethicist's duty "is to be a good, competent, reasonably humble ethicist."[25] While Robertson's intuitions are essentially correct, we can be more explicit today.

Before arguing that the standard of care has been violated, attorneys for Mr. B will need to establish the parameters of such a standard. State licensing standards, board certifications, and a code of professional conduct will not be found, but competent research will reveal signposts of an emerging profession: a professional organization founded more than a decade ago (the SBC); a national organization for bioethicists (the ASBH); regional networks of ethics committees and bioethicists with shared goals; certificate programs with curricula and a course of study; a journal devoted to clinical ethics consultation (*The Journal of Clinical Ethics*); and an extensive and growing literature that openly discusses the goals, standards, evaluation, and other matters in ethics consultation. In short, one strategy would be to compile indications of a consensus about the parameters of generally accepted practice—of what counts as good ethics consultation—as seen by those engaged in the activity itself (perhaps bioethicists in general), and there is ample material to work with. Of course, bioethicists are no strangers to the courtroom and have been qualified to testify as "experts" on numerous occasions.

For convenience we can use as a point of reference the report produced by the SHHV-SBC Task Force on Standards for Bioethics Consultation, *Core Competencies for Health Care Ethics Consultation*.[26] Composed under the stewardship of a diverse task force and with invited scrutiny and review by the bioethics community, this statement may fairly be taken as representative of consensus within the field about the core activities of ethics consultation and the core competencies required to perform these activities well. (This is not to suggest that there is no room for genuine disagreement.) In light of its formal adoption by the ASBH in May 1998, this document would carry substantial weight, perhaps akin to that of a professional code. Similar positions could be constructed from other sources, including the consensus statement on ethics consultation developed at the 1995 Conference on Evaluation of Ethics Case Consultation in Clinical Ethics[27] and detailed review of the literature. This more cumbersome process of reviewing the literature would be part of a thorough case preparation.

The *Core Competencies* report advances an "ethics facilitation model" of ethics consultation and asserts that one of the consultant's functions is "to identify and analyze the nature of the value uncertainty or conflict underlying the consultation." Another function is to "help to address the value uncertainty or conflict by facilitating the building of consensus among involved parties." To identify and analyze the issues, the consultant should (1) gather relevant data from the parties and other sources (the medical record), (2) clarify relevant concepts (autonomy, best interest, family authority), (3) clarify related normative issues (the roles of law, ethics, institutional policy), and (4) identify a range of morally acceptable options. To resolve uncertainty and build consensus the consultant should (1) ensure that concerned parties are heard, (2) help them to clarify their own values, and (3) facilitate shared commitments or understandings that are morally acceptable.[28] Although other conceptual models of clinical ethics consultation have been advanced,[29] there is widespread concurrence that whatever metaphorical descriptor is chosen, a frequent function and goal of case consultation is to facilitate resolution of disagreements.

The ethics facilitation model suggests an important distinction between the process and the substance of ethics consultation—between how the ethicist conducts the activity of consultation and what he or she advises, concludes, or perhaps decides in the course of shaping a resolution. Partaking of both process and substance is the connected matter of how the ethicist defines his or her own authority in the consultative relationship. These distinctions will not be lost on skilled trial attorneys, who may seek to establish deviation from the standard of care on each of these fronts.

The consultation process. Counsel will scrutinize closely the process followed by the consultant for Mrs. B's case. Did the consultant talk to the family, friends, or relatives who came to the bedside? Were these conversations sufficiently probing? Did the family and physician have ample opportunity to openly express their views? Was the medical record consulted? Was evidence of the patient's wishes (an advance directive) or of the patient's religious beliefs pursued? In the effort to clarify relevant conceptual and normative issues, did the consultant look to ethics literature, state and federal law, and institutional policy for guidance? Were these sources accurate and reliable? Did the consultant make sufficient effort to communicate the issues that he or she identified as important to all of the concerned parties, and to work with the parties to help clarify their own values and reach a resolution? In broad terms, did the consultant possess and exercise the requisite skills to perform these activities competently? That is, did the consultant possess and exercise the core skills of ethical assessment, interpersonal communication, and process identified by the *Core Competencies* document and elsewhere in the literature?

Ethical consensus is easily translated into the "reasonableness" language of the law, and into a duty of due care and diligence. The most effective way to make the conceptual and linguistic transition is to call a bioethics expert to the stand. In allowing this testimony, the court need not rule on a question of great moment to bioethicists—"What is a bioethics expert?" It need only determine whether the individual on the stand has the requisite background, education, and experience to testify as a bioethics expert—in other words, "Who is a bioethicist?"[30] One can imagine the response of the ethics expert, asked on the witness stand whether failure to consult the medical record or to speak with a distraught daughter who sat daily in the corridor would be a reasonable thing to have done. Or more pointedly, "If you were uncertain of the patient's wishes, would you have spoken with the patient's spouse a second time?" "As an ethics consultant for the past 10 years, knowing that there was still disagreement, would you have called for a meeting with the family and the attending physician?" "Would you want to know the reasons for the doctor's decision?" While omissions of this sort would be glaring, more subtle facts (such as failure to identify the physician's views about feeding tubes as an issue, failure to return a telephone call) might also reveal a consultant's lack of diligence. One study of decisions about care at the end of life found that almost half of the judges in the study believed testimony from a bioethicist about the ethics of patient care to be "persuasive or useful."[31] There is no reason to believe such testimony to be of less interest when it concerns an ethicist's critique or defense of another ethicist's ethics.

Of related concern is whether there is a duty to be a patient advocate and, if so, whether the facts suggest that this duty was taken seriously. A duty of patient advocacy, perhaps including a duty to protect the patient from harm, might well be found implicit in the fiduciary nature of the consultant-patient-family relationship. To reach this conclusion on the facts and arguments presented by counsel, the court need not resolve (although it might choose to) the more theoretical debate among bioethicists about whether an ethics consultation must be rigorously patient-centered.[32] As discussed above, to proffer in defense that the clinical ethics consultant does not serve the interests of the patient and family would be contrary to common understanding of the consultant's role. There is, however, substantial room for disagreement about the extent to which the ethicist must assume a rigorous advocacy role.

The advice given. More interesting and controversial issues arise when we inquire into the substance of the consultation. Did our consultant give bad advice? Even if we disagree with the advice given, did the consultant act with the level of care we would reasonably expect under the circumstances? It is generally agreed that ethics consultants should have a working knowledge of moral reasoning, common bioethical issues, principles and concepts, relevant laws and legal rules, institutional policy, and clinical information. The list of core areas of knowledge can be given in far greater detail.[33] A critical inquiry might be how the consultant advised the physician and the family regarding the place of autonomy and the legal rights of the patient and family. That family members may make decisions to terminate life support on behalf of incompetent loved ones in PVS is now well settled, and it is expressly recognized as a legal right in the majority of states.[34] Failure to identify and plainly express these principles and to make them a part of the dialogue—perhaps failings in both knowledge and diligence—would make the claim of negligence especially compelling. The stronger, equally compelling assertion is that recommending a course of action that subverts the patient's wishes rather than according patient autonomy and familial authority their rightful priority is "wrong" advice, contrary to prevailing norms. Also significant, physicians have a moral and legal right of professional conscience that may be exercised by arranging an appropriate transfer of care when sincere conflict persists. Was this presented to the physician and family as an option? Did the consultant make clear the (nonbinding) status of his or her recommendations?

Beyond insistence that no deviation from the standard of care occurred, our consultant might respond by invoking the "two schools of thought" exception. Recognized in most states as a valid defense to a charge of medical malpractice, this doctrine holds that the physician who chooses from among two or more accepted courses of treatment will not be liable if the recommendation was consonant with what a "respectable minority" of the profession would have advised. Here the law acknowledges that sometimes there is no single correct course of treatment or "best" choice. The doctrine also implicitly recognizes that there may be genuine disagreement within the medical profession. On either understanding, the physician should not be held liable for exercising sound judgment that can be seen as not having been the best option only with the benefit of hindsight.[35] Again, physicians are not guarantors of good results and cannot be held accountable for reasonable but imperfect judgment. Likewise, the ethics consultant is not expected to demonstrate perfect judgment and true moral wisdom.

The ethicist's assertion that it was reasonable to advise aggressive continuation of Mrs. B's life to be permissible, and that a respectable minority of ethicists would make the same call under the circumstances, is not without support. In a study of ethics consultants' recommendations concerning treatment for patients with PVS, Fox and Stocking found "considerable variability in what ethics consultants say they would recommend for specific hypothetical PVS patients."[36] Respondents, attendees of the 1991 annual meeting of the SBC, were asked what they would recommend in seven hypothetical vignettes. Although none of the vignettes precisely fit Mrs. B's case, 93 percent of those surveyed said they would recommend forgoing life support when both the patient's advance directive and the family refused treatment.[37] Presumably a lesser number would concur with forgoing life support in the case of Mrs. B, where there was no advance directive. The ethics consultant in Mrs. B's case could no doubt find a colleague of like mind to take the witness stand; indeed this would be a critical feature of the claim that his or her advice was in good company, even if not what the majority of ethicists would have done. Chances for a successful defense on this ground are nonetheless slim, as there is little room for disagreement regarding the importance of accurate knowledge and faithful presentation of the moral options, and the substantial weight of authority supports the family's assertion that the ethicist's advice was ethically and legally wrong.

A variation on this theme would be the claim of "mere error in judgment." Rather than claim that the advice given may not, with hindsight, have been the best course but was nonetheless reasonable, our consultant might admit the advice was wrong, but "merely an error of judgment." Those who question the validity of moral expertise might find this line of reasoning superficially appealing. After all, if there are no moral experts, no special claims of ethical authority, and no skills and abilities that the ethicist uniquely possesses, then the ethicist should be held to the same standard as anyone else; honest mistakes are to be forgiven. But even those who harbor such philosophical doubts are unlikely to favor rejection of ethical expertise as a meaningful concept if the consequence is lack of accountability for what ethics consultants do.[38] For similar reasons judges are unlikely to dismiss cavalierly the place of ethics consultation in patient care. Mere error of judgment has become a disfavored doctrine in medical malpractice cases, and would not likely be resurrected to protect the ethics consultant.[39]

At the same time, the fact that reasonable minds may differ on matters of morality and values suggests that ethicists may be at greater risk of legal entanglement for failures of skill and diligence in the process of ethics consultation than for giving substantively erroneous advice. To illustrate the point more clearly, suppose Mrs. B's case was not like Karen Quinlan's, Nancy Cruzan's, or Nancy Ellen Jobes's (cases involving refusal of treatment), but like Helga Wanglie's (in which the family insisted on continuing "futile treatment"). If Mr. B asserts that his wife values life dearly, regardless of its quality, and insists on continued respiratory support, are the physicians caring for Mrs. B obligated to comply, even if they believe such aggressive life support to be "futile"? If our consultant were to advise overriding the patient's and family's wishes, is this recommendation substantively "wrong"?

Siding with patient autonomy, *In re Wanglie* held that indeed there was a professional obligation to honor the patient's and family's request to continue respiratory support, notwithstanding the physicians' objections to doing so for a PVS patient.[40] Given that the case is among the very few to address the futility issue—and hardly represents a legal consensus—Mr. B's attorneys would no doubt rely heavily on this decision. But beyond the task of persuading the court that

Wanglie, a Minnesota trial court decision, was correctly decided and should be followed, counsel face a still more formidable challenge in attempting to establish widespread concurrence among bioethicists to support their claim of negligence.

Respected voices can be found to take a variety of positions. Some contend that physicians should have authority to override the patient's and family's wishes only in very narrow circumstances of physiological futility where, as a matter of science, the treatment will "not produce the effect sought by the one insisting on it."[41] Others support a broader understanding of professional prerogatives that would permit physicians to take into account whether treatment offers a clear benefit, relevant community standards, and fairness in the use of medical resources.[42] There is a compelling argument to be made that there exists no general agreement among bioethicists, professional organizations, and healthcare professionals even on foundational concepts at work in the futility debate, let alone how particular patient care dilemmas should be resolved.[43] Moreover, some notable "consensus" statements, perhaps signposts of an emerging consensus among healthcare professionals, offer at best tenuous support to Mr. B's claims. For example, both a policy statement by the Society of Critical Care Medicine's Ethics Committee[44] and the collaborative policy embraced by a number of hospitals in Houston[45] (which might be construed as evidence of a community standard of care) endorse the general principle that there are some circumstances in the care of dying patients in which physicians and hospitals are justified in saying "no." In fact, a thorough literature review would suggest that our consultant's defense team could well use this very same body of evidence, and the ambiguity and discord it manifests, to establish that a respectable minority of ethicists (perhaps even a majority) would agree that the advice given was reasonable. Bolstering the argument for the defense, the same survey of ethics consultants that found substantial agreement (but not unanimity) on the matter of a PVS patient's refusal of life support also found substantial variation in recommendations for care of the PVS patient when both the patient's prior wishes and the family's wishes are for aggressive life support.[46]

To return to the main point, if the matter of the substantive correctness of our consultant's advice is unsettled, there is far less room for discord about the process to be followed in conducting the consultation. Whether the ethical issue is one of refusal of treatment or insistence on purportedly futile interventions—one of patient autonomy or its limits—it is generally agreed that a competent consultation involves a process of information gathering and communication that facilitates accurate identification of the issues and presentation of a range of morally acceptable options. Failure to exercise due care and diligence in fulfilling these core procedural competencies opens the door to the claim of negligence. The same is true of the many consultations where the issues may be less clear than the two types of end-of-life cases discussed here. (It is worth mentioning that the futility scenario raises other interesting questions of process, as do cases riddled with ambiguity. If the law is silent or unclear—or clear but not widely embraced—does an ethicist have a duty to consult hospital counsel? How would a majority of bioethicists respond to these queries?)

The consultant's authority. The third line of inquiry is whether our consultant acted within the bounds of his or her authority. That ethics consultants have an advisory rather than a decisional role in patient care is widely accepted. The term *consultant* itself implies this understanding. It will (one would hope) be the rare ethicist who manifestly violates Robertson's admonition to be humble,[47] arrogating the decisional authority of patient, family, and physician. There may, however, be more subtle (perhaps even unconscious) ways in which a consultant exercises his or her *de facto* authority.

Legal scrutiny of *de facto* power connects in important ways with bioethical discourse about the ethicist's authority in the clinical setting. Agich identifies at least three types of authority at work in the consultative enterprise: (1) authority of the office (being in authority), (2) epistemic authority (privileged access to a body of knowledge), and (3) competence authority (performance of tasks that engender trust).[48] Just as there are morally licit and illicit ways authority may be used and exercised, so too might these boundaries come to shape a legal standard of reasonableness, short of blatant abuse and arrogance.

As noted earlier, counsel for Mr. B would want to know whether the ethicist made clear to the patient's physician and family that the consultant's role is advisory only and that the decision should be made within the physician-family relationship. Did our consultant assert that he or she was in authority by virtue of the office? Stake a claim to moral wisdom? Allow his or her personal values to interfere with the goal (duty) of objectivity, manipulating the process to reach a corresponding outcome? Counsel would also want to inquire whether the ethicist was aware of, and ignored, signals that he or she was perceived to have moral or decisional authority to which the physician or family felt compelled to defer. Our factual inquiry might pursue, in any number of ways, the question that troubles Agich—did the responsible parties *surrender judgment,* taking a decision on the word of the consultant, even recanting personal responsibility?[49] Does the ethicist have an obligation to disabuse physicians and others of misplaced beliefs about authority, perhaps implied in the duty to present the range of morally (and legally) acceptable options? Here again, the family will be able to look to testimony and literature to make the case that the reasonable ethics consultant would not succumb to such hubris. It would be harder to establish the more discrete claim of a duty of care not to allow excessive deference to perceived authority, but the claim is at least made stronger where there are reasons to believe that others are too willing simply to surrender judgment and the consultant fails to respond appropriately.

CAUSATION

It is tempting to believe that fidelity to the consultant's advisory role shields our ethicist from liability—it was the physician's choice and he assumed the risk of his decision. But to seek shelter baldly in the "I only give advice" defense, denying an influential clinical role and pointing the finger at the physician who ignored the patient's and the family's wishes, is to recant a justificatory feature of the consultative enterprise. Legally speaking, the assertion is not supported by analogous precedent. With more familiar medical consultations, the attending physician retains responsibility for the patient's treatment, but the consultant will also be liable for a negligent consultation. And nonphysician professionals who provide counseling services, such as psychologists and ministers, have on occasion been found liable for negligence. The argument may work to shift the lion's share of responsibility, but it does not exculpate our consultant.

Nonetheless, causation may be difficult to prove when we get down to cases. It must be shown that the consultant's negligence was the cause-in-fact or proximate cause of the patient's injuries. In other words, counsel for Mr. B must establish that *but for* our consultant's negligence, it is likely that the injury would not have occurred—that the patient's and family's wishes would have been honored. Because consultants do not provide hands-on care (recall that our paradigm is the humanist ethicist), the proof will not rely on medical-scientific evidence and testimony as in traditional malpractice, but in far less tangible evidence of the relation between errors of knowledge, judgment, and process, and the decision taken. One fruitful line of inquiry would be akin to that of informed consent, exploring whether there would have been a different outcome had information material to the decision-making process been corrected or accurately imparted. Did our consultant advise that the decision belonged to the doctor, not the family? Did he or she fail to correct a misperception or misapprehension about the basis for the family's wishes, or omit important information? Going to the heart of the matter, if the consultant had given reasonable (if not entirely correct) advice, would the physician have acted differently?

An important inquiry would be whether the attending physician reasonably relied on the ethicist's advice. Even assuming the physician understood that he was not bound to follow the advice given, the social and institutional factors legitimating the ethicist's clinical presence make some degree of reliance reasonable. The ethicist's claim of expertise and that the physician requested the consultation further support this view. The physician arguably has reasonable reasons to take the consultant's advice as highly persuasive, in the same way as other consultations.[50]

The issue of reasonable reliance returns us to the problem of *de facto* authority, and again connects with Agich's challenge to explore the epistemic and institutional bases of the consultant's authority. There is substantial anecdotal evidence that some physicians (and others) believe that "if the ethicist said it, it must be ethical." Others believe that following the ethicist's recommendation shields them from legal liability. If the ethicist has an obligation to "set the record straight"—a duty of fidelity to the rightful bounds of his or her authority—then it follows that failure to do so may result in surrender of judgment and may be the proximate cause of improper patient care. This is not to suggest that whenever bad advice is followed the ethicist is the legal cause. Reasonable reliance and independent judgment are not mutually exclusive. And surrender of judgment may occur through no fault of the ethicist.

The analysis would be different if the law itself augmented the consultant's authority. For example, Maryland mandates consultation and confers decisional power on patient care advisory committees in limited circumstances.[51] Hawaii confers immunity from liability for following a committee's advice—a powerful incentive.[52] Although these laws are directed to institutional ethics committees, consultants in these states whose authority is derivative of the committee's may be governed by different ground rules.

DAMAGES

Once breach of duty and causation have been established, the remaining question is whether the injury is compensable in money damages. How to allocate damages among the parties at fault must also be decided, but it is not important to travel that path here. Suffice it to say that relative to the physician and hospital, the ethicist's exposure is likely to be proportionately small, as is the depth of his or her pocket. That the ultimate act of ignoring the patient's refusal of treatment was the physician's (perhaps with support of hospital administration) shields the ethicist from a substantial percentage.

In one respect, the case of Mrs. B is not a good paradigm for this issue involving the bottom line. This area of law, in contrast to damage actions for medical malpractice, battery, or failure to obtain informed consent, is still in its nascent stages. There are few judicial opinions to look to for guidance, and no true sign of an emerging trend. The best known case, *Estate of Leach v. Shapiro*, involved a patient in a chronic vegetative state whose family refused life support on her behalf.[53] The court recognized a civil cause of action for wrongful continuation of life support, but the litigation ended with an unreported settlement. A subsequent Ohio case, *Anderson v. St. Francis-St. George Hospital* (known as the *Winter* case), which also concerned physicians' refusal to honor a clear treatment refusal, here documented by a do-not-resuscitate (DNR) order, reached a different conclusion.[54] Looking to "wrongful life" cases involving disabled newborns as precedent, the *Winter* court held that "wrongful living" is not a compensable injury. The opinion expressly leaves open the possibility that claims of battery and negligence would be more favorably received, as would, presumably, allegations that the patient's constitutional rights were violated—all of which are available in Mrs. B's case. On the related issue of liability for healthcare costs, courts in New York[55] and North Carolina[56] have refused to force nursing homes to absorb the costs of services wrongly provided to dying patients, ruling in both instances that families must pay the bill even when life support was continued against the patient's and family's wishes. The future direction of damages awarded in end-of-life litigation can hardly be foretold, but the ethicist should take small comfort in the current state of affairs. It may be only a matter of time before the law lives up to its time-honored maxim, "Where there's a right there must be a remedy."

CONCLUSION

The standards and accountability movement is a welcome development in bioethics. Whatever one's view of the ultimate course to be charted, the debate about standards has engendered heightened awareness and important self-reflection concerning the role of the ethics consultant in patient care. In various respects this discourse is an inquiry into what it means to act as a good, competent, reasonable consultant would under the circumstances. (Of course, quality standards aspire to greater heights than reasonableness.)

A central theme of this essay has been that the growth of clinical ethics consultation and the movement toward professionalization lay the groundwork for emergence of legal accountability—for development of a legal standard of reasonable care in the consultative enterprise. Previously received opinion that, in the absence of more familiar standards governing other professions (such as licensure, certification, and professional codes), clinical ethicists cannot be held liable for the services they provide, is no longer tenable. Ethics consultants, like all of us, make mistakes. Ethics consultants, like physicians, lawyers, and others who hold themselves out as experts providing a valuable service, can commit malpractice. Moreover, the very same reasons competence and quality matter to bioethicists, namely growing legitimation of the ethics consultant's role within hospitals and healthcare organizations and the consultant's real and perceived authority at the bedside, offer sound policy reasons to hold the ethicist to legal account.

The analysis suggests that the ethics consultant is at greater risk for failure to exercise due care and diligence with regard to the process of consultation than he or she is for the substantive correctness of recommendations made. For those who take seriously their role as facilitator, mediator, and advisor, and who see the value of their contributions to patient care as predominantly process rather than outcome oriented, this ought to be of some comfort. At the same time, this conclusion points to a troubling irony. Mrs. B's case is most helpful as a tool for understanding the law's possible response to alleged malpractice of consultants precisely because it is a "clean" case. By contrast, clinical ethics consultants are most needed where clinical and social factors are less tidy (uncertainty of medical outcome, differences among medical staff, no obvious patient surrogate), or ethics and law are unclear or immature (ambiguous patient preferences, no legal precedent, strongly divided ethical positions)—in short, when the case is "messy." It is here, where opinion may be legitimately divided and more than one course of action appears reasonable, that the dangers of *de facto* authority loom large. But it is also in these messy situations that the law's ability to hold the ethicist accountable is arguably weakest.

NOTES

1. B. Freedman, "Bringing Codes to Newcastle," in *Clinical Ethics: Theory and Practice,* ed. B. Hoffmaster, B. Freedman, and G. Fraser (Totowa, N.J.: Humana, 1989), 125-39; G.R. Scofield, "Ethics Consultation: The Least Dangerous Profession?" *Cambridge Quarterly of Healthcare Ethics* 2 (1993): 417-26.

2. S. Sherwin, "Certification of Health Care Ethics Consultants: Advantages and Disadvantages," in *The Health Care Ethics Consultant,* ed. F.E. Baylis (Totowa, N.J.: Humana, 1994), 11-24. There are several university-based certificate programs available to those seeking training and employment as clinical ethicists.

3. M.D. Bayles, "The Professions," in *Ethical Issues in Professional Life*, ed. J.C. Callahan (New York: Oxford University Press, 1988), 27-30.

4. B. Barber, "Professions and Emerging Professions," in *Ethical Issues in Professional Life*, ed. J.C. Callahan (New York: Oxford University Press, 1988), 35-9.

5. Society for Health and Human Values-Society for Bioethics Consultation Task Force on Standards for Bioethics Consultation, *Core Competencies for Health Care Ethics Consultation* (Glenview, Ill.: American Society for Bioethics and Humanities, 1998).

6. D.J. Self and J.D. Skeel, "Legal Liability and Clinical Ethics Consultations: Practical and Philosophical Considerations," in *Medical Ethics: A Guide for Health Professionals*, ed. J.F. Monagle and D.C. Thomasma (Rockville, Md.: Aspen, 1988), 408-16.

7. J.A. Robertson, "Clinical Medical Ethics and the Law: The Rights and Duties of Ethics Consultants," in *Ethics Consultation in Health Care*, ed. J.C. Fletcher, N. Quist, and A.R. Jonsen (Ann Arbor, Mich.: Health Administration Press, 1989), 157-72. Robertson offers a discussion of the related question regarding whether there are circumstances in which a physician would have an obligation to seek an ethics consultation.

8. A.L. Merritt, "The Tort Liability of Hospital Ethics Committees," *Southern California Law Review* 60, no. 5 (1987): 1239-97.

9. S. Fry-Revere, *The Accountability of Bioethics Committees and Consultants* (Hagerstown, Md.: University Publishing Group, 1992).

10. The First Amended Complaint for Injunctive Relief and Damages in *Bouvia v. Glenchur*, No. C 583828 (Cal. Super. Ct., Los Angeles Cty., filed Oct. 7, 1986) is discussed in Merritt, 1250-1, see note 8 above.

11. R. Shalit, "When We Were Philosopher Kings," *New Republic*, 28 April 1996, 24-8.

12. D.J. Self and J.D. Skeel, "Professional Liability (Malpractice) Coverage of Humanist Scholars Functioning as Clinical Medical Ethicists," *Journal of Medical Humanities and Bioethics* 9, no. 2 (Fall-Winter 1988): 101-10.

13. See E.P. Richards and K.C. Rathbun, *Law and the Physician: A Practical Guide* (New York: Little, Brown and Co., 1993), 113-27.

14. A. Holder, *Medical Malpractice Law* (New York: John Wiley & Sons, 1975), 43.

15. See B.R. Furrow et al., *Health Law* (St. Paul, Minn.: West Publishing Co., 1995), 1: 351-409.

16. Ibid.

17. For a concise review of early cases, see R. Weir, *Selective Nontreatment of Handicapped Newborns* (New York: Oxford University Press, 1984), 116-27. For more recent analysis see F.A. Hanson, "Suits for Wrongful Life, Counterfactuals, and the Nonexistence Problem," *Southern California Interdisciplinary Law Journal* 5 (Winter 1996): 1-24.

18. Ibid.

19. J.A. Tulsky and E. Fox, "Evaluating Ethics Consultation: Framing the Questions," *The Journal of Clinical Ethics* 7, no. 2 (Summer 1996): 110-1.

20. M. Yeo, "Prolegomena to Any Future Code of Ethics for Bioethicists," *Cambridge Quarterly of Healthcare Ethics* 2 (1993): 402-15.

21. See note 6 above.

22. See note 20 above, pp. 411-2.

23. G. Duval, "Liability of Ethics Consultants: A Case Analysis," *Cambridge Quarterly of Healthcare Ethics* 6 (1997): 272. (Duval reaches the same conclusion on a somewhat different analysis, emphasizing the consultant's fiduciary responsibilities).

24. See note 7 above, pp. 165-8.

25. Ibid., 166.

26. See note 5 above.

27. J.C. Fletcher and M. Siegler, "What Are the Goals of Ethics Consultation? A Consensus Statement," *The Journal of Clinical Ethics* 7, no. 2 (Summer 1996): 122-6.

28. See note 5 above, pp. 6-7.

29. J. La Puma and E.R. Priest, "Medical Staff Privileges for Ethics Consultants: An Institutional Model," *Quality Review Bulletin* (January 1992): 17-20.

30. D.B. Mishkin, "Proffering Bioethicists as Experts," *Judges' Journal* 36 (Summer 1997): 50-1.

31. T.L. Hafemeister and D.M. Robinson, "The Views of the Judiciary Regarding Life-Sustaining Medical Treatment Decisions," *Law & Psychology Review* 18 (Spring 1994): 189.

32. R.M. Veatch, *The Patient-Physician Relation: The Patient as Partner, Part 2* (Bloomington, Ind.: Indiana University Press, 1991), 250-60; S.M. Wolf, "Ethics Committees and Due Process: Nesting Rights in a Community of Caring," *Maryland Law Review* 50, no. 3 (1991): 798-858.

33. See note 5 above, pp. 16-21.

34. For a recent review of jurisprudence regarding treatment refusal, see L.O. Gostin, "Deciding Life and Death in the Courtroom: From *Quinlan* to *Cruzan, Glucksberg* and *Vacco*—A Brief History and Analysis of Constitutional Protection of the 'Right to Die,' " *Journal of the American Medical Association* 278, no. 18 (12 November 1997): 1523-8.

35. See note 15 above.

36. E. Fox and C. Stocking, "Ethics Consultants' Recommendations for Life-Prolonging Treatment of Patients in a Persistent Vegetative State," *Journal of the American Medical Association* 270, no. 21 (1 December 1993): 2581.

37. Ibid., 2580.

38. Scofield, "Ethics Consultation," see note 1 above.

39. *Rogers v. Meridian Park Hosp.*, 307 Or. 612, 772 P.2d 929 (Or. 1989).

40. *In re Wanglie,* no. PX-91-283, slip op. (4th Dist. Ct., Hennepin Cty., Minn., 1 July 1991).

41. R.M. Veatch and C.M. Spicer, "Futile Care: Physicians Should Not Be Allowed to Refuse to Treat," *Health Progress* 74, no. 10 (December 1993): 22-7.

42. S.H. Miles, "Informed Demand for 'Non-Beneficial' Medical Treatment," *New England Journal of Medicine* 325 (1991): 512-5.

43. S.B. Rubin, *When Doctors Say No: The Battleground of Medical Futility* (Bloomington, Ind.: Indiana University Press, 1998).

44. Society of Critical Care Medicine, Ethics Committee, "Consensus Statement of the Society of Critical Care Medicine's Ethics Committee Regarding Futile and Other Possibly Inadvisable Treatments," *Critical Care Medicine* 25, no. 5 (1997): 887-91.

45. A. Halevy and B.A. Brody, "A Multi-Institution Collaborative Policy on Medical Futility," *Journal of the American Medical Association* 276, no. 7 (21 August 1996): 571-4.

46. See note 37 above, p. 2580.

47. See note 7 above, p. 116.

48. G. Agich, "Authority in Ethics Consultation," *Journal of Law, Medicine & Ethics* 23 (1995): 273-83.

49. Ibid.

50. See note 23 above, p. 276.

51. Ann. Code of Md., Health-General, secs. 5-605(b); 5-612 (Michie 1996).

52. *Haw. Rev. Stat.,* sec. 663-1.7.

53. *Estate of Leach v. Shapiro*, 13 Ohio App.3d 393, 469 N.E.2d 1047 (1984).

54. *Anderson v. St. Francis-St. George Hospital*, 77 Ohio St.3d 82, 671 N.E.2d 225 (1996).

55. *Grace Plaza of Great Neck, Inc., v. Elbaum*, 82 N.Y.2d 10, 603 N.Y.S.2d 386, 623 N.E.2d 513 (1993).

56. *First Healthcare Corp. v. Rettinger,* 342 N.C. 886, 467 S.E.2d 243 (1996), affirming, 118 N.C.App. 600, 456 S.E.2d 347 (1995).

19

Continuous Quality Improvement in Case Reviews Facilitated by Hospital Ethics Committees

Bruce E. Zawacki and William May

INTRODUCTION

Primum non nocere (above all, do no harm) is among the earliest, most honored, and most perennially expressed goals of Western medicine. In the relatively brief history of hospital ethics committees (HECs), the goal "to serve patients and protect their interests" has held a similar status.[1] Physicians and HECs can hardly say no or be indifferent to reasonable and constructive efforts to identify and correct mistakes and thereby improve the quality of what they do. Indeed, their authority and standing depend not only on submitting to such efforts, but on being credible leaders. But there are problems.

Many physicians and other caregivers doubt that the current emphasis on "quality of care" is really capable of improving the quality of their patients' lives. Rarely do such efforts even try, much less succeed, to improve health directly. Traditional in-hospital quality assurance (QA) programs usually focus on issues identified by regulatory or accreditation organizations—such as checking documentation, studying credentialing processes, reviewing the work of oversight committees in hospitals, and the like.[2] Other efforts focused on statistics from many institutions have regularly failed to make a difference in the care of individual patients. A Medicare-sponsored study of mortality rates among hospitalized patients was abandoned when it was found to be, on balance, unsuccessful.[3] More recently, the Health Plan Employer Data and Information Set (HEDIS) developed by the National Committee for Quality Assurance, with only nine of 60 measures focusing on quality of care, has been seen as unlikely to satisfy the needs of physicians because of its scant information on medical services provided to individual patients with acute and chronic illnesses.[4] The consistent belief underlying large and expensive surveillance programs like these seems to be that only statistical analysis of extensive data banks can be trusted to warrant changed behavior and improve quality.[5] Of course there are exceptions, but meaningful progress based on this assumption has been disappointingly slow.

Another problem is doubtful motives. Much of what is called quality improvement is viewed by physicians and other caregivers as thinly veiled cost containment—especially when quality improvement efforts focus mostly on outcomes such as reducing length of hospital stay. The development and widespread application of guidelines, computerized medical-information systems, and methods of total quality management have coincided with the commercialization of the medical marketplace and have been motivated, at least in part, by an unspoken desire to increase profits.[6] A similar "implicit agenda" has been discerned in the fact that only "over time [did] the surgeons responsible for data collection [for the New York State Department of Health Cardiac Surgery Reporting System become] . . . increasingly aware that they were the principal subjects of the investigation."[7] For many physicians, this and similar efforts to develop report cards on particular healthcare providers seem to have been based on the assumption that an overridingly important way to improve care is by hunting for and eliminating "bad apples" from the ranks of practitioners, or at least by giving purchasers of healthcare sufficient information about inadequate performance that they can "vote with their feet."[8]

Because of widespread misgivings about the effectiveness and motivation of quality improvement efforts, the physicians, nurses, and other caregivers serving on HECs can hardly be faulted for having reservations about efforts to improve what they do, especially in view of the stridency of some calls for accountability of ethics committees and consultants.[9] Moreover, two practical problems appear to compound their reservations. First, HECs, on average, conduct no more than 10 to 15 case reviews per year. With such a light caseload, how could any quality improvement study by a single HEC achieve statistical validity? Second, it is an axiom of modern quality improvement that error can be minimized only by protecting disclosure of error against sanction.[10] However, fear of public embarrassment, disparagement by peers, and litigation by patients can make it almost as difficult for HECs to disclose their deficiencies as it is for physicians to admit theirs. How can HEC members be assured that honesty in revealing their own errors or deficiencies in conducting case reviews will be used to improve what they do and not to harm or humiliate them unnecessarily, perhaps by inviting into their lives a "distant-and-therefore-objective-and-trustworthy" bureaucracy bent on finding and chastising "bad apples?"[11]

As indicated above, there is a widely held assumption that, to be defensible, efforts to reduce error must be validated by methods of sufficient scientific merit that they will be suitable for publication or at least applicable in other settings. This assumption is contradicted by the continuous quality improvement (CQI) movement, which has worked remarkably well in industry and is beginning to demonstrate success in medicine.[12] Whether the activity examined is playing golf, performing surgery, preventing airplane crashes, or performing ethics consultations, it is not always possible or necessary to collect statistically significant proof in order to achieve meaningful (and at times lifesaving) improvement by correcting discerned error. In informal bedside discussions, and in formal mortality and morbidity (M&M) conferences held in their own medical departments, surgeons and other physicians have for generations revealed, scrutinized, corrected, and confirmed their deficiencies and mistakes in care; in this manner they have improved their own performance, one case at a time, and very often without statistical proof. In answer to the question about how to make good-faith self-revelation of error immune to unnecessary harm or embarrassment, the proceedings of M&M conferences, like many other formal QA activities, have been made legally undiscoverable precisely because society values such peer-reviewed self-criticism. Mechanisms for achieving accountability in medical practice (such as accreditation, certification, licensure, professional discipline, and tort claims) have not been so intrusive that the confidentiality of peer review has been significantly violated by "impartial" third-party bureaucrats. Some similar accommodation between accountability for procedural fairness and peer-review confidentiality should be achievable for ethics case review by HECs.[13]

HECs can develop a readily available, realistic, and effective program for discernment of and response to their own deficiencies in case review if (1) they organize a CQI process in a legally undiscoverable setting like that used in M&M and similar QA conferences; and (2) they recognize that, just as in M&M conferences or investigations of airplane crashes, changes in structure or process can lead to improvement after review of a problem case or a problematic system even before they can accumulate numbers necessary for statistical significance. Such CQI processes have become accepted, familiar, nonstigmatizing sources of enthusiastic self-improvement of both individuals and systems in hospitals throughout the United States. Despite widespread "bad-apple hunting," we believe now is an especially opportune time for HECs to turn to CQI. Performance report cards may or may not be developed to evaluate HECs through scrutiny of computerized data by impartial third parties. If these activities prove to be more than briefly fashionable methodological failures, they may or may not prove to be valid and useful and they may or may not change the behavior of HECs.[14] Professional medical caregivers and HECs who are truly committed to protecting, honoring, and doing no unnecessary harm to those who seek their help have not waited in the past, and will not wait in the future, to learn if such surveillance activities succeed or fail before participating in their own programs of error discovery and quality improvement. Out of their concern and commitment to patients and other stakeholders, HECs will continue or will inaugurate the self-policing efforts that distinguish professionals and continually seek to improve quality—no matter how, when, why, where, and by whom it is measured. CQI can become a reasonable and relatively inexpensive means for HECs to fulfill that professional duty and create the improvement that is their privilege to seek and achieve, even if others choose to measure the efforts and outcomes for themselves.

THE ROLE OF HECS IN CARRYING OUT CQI

To discern an appropriate role for HECs in continually correcting their mistakes or problems in case review, it is useful to look at how new and more adequate answers to problems are developed in science—a field of study much more familiar to most people than bioethics.[15] In trying to resolve problems and bring reason into our view of the physical world, several levels of investigation or research may be necessary (see Exhibit 19-1). We are all able to handle small day-to-day problems in the physical world by ourselves, but from time to time we may encounter an anomaly beyond our skill to correct (such as an electric light switch or a plumbing arrangement we simply cannot get to work properly). We usually turn to a skilled technician, such as an electrician or plumber, who, after appropriate investigation, is able to provide an answer to the problem based on his or her superior training and experience with the rules of how such things work. Perhaps some problems will prove so difficult as to require assistance from an electrical or hydraulic engineer, who has a richer and deeper knowledge of the principles of electricity or hydraulics than a technician. But what happens when technicians and engineers encounter an anomaly that they cannot understand and resolve? They may well be able to devise ways to accomplish what they want without understanding and explaining the anomaly, but at this point the new problem—that of an unexplained problem or anomaly—

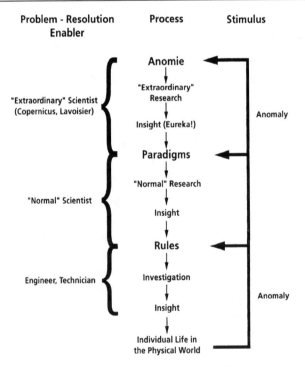

Exhibit 19-1. Schematic outline of the process of problem solving in science.
BEZ created this graphic adapting material from T.S. Kuhn, *The Structure of Scientific Revolutions,* 2nd ed. (Chicago: University of Chicago Press, 1970); the graphic first appeared in B. Zawacki, "The Structure of Progress in Burn Immunology," in *The Immune Consequences of Thermal Injury,* ed. J.S. Ninemann (Baltimore: Williams & Wilkins, 1983); ©1983 by Lippincott Williams & Wilkins. Used with permission.

becomes the province of the "normal" scientist (see Exhibit 19-1). Knowing not just the rules, but the principles (of electricity or hydrodynamics) from which the rules are derived, such individuals are professional scholars in their fields who, by their work, enable others to solve problems in those fields. The problem these scholars solve is how to explain or resolve anomalies using the principles or paradigms accepted by the community of scientists. In fact, that is what the vast majority of scientists normally do. Normal scientists specializing in electricity use and take for granted the paradigms established by "extraordinary" scientists such as Benjamin Franklin, André-Marie Ampère, and Max Planck. According to Kuhn, normal scientists actualize the promise of an already existing paradigm "by extending the knowledge of those facts that the paradigm displays as particularly revealing, by increasing the extent of match between those facts and the paradigm predictions, and by further articulation of the paradigm."[16]

The term *normal science* is appropriate in describing the activities of these scholars for two reasons: (1) such activities usually (that is, normally) constitute what most scientists do most of the time; and (2) normal research is based on accepted paradigms or norms. As Kuhn points out, however, anomalies occasionally turn up that prove refractory to science as it is ordinarily practiced—that is, they are not explicable or manageable by currently accepted paradigms. The resulting condition might well be termed *anomie*—a condition in which satisfactorily stable or integrating paradigms or norms are lacking. This sets the stage for scientific revolution—the struggle to give birth to new and more adequate paradigms. In this way Galileo's views of motion replaced those of Aristotle, Lavoisier's theories regarding oxygen replaced the phlogiston theory, and Pasteur proposed the germ theory of disease.

In the realm of bioethics, the system for solving problems and handling anomalies is in some ways similar to that described by Kuhn for science (see Exhibit 19-2). In their individual, day-to-day moral life, physicians, nurses, and their patients are able to deal with most clinical ethics problems by themselves. Informed consent is obtained, the process of death is dealt with tolerably, and confidentiality is preserved with little trouble. Occasionally (no more than twice a month in most hospitals), stakeholders encounter an ethics problem that just will not work out as they would like, and they turn to the HEC with their problem by asking for a case review. In most circumstances, HECs or their subcommittees can facilitate resolution of problems by acting like ethics technicians (for example, by reading or explaining an institution's guidelines on foregoing life-support to those who call for help and allowing them to act accordingly). On other occasions, merely reading the rules is too superficial an answer. A formal meeting of stakeholders must be held with all or a portion of the committee. After information gathering and preparatory planning, the committee arranges a meeting with stakeholders beginning with a previously prepared "preamble," followed by a structured clarification and discerning process, during which, ideally, the goals of case review are sought using an appropriate structure and process.[17] In these circumstances, HEC members probe below superficial rules and act in a more sophisticated role analogous to that of an experienced engineer in science. At this level they seek to discover and verify empirical facts, clarify concepts, elicit options, and help stakeholders deliberate using various principles or other discerning skills in deciding which option to pursue. Usually this seems to work out quite well. Yet, in recent years, there has been growing dissatisfaction with both the processes and the outcomes of case review.[18] The uncertainties giving rise to this dissatisfaction are reflected not only in the literature, but in the great variability with which HECs answer questions such as the following: Should patients be allowed to request case review? Should they be present during deliberations? Should HECs give recommendations or not? Should they make decisions or not? Is case review more successful when conducted by an HEC or when conducted by an individual ethics consultant?

At this point in history, these and other persistent problems with case review have required the work of those further up the ladder of problem solving in bioethics (see Exhibit 19-2). Scholars in normative ethics have responded recently by forming three task forces designed to formulate and put into practice standards for bioethics case review (or case consultation, as it is often called).[19] Their work has been analogous to that of "normal" scientists in science, that is,

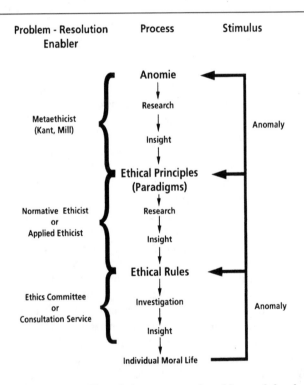

Exhibit 19-2. Schematic outline of the process of problem solving in bioethics.
Adapted from a graphic that first appeared in B. Zawacki, "The Structure of Progress in Burn Immunology," in *The Immune Consequences of Thermal Injury,* ed. J.S. Ninemann (Baltimore: Williams & Wilkins, 1983); ©1983 by Lippincott Williams & Wilkins. Used with permission.

it does not develop new paradigms of ethics by replacing the revolutionary work of Plato, Aristotle, Kant, and Mill, but improves case review "by extending the knowledge of those facts that . . . [the currently accepted paradigms of Western ethics] display as particularly revealing, by increasing the extent of match between those facts and the paradigm predictions, and by further articulations of the paradigm[s themselves]."[20] The work of these task forces is similar to the normal work of normative ethicists; it articulated what case review *ought* to be, what core competencies *should* be available, and so forth. The argument-supported insights of the task forces were designed to enable empirical research in, and to improve the clinical practice of, ethics case review by HECs and others. Of course their efforts may fail, or we may find that the goals of case review are better achieved by other methods, such as better education, better policies and/ or laws, and so forth. In fact, some of the problems of case review faced by HECs and others (such as the problem of "futile" interventions) may actually require fundamentally new paradigms or combinations of paradigms (such as casuistry, narrative ethics, and/or communitarian ethics, among others) to be developed by the visionary "extraordinary ethicists" who occupy the top of the ladder in Exhibit 19-2. Only history will tell which of these ethicists (if any) might turn out to be the Mill or Kant of his or her day.

Right now, however, the next step is not that steep. HECs and others who do clinical ethics case reviews are called to work out the rules or standards articulated by the expert task forces cited above. The SHHV-SBC Task Force on Standards for Bioethics Consultation indicates it "attaches great importance to evaluation [of ethics consultants, the consulting process, and the outcomes of consultation] . . . as an area that should be actively pursued. . . ."[21] These are the kinds of tasks CQI was invented to handle.

HOW DOES CQI WORK?

The concept of CQI is quite simple. We will begin this discussion with some illustrations involving hospital care (see Exhibit 19-3). Conventionally, quality of care has been evaluated on the basis of structure, process, or outcome.[22] *Structure* includes the individuals, institutions, and resources put into the care provided (the caregivers, their competencies, and the equipment they use). *Process* refers to the components of the interaction between healthcare providers and patients (what the provider says, how he or she arrives at a diagnosis, the tests and drugs ordered, and so forth). *Outcome* usually refers to the resultant bio-psycho-social health status of the patient and the patient's subjective attitudes about the care received (satisfaction or dissatisfaction). In an imperfect world, outcomes regularly fall short of desired goals. The extent by which an outcome falls short of a goal is a convenient measure of an "error" made. Even an error in process (such as taking an inadequate medical history) can be conveniently construed as falling short of a goal. In CQI, caregivers are more likely to honestly and enthusiastically collaborate when falling short of a goal is referred to as a "problem" rather than an "error" or "mistake." It is for this reason—and not because we expect those responsible for CQI to be naïvely blind and unresponsive to the possibility of dangerous or damaging negligence, blunders, or crimes—that we prefer the word "problem" instead of "error."

When a problem is identified, it is evaluated, and improvement can be planned (see Exhibit 19-3). Improvements in structure and/or process can then be carried out, and their success measured. Measurement of any subsequent problem (that is, a significant shortfall from a goal) is followed by one or more subsequent cycles, leading to resolution of the problem.

MICRO-ORGANIZATIONAL CHANGE

Consider the following surgical case, in which a single event triggered a CQI process has continued to be successful. Young children with severely burned faces often must have a tube inserted into their airways through the nose or mouth to allow them to continue to breathe when their airway swells because they have inhaled smoke. Because moisture gathers on the surface of burned

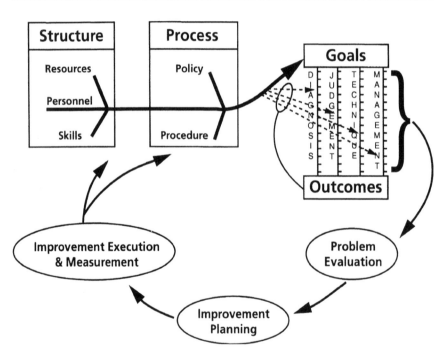

Exhibit 19-3. The cycle of continuous quality improvement as applied in a medical setting.

Structure and process are represented as components of a typical "fishbone" or "Isikawa" CQI diagram. As indicated by the solid bold arrow, they are designed to achieve goals. Outcomes are indicated by hatched arrows pointing in graduating scales. First published privately in 1917, and used for generations at all Massachusetts General Hospital General Surgical M&M conferences, the four outcome measures cited here were modified from E.A. Codman, *A Study in Hospital Efficiency as Demonstrated by the Case Reports of the First Five Years of a Private Hospital* (Oakbrook Terrace, Ill.: Joint Commission on Accreditation of Healthcare Organizations, 1996), 59.

skin, burns of the face make it difficult to hold breathing tubes in place using adhesive tape. Displacement of a tube too far up or down in the trachea can be dangerous, and displacement out of the trachea may be immediately life-threatening. There is no room for error in displacing a tube in or out of such a child's trachea—a displacement can be fatal, or perhaps even worse, if severe neurological damage results. A single dramatic episode of tube displacement out of the trachea so concerned the care team at the Los Angeles County + University of Southern California (LAC + USC) Burn Center, even though the tube was promptly replaced, that the team formally declared the procedure a "problem in technique" and established a process-improvement planning team. After reviewing the literature and considering and trying several options, the Burn Center implemented a policy for securing tubes inserted through the nose by lashing them securely in place (using a second, softer, and more slender tube to encircle an internal nasal bone). The Burn Center achieved the goal of 0 percent significant displacements of breathing tubes inserted through the nose.

MESO-ORGANIZATIONAL CHANGE

The Burn Center's continued response to the displacement of a child's tube demonstrates how the process of CQI is not necessarily limited to the review of a single case requiring micro-organizational change in process by one or a few members of one care team. Often the scope of CQI must be expanded to the review of several cases or may require meso-organizational changes (that is, changes in structure or process for several departments in the hospital). To continue the examination of this example: although the "nasal lashing procedure" permanently stopped significant displacement of tubes inserted through the nose, significant displacements of tubes inserted through the mouth continued to occur. The Burn Center made a temporary structural change by adding a pediatric intensivist, an otolaryngologist, and an anesthesiologist to the process-improvement planning team and the execution team. Holding structure and process otherwise stable, the teams found that two cycles of explicitly measured process change (adding wire-suture fixation of the tube to the teeth and applying a movement-limiting neck collar) were necessary before the problem was at last completely resolved.

An example of meso-organizational CQI involving many cases and many departments occurred between January 1984 and December 1988.[23] During that period, 943 skin-grafting procedures were performed at the LAC + USC Burn Center. Following surgery, the wound cultures of 35 patients were found to be positive for *Aspergillus* (a kind of fungus "almost ubiquitous on the planet," but potentially dangerous on a large burn wound). Invasive infection of the burn wound occurred in 63 percent of these culture-positive cases, and death in 54 percent. These outcome percentages fell short of the Burn Center's goal of 0 percent contamination, infection, or death. The Burn Center chose to use these unsatisfactory outcome percentages as measures of its problems in technique and management. Holding structure and process otherwise stable, the Burn Center sequentially made several carefully researched and planned structural changes of the air-duct system (such as installation of new ducts and high-efficiency antimicrobial filters) and several process changes (such as changes in the antimicrobial drugs applied to the surface of the burns). The effectiveness of each change was measured using the number of contaminations, infections, or deaths associated with *Aspergillus* in patients with burn wounds as an outcome. It took a little more than four years, a total of four planned and verified improvements in the air-duct system, and five planned and verified changes in the antimicrobial drugs applied to the burns to reach and thereafter maintain the goal of 0 percent contamination, infection, or death associated with *Aspergillus.* Epidemiology, infectious disease, hospital engineering, and several other departments were involved for years. During that time, the Burn Center staff knew from the ongoing data collection that the problem was diminishing, but they could prove it with statistical significance only in retrospect.

MACRO-ORGANIZATIONAL CHANGE

In dealing with another clinical problem, macro-organizational changes were needed that involved an entire healthcare system. About two years ago, burned patients with large burns frequently arrived at the LAC+USC Burn Center from institutions across the county having lost significant amounts of body heat (hypothermia). Investigation revealed that the patients had not had adequate heat-conserving measures applied before and during transfer. Letters to the transferring institutions and teams seemed to make little difference. Finally, with the help of a sister institution, the Burn Center developed a large, colorful, attractive poster giving emergency burn-care instructions, including prominent warnings about preventing heat loss before and during transfer. With the additional help of the appropriate county agency, the poster was delivered to every emergency department in the county. For a period of time, this macro-organizational problem greatly diminished.

IS CQI REASONABLE?

Was the team that prevented displacement of breathing tubes from the noses, mouths, and tracheas of children with burned faces acting rashly by responding so extremely to a single case, even though proof of statistical significance in a single case was impossible? Hardly. Was the team that struggled to eliminate *Aspergillus* unreasonable to make the changes it did, even though the changes could be statistically verified as improvements only after the fact? Of course not. Such problems develop constantly in the services of every hospital on earth. Must they all be referred to bureaucratic, "objective" outside agencies for monitoring? We think not, if only because there simply are not enough bureaucrats. Moreover, efforts at self-monitoring and self-improvement are seen as so effective that they are even required by the Joint Commission on Accreditation of Healthcare Organizations (JCAHO). Finally, was it strained and unnatural to extend the CQI process to several departments in order to control *Aspergillus,* or to several institutions and the entire county emergency healthcare system to reduce burn-associated hypothermia? Not at all. The process was similar, natural, efficient, and reasonable when applied after a single case in a single unit, or to many widely scattered cases. Whether the problem proved to be micro-organizational, meso-organizational, or macro-organizational in scope, the CQI process was quite naturally and with relatively little difficulty collaboratively expanded so that correction and improvement could occur.

WHY HECS RARELY USE
A FORMAL SYSTEM OF CQI

After reading the examples of CQI cited above, we expect readers to react much like the character in Moliere's play who discovered that he had been speaking prose for more than 40 years without knowing it. Application of informal CQI efforts to significant medical problems like those cited above seem natural and common-sensical—even automatic. Texts about CQI are filled with more ambitious examples using sophisticated statistical techniques and numerous variables that are definitely not automatic or mere common sense, and such examples can be very daunting.[24] But CQI, formally identified as such, is very popular in medicine. Although quality assessment is recommended not infrequently in the literature related to HECs,[25] we have nevertheless found only one publication reporting the explicit use of CQI for assessment and improvement of case review as conducted by an HEC.[26] Why hasn't it been applied to improvement of case review by HECs more often?

The answer to this question may be related to the fact that, unlike the practice of HECs, the practice of medicine is ancient in origin, it is seen as valuable in virtually all known societies, and there is consensus throughout the civilized world regarding its appropriate means and ends. Moreover, the scope of medicine is relatively concrete, particular, and scientific, while that of ethics case review is more abstract, general, and humanistic. The goals and mission statements of ethics committees in regard to case review published before 1986 cite vague, variable, general, and virtually unmeasurable end points.[27] In retrospect, they were "good guesses" expressed at the time when HECs first explored new ways of acting. Early committees believed they existed "primarily to serve patients and protect their interests."[28] Early efforts at self-evaluation focused on the frequency and subjects of case reviews, process, satisfaction surveys, and so forth.[29] Now, with several years of experience, HECs and scholars on the subject of ethics case review find that they have moved into new ways of thinking.

As indicated above, after almost two years of work, a task force of distinguished and respected scholars from the Society for Health and Human Values and the Society for Bioethics Consultation Task Force on Standards for Bioethics Consultation (the Task Force for short) made widely available a consensus document detailing with considerable clarity the definition and goals of, as well as the "core competencies" and procedural model recommended for, healthcare ethics consultation.[30] At approximately the same time, a similarly distinguished conference (involving some of the same scholars) on the Evaluation of Care Consultation in Clinical Ethics (ECCCE) published its work.[31] The work sought, among other things, to "enumerate the goals of" and "specify appropriate and workable outcomes for evaluating ethics consultation" and to "devise research strategies to evaluate such consultations."[32] For the first time, these experts provided for this field of study a significant consensus about (1) major characteristics of structure (that is, the organization and competencies of the practitioners); (2) the goals to be sought, expressed in such a way that outcomes could be measured against them; and (3) the details of the recommended process ("ethics-facilitation approach"), sufficient to allow its characteristics to be specified as goals. By this work, significant portions of the beginning and end of the CQI sequence (from structure through process to goals and outcomes) appear to have been fixed by an adequate consensus about ethics case review. This may at last provide sufficient stability to the "wheel of the CQI unicycle" (illustrated in an application to clinical medicine in Exhibit 19-3) that it can be applied, repetitively turned, and "ridden" by HECs seeking continuous improvement in their efforts to reduce the problems and achieve the goals of ethics case review.

CQI APPLIED TO CASE REVIEW BY HECs

The goals of healthcare ethics consultation as described by the Task Force are presented in Exhibit 19-4. Except for small and, we believe, insignificant changes in language, it is identical to that previously published by Fletcher and Siegler[33] and has unequaled status and authority as a statement of consensus. Unfortunately, there is not yet the same quality and extent of consensus about how to operationalize these goals for purposes of research and quality-improvement studies of outcome. After reflecting on these statements of goals, and after input from still other experts, Fox and Arnold[34] and later Andre[35] sought to simplify and operationalize the goals of healthcare ethics consultation. Readers will profit by consulting the original articles. Because, in our judgment, Andre's operationalizing language adds the most "clarity, utility, and fidelity" to the Task Force's goals statement, we summarize it in Exhibit 19-5 to illustrate the relation of goals to outcomes and problem measurement in ethics case review. To the four *goals of moral quality*—that is, (1) optimum ethicality of process, (2) optimum stakeholder education, (3) optimum stakeholder empowerment, and (4) optimum ethicality of outcome (resolution)—we have added (5) *et cetera*, which includes optimum cost-effectiveness, satisfaction, and conflict resolution— the *goals of nonmoral quality* recommended by others.[36] In analogy to Exhibit 19-3, the problems (that is, outcome shortfalls from goals) for ethics case review in Exhibit 19-5 are, for convenience, listed in the temporal order in which they typically occur in a given case.

1. Optimum ethicality of process reflects the Task Force's goal (expressed in Exhibit 19-4) to "facilitate resolution of conflicts in a respectful atmosphere with attention to the interests, rights, and responsibilities of those involved." Included among the measures to be examined under this heading might be inclusion of all relevant stakeholders in discussion and completeness of medical, psychosocial, legal, and other relevant information; consideration of the patient's preferences and input by staff, family, and relevant agencies; adequate review of options and consideration of all relevant values to assist in choosing an option;[37] and the explicit seeking of win-win resolutions.

2. *Optimum education of stakeholders* reflects the SHHV-SBC Task Force's goals (see Exhibit 19-4) to "assist individuals in handling current and future ethical problems by providing education" and "inform institutional efforts at policy development, quality improvement, and appropriate utilization of resources. . . ." Relevant under this heading are measures of stakeholders' knowledge about ethics and relevant law, ethnic pluralism, and so forth; evidence of transfer to stakeholders of skills in applying ethical categories, analysis of issues and arguments, and mediation in their ethical dialogues. Tests of progress in "moral development" of the attending physician and house staff and of the HEC itself would be of great interest, if these prove to be testable with reasonable reliability and expense.[38]

3. *Optimum empowerment of stakeholders* reflects the spirit of the Task Force's consensus expressed in words like "help," "facilitate," "promote," and "assist" (see Exhibit 19-4). It is also reflected in its statement that ethics consultants "should not usurp moral decision-making authority or impose their values on other involved parties."[39] Documented efforts to "help those involved learn to work through ethical uncertainties and disagreements on their own"[40] would be measures of relative achievement of this goal.

4. *Optimum ethicality of resolution* reflects the Task Force's consensus that a primary goal of case review is to "promote practices consistent with ethical norms and standards," and the need to "identify and analyze the nature of the value uncertainty or conflict that underlies the consultation" (see Exhibit 19-4).

Exhibit 19-4. Task Force's Goals of Health Care Ethics Consultation

---

The general goal of health care ethics consultation[a] is to:
- improve the provision of health care and its outcome through identification, analysis, and resolution of ethical issues as they emerge in consultation regarding particular clinical cases in health care institutions.

This general goal is more likely to be achieved if consultation accomplishes the intermediary goals of helping to:
- identify and analyze the nature of the value uncertainty or conflict that underlies the consultation
- facilitate resolution of conflicts in a respectful atmosphere with attention to the interests, rights, and responsibilities of those involved.

Successful health care ethics consultation will also serve the goal of helping to:
- inform institutional efforts at policy development, quality improvement, and appropriate utilization of resources by identifying the causes of ethical problems and promoting practices consistent with ethical norms and standards
- assist individuals in handling current and future ethical problems by providing education in health care ethics.

---

[a] The word "consultation" appears in the original document. We believe the words "case review" or "case counseling" to be more appropriate and less confusing. Source: SHHV-SBC Task Force on Standards for Bioethics Consultation, *Core Competencies for Health Care Ethics Consultation* (Glenview, Ill.: ASBH, 1998).

Measures suitable for outcome study are those "about which agreement is currently sufficient to make the definition of meaningful outcome measures a realistic possibility."[41] Examples would include American society's consensus about norms of self-determination by the patient, informed consent, decision making for incompetent patients, decisions at the end of life, and confidentiality.[42] Items that could be used as measures include compliance with institutional policies; local standards of care; relevant legislation; published county, state, and national medical association guidelines; and specialty guidelines.

5. Et cetera. Although usually desirable and recommended strongly by some authors, nonmoral goods such as optimum "cost-effectiveness," "conflict reduction," "satisfaction,"[43] and "comfortable . . . communication among the parties involved [during resolution]"[44] are not present in the Task Force's goals statement, and are not necessarily measures of *ethicality* of resolution if *ethically* unjustified. Measures of the frequency of lawsuits or costs of "unnecessary" stays in the intensive care unit might be appropriate under this heading. The goal of reduction of conflict might be numerically graded with win-win as 4 +, compromise as 3 +, success for one party and failure of the other as 2 +, stalemate as 1 +, court settlement as 0, and physical battle as -1.[45] Semiquantitative Likert scales could be used to measure satisfaction with outcome and perceived comfort and respectfulness during case review.

A few explanatory remarks are appropriate here. "Ethicality" is to ethics as "legality" is to law. It is an outcome not conventionally considered in business or medicine, but in ethics case review by HECs it is a major dimension of the activity to be focused on and improved. Ethicality of resolution and ethicality of process must both be addressed, because it is obviously self-defeating for an HEC to facilitate an ethical resolution using unethical means. Our reference to ethicality of process might be construed *prima facie* as a process measure rather than an outcome measure. We recognize this ambiguity, but persist in listing it as an outcome measure because it may be more or less well achieved as an end or outcome, depending on which policies or procedures (that is, on which interventions or processes) are chosen as means to achieve it. If, for example, corrective changes in process were inadequate to improve outcomes, measures properly labeled as "process measures" would be necessary to ensure that process changes had occurred. Another concern is how to classify a case if its outcome fails to meet the goal set for it. For example, consider the conflict between an ICU chief physician and the children of his patient, a Japanese woman, from whom the children have hidden the diagnosis of cancer. After meeting with the HEC, the physician and the family agreed to keep the patient ignorant of her diagnosis. The HEC did not advise the physician that he could first ask the patient privately about how she wished important decisions to be made before honoring her family's wishes. At first glance, it appears that the HEC did not meet its goal of empowering the patient to make her own decision, if she chose to do so. On further reflection, perhaps the HEC did not meet its goal of adequately educating the physician. Asking more than once, if necessary, the open question "And why did *that* happen?" may help in determining under which goal the shortfall should be located.

After problems in ethics case review are identified and measured, they are subjected to problem evaluation, which logically begins with classification of the measured shortfall from the goal as preventable or not (see Exhibit 19-5). Severe emergency situations, for example, may make normally mandatory education or empowerment not humanly possible. Other problems—such as inadequate resolution of case review due to lack of consensus about how long a case of anoxic persistent vegetative state must persist before anticipated recovery approaches 0 percent—may be preventable in the future, but only after further research. The persistently insoluble problem of how HECs should deal with cases that meet any of several available definitions of futility, for another example, may well require more formal research by pushing it up the ethics ladder (illustrated in Exhibit 19-2), although at least two authors believe the problem of futility to be manageable by improving on currently available methods.[46] Most problems, however, will be judged by the process of HEC self-evaluation as preventable. Because of resource limitations, not all preventable problems are worth preventing. HECs may use a "Pareto determination" to identify which problems are most likely to be successfully prevented with the most impact; such a determination can be used to indicate which problems are "worth" the expenditure of limited resources to control or prevent them. This may be im-

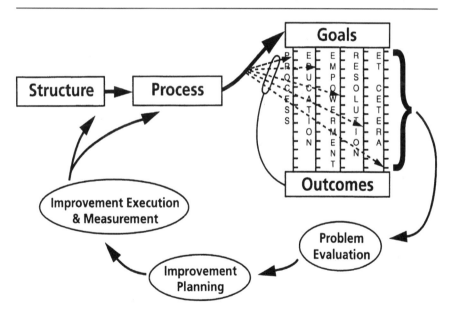

Exhibit 19-5. The cycle of continuous quality improvement as applied to case review by HECs.

Some shortfalls from goals may permit only semiquantitative estimates of their gravity and/or magnitude, and some will be refractory to quantification. The latter maybe noted "present" or "absent" in a given case and occurence rate in accumulated cases used as a measure of the problem. Adapted from J. Andre, "Goals of Ethics Consultation: Toward Clarity, Utility, and Fidelity," *The Journal of Clinical Ethics* 8, no. 2 (Summer 1997): 193-8; © 1997 by *The Journal of Clinical Ethics.* Used with permission.

mediately obvious (as in an instance of active involuntary euthanasia occurring after HEC evaluation), or it may not be evident until a series of similar cases is appreciated only in retrospect. Hence the need for accurate record keeping by HECs. Texts and courses devoted to CQI offer methods to help with Pareto discernment in difficult cases.[47]

At this point, "preventable problems worth preventing" are moved to the "improvement planning" step in the feedback loop (see Exhibit 19-5). The members of the task force of stakeholders who will address the problem should be based on who will be responsible for preventing the problem in the future. Consider again the case in which the HEC failed to inform the physician that he could ask the Japanese cancer patient privately how she wanted decisions to be made. If, on further inquiry, it was found that the chair of the HEC had assigned only new and untrained members to the case, improvement would require micro-organizational correction (that is, correction of only one or a few individual members of the HEC). If this lack of cultural awareness occurred because not only the HEC chairperson, but the hospital, was culturally unaware and required corrective education, improvement would require meso-organizational correction of not just a few stakeholders, but the whole hospital staff. If, on still further investigation, the whole health-maintenance organization or the whole healthcare system of a city was found to be unaware, macro-organizational correction (correction of and by many institutions) would be needed. A corrective action requiring mega-organizational responsibility and action refers to a problem involving an entire society. For example, lack of a consensus on a system to achieve equitable distribution of organs for transplantation throughout the country has long been an example of needed mega-organizational action.

Improvement planning continues with formation of a task force of responsible stakeholders. The makeup of the task force will obviously vary with the type of problem and how it is classified. It should be made up of HEC members and other responsible stakeholders or their appropriate representatives. If *prima facie* estimates of who should be involved prove incorrect, task force members should be changed as necessary. The last step in the feedback limb of the CQI loop (illustrated in Exhibit 19-5) indicates that the improvement that is planned must be not only executed, but measured as actually occurring; then outcome versus goals must be measured once again. A micro-organizational corrective plan seeking to improve the sensitivity of a single HEC to ethnic differences in decision making at the end-of-life by Japanese-Americans, Japanese in America, and others might require only assignment of some reading[48] and role playing annually by the educational subcommittee of the HEC to resolve satisfactorily any deficiency in that area of knowledge. This would be an example of building new skills into the structure of the HEC, the effectiveness of which would require a subsequent measurement of appropriate outcomes versus goals. As an example of a problem of larger scope, it was shortly after the *Barber v. Superior Court* case arose in one of its hospitals during 1983 that the Kaiser Permanente Health Care System of Southern California undertook a macro-organizational improvement planning process to improve the ability of its HECs to facilitate ethicality of resolution and process in ethics case review.[49] One outcome of the effort was that Kaiser contracted with professional medical ethics firms to provide ongoing education and skill building for all its HEC members. This represented a major change in structure. Policies and procedures for HECs were developed and promulgated as part of this process. To discover what effects these ethics educational events have had on outcomes, follow-up evaluation reports are appropriate.

Articulation of details can be offputting. Descriptions of driving a car are lengthy and boring; driving it, again and again, with coaching, is much more attractive and productive. The clinical examples of CQI in medical care cited above were natural, helpful, hopeful, and satisfying once we were used to them. However, they were difficult and unnatural at first. The more we do CQI in case review, the easier and more successful it will become; that has been the case with many other applications of the technique. What HECs need to do now is to get started.

HOW SHOULD HECS BEGIN NOW TO CARRY OUT CQI EFFORTS?

Of course this will vary with each HEC. Probably, like most HECs, ours at the LAC+USC Medical Center started its journey toward case review with a mission statement or charge that pointed us toward the goals of protecting patients and helping to resolve conflicts. In terms of CQI, we had some poorly defined goals, and no structure, process, or outcomes. "Cranking" for the first time through the cycle of CQI, our earliest efforts identified our initial problem as lack of a structure and process, and measured the problem as "large." Problem evaluation led to improvement planning and then improvement execution, and a committee of a particular size, makeup, competency, and resources (that is, structure) was developed. After further self-education, the HEC implemented policies and procedures for case review (that is, processes) and experienced some outcomes. To adjust toward what we judged (with no evidence) to be a more balanced representation of stakeholders on the committee, we added one African-American, one Mexican-American, and one European-American as lay members of the committee. With no evidence available pro or con, we arranged for subcommittees of three members (usually a physician, a nurse, and one "other" such as a clergy person, social worker, lawyer, ethicist, or layperson) to review cases at the bedside, rather than asking stakeholders to sit with the whole committee of 25 members. With no evidence pro or con, we committed, almost fanatically, to an education-counseling model rather than a medical or judicial model of case review.[50] Accordingly, we labeled our committee the Ethics Resource Committee, and we called our bedside case review subcommittees Case Clarification and Counseling subcommittees, or CCC subcommittees for short. We decided that, with the sole exception of lawyers representing parties to a case, anyone in the LAC+USC Medical Center who had a legitimate purpose could ask for and expect to receive the committee's help with case review. We distributed satisfaction surveys to all stakeholders after CCC sessions; almost uniformly high satisfaction was expressed, so we eventually lost interest in continuing the survey. After a decade of orientation of all new house staff and sporadic medical and surgical grand-rounds presentations, residents and attending physicians generally know about the committee, but remain unknowledgeable about our hospital ethics policies. We know nothing of how much our patients know of our service and can only guess what any new educational intervention might accomplish.

Our HEC has used the continuous improvement cycle depicted in this chapter informally and intuitively from the very beginning, closing the feedback loop with information from our satisfaction surveys. Yet without more detailed and ethically relevant outcome measures, we had no way to determine how ethically effective our process was. To remedy that problem, we have begun to incorporate into our self-evaluation effort portions of the detailed Task Force's consensus recommendations about competencies (structure) and goals (the latter greatly enabling measures of outcome). We believe the SHHV-SBC *Care Competencies for Health Care Ethics Consultation* Task Force report should give our HEC and others sufficient grounding and foundation to undertake a formal process of CQI. But where should we start, especially if we do not have, and do not anticipate receiving in the near future, the research funds needed for scientifically validated research?

We believe we should start with the 12 to 24 formally reviewed cases we see each year. Unlike the hundreds of medical and surgical M&M cases that must be reviewed each year, the smaller number of ethics case reviews we perform makes it possible for us to conduct an extensive and in-depth examination of each to discover where each case could be improved in terms of the five outcome measures noted in Exhibit 19-5. From clinical M&M experience we have found it convenient—but self-destructive—to classify dysfunctional events under categories of "errors." As noted previously, we have found the parties involved more willing to look at and take responsibility for such events when the events are labeled as "problems," classified by proposed method of improvement, rather than as "problems" classified by the category in which goals were not achieved. For example, a problem in which CCC subcommittees are found regularly to take over decision making from stakeholders (because there is no policy against it) would, for CQI purposes, be better classified as a "problem in micro-organizational policy" than a "problem in stakeholder empowerment," even though it is *measured* as a shortfall from the goal of full stakeholder empowerment. A CCC meeting from which a "difficult" family was excluded from participation in a particular case—contrary to policy—would be better classified a "problem in micro-organizational procedure" (regarding who is to be present at the conference) rather than as a "problem in ethicality of process," even though its correction must be measured by a subsequent reduction in shortfall from that goal. After a period of time, it usually becomes clear where the most frequent and most significant opportunities for improvement lie. Pareto-like techniques for discerning the 20 percent of the opportunities most likely to give an 80 percent improvement are available in the CQI literature, if needed. Holding the rest of process and structure stable, the HEC can plan an intervention and CCC subcommittee chairs can document it as ongoing, and the HEC can make preplanned outcome measurements in the chosen area or areas where outcomes have fallen short of goals.

As the scope of our HEC's activity enlarges from micro-organizational toward meso-, macro-, and perhaps mega-organizational management of cases and problems, our CQI process should enable us to clarify, in an organized way, what augmentations in personnel, skills, resources, policies, and procedures will be required. We anticipate that expanded use of our educational-counseling and stakeholder-enabling model of ethical discourse will entail much less risk of unnecessary duplication of expertise and expense than that required by a consulting-expert or judicial-expert model committee (which assumes that *the committee* should provide all the expertise required for offering and/or making decisions).

Most of what we recommend here represents an untested hypothesis when applied to HECs. Optimally, this and alternative approaches to quality improvement in case review should be prospectively tested against one another. Moreover, there are significant practical "start-up" problems that must be faced. Our HEC's ability to guide the CCC panels drawn from its membership is limited by the fact that many of its members are busy volunteers who lack either medical-professional knowledge or a solid background in ethics. Members are quite often unable to attend every meeting, resulting in gaps in the knowledge of individual members and inconsistency in assessment and evaluation of CCC subcommittee performance. Institutional memory is short, and the experience and knowledge gained by HECs is often collected in the heads of longtime staff members rather than in a permanent, printed form designed to display efficiently the status of ongoing CQI-identified problems. Most hospitals and medical centers, however, already have significant resources dedicated to quality-improvement activities. There is now a reasonable rationale available for similar resources to be made available to HECs. Significant increase in financial and other resources, as well as several revolutions of the CQI cycle illustrated in Exhibit 19-5, will obviously be necessary.

DISCUSSION

At our institution, each small CCC subcommittee that conducts an ethics case review submits a report of its work for critique at the next scheduled meeting of the full Ethics Resource Committee, which serves as a reviewing committee of peers. The chief of staff and executive committee of the medical center review the details of each case and the minutes of the meeting, critiquing each case review monthly, and they review a detailed annual report describing the year's activities, accomplishments, and problems, and the plans for the next year. We believe that proper application of the scheme of CQI described above to this routine could (1) enable continuous and authentic improvement in quality by meaningful and credible self- and peer-identification of problems and measurement and monitoring of their correction; and (2) meet JCAHO peer-review standards requiring that "each clinical department or major clinical service (or medical staff, for a nondepartmentalized medical staff) hold . . . monthly meetings to consider findings from the ongoing monitoring and evaluation of the quality and appropriateness of the care and treatment provided to patients."[51] It would not, however, necessarily meet the demands of critics for accountability—that is, assurance of maintenance of an appropriate degree "of procedural fairness in how bioethics consultations are granted and conducted . . . allowing equal access and equality of processes for like cases . . . [because] society should not want to leave the resolution of ethical dilemmas to committees and consultants whose deliberations are secret and who are only kept in check by their hospitals or professional organizations."[52] We believe that the demands for strict public policing of case review to achieve this kind of accountability would diminish greatly if HECs stopped acting in the role of consultants making recommendations as a matter of policy.

Since its inception, our committee has required, whenever possible, the presence of all available stakeholders at CCC meetings at the bedside, especially the patient and family or other surrogates. Our HEC has always required that no recommendations be given by the CCC subcommittee and that all decisions be crafted or negotiated by the stakeholders only so that no "secret recommendation or decision-making deliberations by committees or consultants" occur.[53] The *Core Competencies* document appears to ratify this approach. It recommends that consultants "ensure that involved parties have their voices heard, assist involved individuals in clarifying their own values, [and] help facilitate the building of morally acceptable shared commitments or understandings," yet "not usurp moral decision-making authority or impose their values on other involved parties."[54] This indicates a shift toward an educational-counseling model (in which, typically, stakeholder discernment and judgment are facilitated and recommendations by the HEC are avoided) from a medical-consulting model (in which stakeholder decision making and action are facilitated by the discernment, judgment, and recommendations of an individual or committee who are seen as experts).[55] We believe the former heuristic model to be superior for adult education: it tends to be psychogogic, growth-promoting, and empowering rather than pedagogic, paternalistic, and overpowering. By its action, the *Core Competencies* report appears, in effect and in one stroke, (1) to endorse a model of case review that is more congruent with the deliberation-enhancing role of ethics than with the recommendation-making (that is, decision-offering) role of the medical consultant, or the decision-making role of the judge; and (2) to remove, or at least greatly reduce, the likelihood of significant violation or abridgment of due process that is so repugnant to those demanding "maintenance of an [at least legally] acceptable degree of procedural fairness in how bioethics consultations are granted and conducted."[56] We visualize achievement of an educational-counseling model to be a major internal CQI project for HECs that could also be routinely "spot-checked" (or examined in detail in response to any complaints) by whatever accountability scheme society and its representatives determine to be worthwhile.

Why should CQI be expected to change the behavior of HEC members when so many other larger, more sophisticated, and better-financed quality improvement schemes have failed in their efforts to change other behaviors in medical practice? To our knowledge, outside of industrial applications, so far only uncontrolled observations suggest that CQI can improve the quality of care,[57] patient outcomes (see examples above), and ethics case review.[58] Greco and Eisenberg, however, indicate that six general methods for changing medical-practitioner behavior have been described: education, feedback, participation by practitioners in efforts to bring about change, administrative rules, financial incentives, and financial penalties.[59] As demonstrated by the clinical examples noted above, CQI focuses strongly on the first three. Administrative interventions to force behaviors and financial sanctions to reinforce behaviors should be used only after reasonable alternatives have been tried, and CQI is such an alternative. As far as meeting the several recommendations for success cited by Greco and Eisenberg, CQI has the advantage of combining several methods rather than depending only on one; it allows the appropriateness of interventions to be discerned by feedback, avoids cost reduction as its primary goal, and avoids the perception of feedback as a threat. CQI gets good marks on these predictive scores, but, ultimately, practice and not theory will be necessary to verify success as applied to case review by HECs.

Is the effort to continually improve case review misplaced? One very creative, thoughtful, and influential group has indicated that "the next generation" of healthcare ethics committees "should emphasize [the HEC's] educational function, not its consultative one."[60] In an original and creative report entitled "A Paradigm Shift for Ethics Committees and Case Consultation: A Modest Proposal," Glaser and Miller, from the same group, have said: "Case consultation by an ethics committee should be recognized as an institutional embarrassment to be eliminated as soon as possible and replaced by consistent, effective patterns of case conferencing by staff as a routine part of patient care."[61] Have the consensus reports cited above recommended and articulated the foundation necessary for continuous improvement of case review just in time for application to an activity that is no longer necessary or even desirable?

We think not, and we believe a careful reading of this apparent condemnation of ethics case review will confirm our opinion. Glaser and Miller state that ethics case consultation was a "stop-gap intervention" invented only because of the "chronic . . . absence of adequate discussion of patient care by key stakeholders in the case."[62] What we understand them to condemn and demand cease is case *consultations*, which disenfranchise and diminish full participation of stakeholders in bedside decision making. What we understand them to advocate and wish to enable through education and institutional change are routine case *conferences*, at which "the primary care community (patient, loved one, and the clinical professionals involved in giving care) discuss the ethical dimensions of cases effectively, consistently, and adequately in the setting of care."[63] As indicated above, we believe that this is a major end of case review as stipulated by the goals of stakeholder empowerment and ethicality of process, as well as by our advocacy for the educational-counseling model of case review as a replacement for the medical-consultation model. Glaser and Miller further indicate that when HECs participate in case review, they should "build explicit institutional examination into every case conference" with a view to changing institutional systems or patterns "to better meet the needs uncovered" by the case conference.[64] This is very similar to the CQI approach we recommend: whatever the problem or "need uncovered" at first appears to be, HEC members should ask, repetitively, the open question: "And why did that happen?". Thereafter, they should follow the causal trail and the search for improvement from the micro-organizational through the meso-, macro- and mega-organizational levels, if necessary. After a closer reading, the apparent conflict appears to be not a contradiction, but different language and different images foreshadowing and confirming the consensus conference documents we have cited, the "great importance" the Task Force attaches "to evaluation [of consultants, process, and outcomes] . . . as an area that should be actively pursued through research and practice,"[65] and, in principle, the CQI process as we have outlined it. In fact, although we are convinced that the term and process of "case consultation" have outlived their usefulness, we believe the dialogical, educational-counseling model of case review has great value and promise, not only in one-on-one ethical discussions, but in meso-organizational and macro-organizational ethics discussions. From its inception, our HEC has extended this noncontrolling, enabling, and educational methodology to the development of ethics policy by stipulating that "ethics policies must be written by those [individuals, departments, and so forth] who will be most affected by them," and not by some committee of remote or less-than-maximally involved experts. Our HEC's role has been to provide information, education, organization, and dialogical and mediation skills to the policy writers. This has worked quite well, although we look forward to use of the above-described CQI scheme to be sure that stakeholder empowerment, stakeholder education, and ethicality of process are improved and maintained in future efforts to enable policy making.

Using other metaphors, Ross and colleagues recommend that the "next generation" of HECs not be "hobby clubs" that are poorly integrated into the community and are interested primarily in their own moral authority, growth, and development from which they might be willing to share a bit, if requested.[66] We agree and hope that, rather like Socrates, HECs will come to admit, and by CQI efforts demonstrate, that they are struggling to become aware of and work on our own moral inadequacies. We hope that, like Socrates, they will be eager to communicate and work with other similarly struggling individuals and groups, to learn with and from them, and to discover, as Socrates did, that moral growth and maturity will be found to be not a condition but a byproduct of enabling moral growth in others.

Using another metaphor, this time biological one, for its role in the moral life of the hospital, the HEC in its case consultation role has been, in the past, rather like the human pancreas—hidden, behind the scenes, perhaps dangerous for physicians to approach directly from the outside, and, because immobile, requiring that the raw materials it deals with be brought to it for processing and subsequent distribution throughout the system of which it is part. We suggest that this receptive and relatively passive posture of the HEC should be supplemented in the future by an analogue to a second, probably more recent and more important role of the pancreas: that of producing insulin. Insulin is a "chemical messenger and enabler of change" that is distributed to, empowers, and enhances the life of virtually all the cells and cell groups of the body, by altering their readiness to be open to—and to use where, when, and how it is most needed—that nutrient (glucose) without which physical life and flourishing would be impossible. By analogy, the HEC can continue to act as a separate, specialized, and immobile organ within the organization, charged to remain in that locus, to react only to problems delivered to it, and to receive, prepare, and customize educational and other ethics-oriented materials for distribution and use by the whole organization. Or it can become mobile and move to perform its most important function at the locus of moral life wherever it is. But where is the locus of moral life in the healthcare system? At the micro-organizational level, it is in the head of each individual and in the heads of the few individuals who comprise the small groups of caregivers and patients/surrogates working at the bedside in a given department of the healthcare institution. At the meso-organizational level, it is in the heads of the larger groups of individuals who make up the departments of a hospital, medical center, or similar healthcare institution. At the macro-organizational level, it is in the heads of the individuals who represent different healthcare institutions. At the mega-organizational level, the locus of moral life is in the heads of the members of society and/or their representatives.

Depending on the problem, members of an HEC usually should focus their energies on the first three of these loci, by acting as empowering moral messengers and enablers of change. In this role, an HEC should remain an HEC, and not become a "PAC (political action committee) in HEC's clothing" using political maneuvering and power in dealing with larger groups. That might indeed constitute a kind of "paradigm shift" from Aristotle and Kant to Alinsky and Kissinger (that is, from ethics to community organizing or politics).[67] Rather it should seek to be a catalyst for moral change by doing what HECs are already valued for and trained to do (by counsel, education, and collaborative moral dialogue): to "build up the individual [the individuals who make up healthcare institutions] and society, by the cultivation and enrichment of their intellectual and spiritual lives."[68] This would not constitute a paradigm change, but an ordinary or normal extension and further articulation of the paradigm of dialogical moral discourse from small to large groups.

Like any chemical reaction, the chemistry sought by dialogical moral discourse works best when the properly prepared catalysts, cofactors, and ingredients (the structures) are well dispersed where change is necessary, when change is most likely, and when the proper conditions and procedures (the processes) are used and continually improved in an effort to achieve the goals desired. We have been told that, as much as 85 percent of the time, the locus of needed change in medical CQI may be in systems rather than individuals and small groups.[69] If the same proves also to be true of CQI in HEC activities, extension of the dialogical-moral-discourse paradigm from micro-organizational cases to problems of larger scope could be expected to be associated with a marked increase in frequency and relevance of HEC activities in dealing with such difficulties. Just as the presence and actions of insulin in the blood stream require tempering by constant feedback to avoid a dangerous overreaction and swing from too little to too much activity, so too the CQI cycle will be necessary for HECs to ever more nearly approximate their goals and avoid intemperate or premature changes in structure, process, or paradigm. This essay is meant to be a constructive contribution to that endeavor, and to whatever evolutionary processes lead to the next and subsequent generations of HECs or similar structures designed to reify the ethical dimensions and enrich the moral life of healthcare institutions.

ACKNOWLEDGMENTS

The authors are grateful to Callene Buck, MA, for her help in this research effort and to Lois Ramer, PhD, for her review of the CQI portions of this essay.

NOTES

1. J.W. Ross et al., *Handbook for Hospital Ethics Committees* (Chicago: American Hospital Publishing, 1986), x.

2. M.R. Chassin, "Part 3: Improving the Quality of Care," in *Quality of Care: Selections from the New England Journal of Medicine,* ed. J.P. Kassirer and M. Angell (Waltham, Mass.: Massachusetts Medical Society, 1997), 57-60.

3. D. Blumenthal and A.M. Epstein, "Part 6: The Role of Physicians in the Future of Quality Management," in *Quality of Care: Selections from the New England Journal of Medicine,* see note 2 above, pp. 70-3.

4. Ibid.

5. S.J. Tanenbaum, "Sounding Board: What Physicians Know," in *Quality of Care: Selections from the New England Journal of Medicine,* see note 2 above, pp. 9-11.

6. See note 3 above.

7. J. Green and N. Winfeld, "Report Cards on Cardiac Surgeons," in *Quality of Care: Selections from the New England Journal of Medicine,* see note 2 above, pp. 25-8.

8. M. Angell and J.P. Kassirer, "Quality and the Medical Marketplace: Following Elephants," in *Quality of Care: Selections from the New England Journal of Medicine, see* note 2 above, pp. 45-7.

9. S.M. Wolfe, "Ethics Committees and Due Process: Nesting Rights in a Community of Caring," *Maryland Law Review* 50, no. 3 (1991): 798-858; G.S. Scofield, "Ethics Consultation: The Least Dangerous Profession," *Cambridge Quarterly of Healthcare Ethics* 2, no. 4 (1993): 417-26; S.M. Wolfe, "Quality Assessment of Ethics in Health Care: The Accountability Revolution," *American Journal of Law & Medicine* 20, no. 1 & 2 (1994): 105-28.

10. D.M. Berwick, "Continuous Improvement as an Ideal in Health Care," *New England Journal of Medicine* 320 (1989): 53-6; L.L. Leape, "Error in Medicine," *Journal of the American Medical Association* 272, no. 23 (1994): 1851-7 [Leape's article is reprinted as chapter 7 of this book—*ED.*]; D. Blumenthal, "Making Medical Errors into 'Medical Treasures', " *Journal of the American Medical Association* 272, no. 23 (1994): 1867-8.

11. Berwick, "Continuous Improvement," see note 10 above.

12. See note 3 above.

13. S. Fry-Revere, *The Accountability of Bioethics Committees and Consultants* (Frederick, Md.: University Publishing Group, 1992): 73-7.

14. A. Epstein, "Performance Reports on Quality: Prototypes, Problems, and Prospects," in *Quality of Care: Selections from the New England Journal of Medicine,* see note 2 above, pp. 29-33.

15. T.S. Kuhn, *The Structure of Scientific Revolutions,* 2nd ed. (Chicago: University of Chicago Press, 1970).

16. Ibid., 24.

17. For a detailed methodology of case review seasoned by many years of use, readily converted from a medical-consulting to an educational-counseling model, and readily applicable at the meso- and macro- as well the micro-organizational level, see Bioethics Consultation Group, *Forming a Moral Community: A Resource for Healthcare Ethics Committees* (Berkeley, Calif.: General Printing, 1992), 28-62.

18. B. Lo, "Behind Closed Doors: Promise and Pitfalls of Ethics Committees," *New England Journal of Medicine* 317, no. 1 (1988): 46-50; J. Moreno, "Ethics Committees: Proceed with Caution," *Maryland Law Review* 50, no. 3 (1991): 895-903; D. Blake, "The Hospital Ethics Committee: Health Care's Moral Conscience or White Elephant?" *Hastings Center Report* 22, no. 1 (1992): 6-11; Wolfe, "Ethics Committees and Due Process," see note 9 above; and Scofield, "Ethics Consultation," see note 9 above.

19. The three task forces include the Society for Health and Human Values-Society for Bioethics Consultation (SHHV-SBC) Task Force on Standards for Bioethics Consultation, participants in the Evaluation of Care Consultation in Clinical Ethics (ECCCE) conference, and the Sparrow Hospital Task Force. See SHHV-SBC Task Force on Standards for Bioethics Consultation, *Core Competencies for Health Care Ethics Consultation* (Glenview, Ill.: American Society for Bioethics and Humanities, 1998).

J.A. Tulsky and E. Fox, "Evaluating Ethics Consultation: Framing the Questions," *The Journal of Clinical Ethics* 7, no. 2 (Summer 1996): 109-15; E. Fox, "Concepts in Evaluation Applied to Ethics Consultation Research," *The Journal of Clinical Ethics* 7, no. 2 (Summer 1996): 116-21; J.C. Fletcher and M. Siegler, "What Are the Goals of Ethics Consultation? A Consensus Statement," *The Journal of Clinical Ethics* 7, no. 2 (Summer 1996): 122-6; E. Fox and R.M. Arnold, "Evaluating Outcomes in Ethics Consultation Research," *The Journal of Clinical Ethics* 7, no. 2 (Summer 1996): 127-38; J.A. Tulsky and C.B. Stocking, "Obstacles and Opportunities in the Design of Ethics Consultation Evaluation," *The Journal of Clinical Ethics* 7, no. 2 (Summer 1996): 139-45; E. Fox and J.A. Tulsky, "Evaluation Research and the Future of Ethics Consultation," *The Journal of Clinical Ethics* 7, no. 2 (Summer 1996): 146-9. These articles report the findings of the ECCCE conference which first met on 21-23 September 1995.

J. Andre, "Goals of Ethics Consultation: Toward Clarity, Utility, and Fidelity," *The Journal of Clinical Ethics* 8, no. 2 (Summer 1997): 193-8. This publication reports the findings of the Sparrow Hospital Task Force, which engaged in a year-long evaluation of its own ethics consultations at the same time that the ECCCE conference did its work.

20. Modified, as indicated by brackets, from Kuhn, see note 15 above, p. 24.

21. SHHV-SBC Task Force, *Core Competencies*, see note 19 above, p. 27.

22. A. Donabedian, *The Definition of Quality and Approaches to Its Assessment*, 1st ed. (Ann Arbor, Mich.: Health Administration Press, 1980); D.E. Hoffmann, "Evaluating Ethics Committees: A View from the Outside," *Milbank Quarterly* 70, no. 4 (1993): 677-701; R.H. Brook and P.D. Cleary, "Part 2: Measuring Quality of Care," in *Quality of Care: Selections from the New England Journal of Medicine*, see note 2 above, pp. 52-6. Brook and Cleary indicate that quality measurement in medical care should depend "more on process data than on outcome data," but only if we use "process measures for which we have sound scientific evidence or a formal consensus of experts that the criteria we are using do indeed, when applied, lead to an improvement in health care." To our knowledge, there are as yet no scientifically validated process measures available for evaluating ethics case review, and the "ethics facilitation approach" of process recommended by the SHHV-SBC Task Force is only sketchily outlined in its report (see SHHV-SBC Task Force, *Core Competencies*, note 19 above, pp. 6-7). There is, on the other hand, what amounts to an expert consensus about the goals (that is, outcomes sought) in ethics case review expressed by the extensive overlap of three task force reports referred to in note 19 above. This overlap-based consensus includes the goal of procedural fairness (expressed in this essay under the heading "ethicality of process") precisely because the best means (processes) to that end (goal) are as yet uncertain.

23. C. Levenson et al., "Preventing Postoperative Burn Wound Aspergillosis," *Journal of Burn Care & Rehabilitation* 12, no. 2 (1991): 1321-35.

24. C.G. Meisenheimer, *Improving Quality: A Guide to Effective Programs*, 2nd ed. (Gaithersburg Md.: Aspen Publishers, 1997); D. Blumenthal and A.C. Sheck, ed., *Improving Clinical Practice: Total Quality Management and the Physician* (San Francisco: Jossey-Bass, 1995).

25. M. Neff-Smith, "Part II, Ethics Program Evaluation: The Virginia Hospital Ethics Fellows

Example," *Healthcare Ethics Committee Forum* 9, no. 4 (1997): 375-88; SHHV-SBC Task Force, *Core Competencies,* see note 19 above, p. 27.

26. J.C. White, P.M. Dunn, and L. Homer, "A Practical Instrument to Evaluate Ethics Consultations," *Healthcare Ethics Committee Forum* 9, no. 3 (1997): 228-56.

27. See note 1 above, pp. 115-23; B. Hosford, *Bioethics Committees: The Health Care Provider's Guide* (Rockville, Md., Aspen Systems, 1986), 185-96.

28. See note 1 above.

29. T.A. Brennan, "Ethics Committees and Decisions to Limit Care: The Experience at the Massachusetts General Hospital," *Journal of the American Medical Association* 260, no. 6 (1988): 803-7; J. La Puma, "Consultation in Clinical Ethics: Issues and Questions in 27 cases," *Western Journal of Medicine* 146, no. 5 (1987): 633-7; J. La Puma et al., "An Ethics Consultation Service in a Teaching Hospital: Utilization and Evaluation," *Journal of the American Medical Association* 260, no. 6 (1988): 808-11; H.S. Perkins and B.S. Saathoff, "Impact of Medical Ethics Consultations on Physicians: An Exploratory Study," *American Journal of Medicine* 85 (1988): 761-5.

30. SHHV-SBC Task Force, *Core Competencies,* see note 19 above.

31. Tulsky and Fox, "Evaluating Ethics Consultation"; Fox, "Concepts in Evaluation"; Fletcher and Siegler, "What Are the Goals of Ethics Consultation"; Fox and Arnold, "Evaluating Outcomes"; Tulsky and Stocking, "Obstacles and Opportunities"; and Fox and Tulsky, "Evaluation Research," see note 19 above.

32. Tulsky and Fox, "Evaluating Ethics Consultation," see note 19 above.

33. Fletcher and Siegler, "What Are the Goals of Ethics Consultation?" see note 19 above.

34. Fox and Arnold, "Evaluating Outcomes," see note 19 above.

35. Andre, "Goals of Ethics Consultation," see note 19 above.

36. Hoffman, "Evaluating Ethics Committees," see note 22 above; Fox and Arnold, "Evaluating Outcomes," see note 19 above.

37. See note 17 above, pp. 28-62.

38. D.J. Self and J.D. Skeel, "The Moral Reasoning of HEC Members," *Healthcare Ethics Committee Forum* 10, no. 1 (1998): 43-54.

39. SHHV-SBC Task Force, *Core Competencies,* see note 19 above, p. 9.

40. Andre, "Goals of Ethics Consultation," see note 19 above.

41. Fox and Arnold, "Evaluating Outcomes," see note 19 above.

42. Ibid.

43. Ibid.

44. Andre, "Goals of Ethics Consultation," see note 19 above.

45. Modified from Fox and Arnold, "Evaluating Outcomes," see note 19 above.

46. B.E. Zawacki, "The 'Futility Debate' and the Management of Gordian Knots," *The Journal of Clinical Ethics* 6, no. 2 (Summer 1995): 112-27; S.B. Rubin, *Futility: An Insufficient Ground for Physician Unilateral Decision-Making* (Washington, D.C.: UMI Dissertation Services, 1996).

47. Meisenheimer, *Improving Quality,* see note 24 above, pp. 53-6.

48. L. Blackhall et al., "Ethnicity and Attitudes Towards Patient Autonomy," *Journal of the American Medical Association* 274 (1995): 820-5.

49. *Barber v. Superior Court,* 147 Cal.App.3d 1006, 195 Cal. Rptr. 484 (1983).

50. J.W. Ross, "Why Cases Sometimes Go Wrong," *Hastings Center Report* 19, no. 1 (1989): 22-3.

51. Joint Commission on Accreditation of Healthcare Organizations, *The Joint Commission 1990 AMH: Accreditation Manual for Hospitals* (Chicago: Joint Commission, 1989): MS.3.7, quoted in Fry-Revere, *The Accountability,* see note 13 above, p. 74.

52. Fry-Revere, *The Accountability,* see note 13 above, 77. In this discussion, we have recounted how a report is submitted and critiqued, then submitted to the chief of staff and executive committee of the medical center. Yet, in a shortcoming of ethicality of process, we recognize that the case reports are uneven; that the minutes critiquing the case are brief and, on occasion, inadequate; and that there is no assurance that the chief of staff and executive committee have reflected on the monthly minutes or annual report. Each of these components of our process, when submitted to CQI, will be improved, we believe.

53. Ibid.

54. SHHV-SBC Task Force, *Core Competencies*; Fletcher and Siegler, "What Are the Goals of Ethics Consultation?" see note 19 above.

55. See note 49 above.

56. See note 13 above, p. 8.

57. See note 3 above.

58. See note 26 above.

59. P.J. Greco and J.M. Eisenberg, "Changing Physicians' Practices," in *Quality of Care: Selections from the New England Journal of Medicine,* see note 2 above, pp. 12-6.

60. J.W. Ross et al., *Health Care Ethics Committees: The Next Generation* (Chicago: American Hospital Publishing, 1993), 186.

61. J.W. Glaser and R.B. Miller, "A Paradigm Shift for Ethics Committees and Case Consultation: A Modest Proposal," *Healthcare Ethics Committee Forum* 5, no. 2 (1993): 83-8.

62. Ibid.

63. Ibid.

64. Ibid.

65. SHHV-SBC Task Force, *Core Competencies,* see note 19 above.

66. See note 60 above, p. 113.

67. In some circumstances it might appear normal, prudent, or even morally obligatory for an HEC to make an implicit or explicit paradigm shift from the use of ethical dialogue for seeking education, consensus, and/or compromise, to the use of sociological power, community organizing, or political power. Such a paradigm shift might appear especially attractive to an HEC seeking to enable stakeholders to resolve meso-, macro-, or mega-organizational problems. It would be naïve to believe that education and ethical dialogue alone will always suffice to undo problems caused, for example, by power imbalances or fiscal constraints. It would be destructive for ethics, however, were HECs to abandon reliance on ethical dialogue prematurely, or even unconsciously, in exchange for such alternatives.

68. Modified slightly from the mission statement of the University of Southern California.

69. Lois Ramer, PhD, personal communication with the authors; Leape, "Error in Medicine," see note 10 above.

20

Why Medical Ethicists Don't (and Won't) Share Uncertainty

Giles R. Scofield

FROM THE ABSURD

Because uncertainty lies at the heart of every ethical dilemma, the suggestion that ethics consultants do not and will not share uncertainty with others must seem utterly absurd. Not only do ethics consultants share uncertainty; uncertainty brings ethics consultants and others together. To suggest that ethics consultants do not and will not share uncertainty reveals—if it does not confirm—that I do not know what I am talking about when it comes to ethics consultation.

Although these sentiments are true as far as they go, the problem is that they do not go nearly far enough. In addition to sharing *uncertainty,* there is sharing *Uncertainty.* And the two could not be more different from each other.

It goes without saying that ethics consultants share uncertainty with others. Indeed, one of the ethics consultant's tasks is to identify and do something about uncertainties that others are unaware of. Without getting into the psychological, financial, and political dimensions of the ethics consultant-client relationship, it is fair to say (and dishonest to deny) that, when it comes to uncertainty, ethicists don't hold back.

When it comes to Uncertainty, on the other hand, ethics consultants are more parsimonious than they are generous, reflecting the love-hate relationship they have with Uncertainty. Thus, they offer others a glimpse of Uncertainty and otherwise conceal Uncertainty from others for one reason: to give others some good reasons, and perhaps some even more powerful nonreasons, to believe that ethics consultants can save us from the perils of Uncertainty.

Why do ethics consultants behave as they do? One way about uncertainty; another about Uncertainty? Because to reveal too much about Uncertainty would reveal something unbearable about the foundations of ethics, which would cast into doubt our faith in it and in ethics consultation. To share honestly what they know about Uncertainty with others would cause the world as we know it to come crashing down like the proverbial house of cards. Because this would be a dreadful result—for us as well as for them—ethics consultants must keep what they know about Uncertainty largely under wraps. Thus, the art of ethics consultation, the knack to being the successful ethicist, lies in being generous with uncertainty, but parsimonious about Uncertainty. To understand how and why this is so, we must examine ethics consultation, uncertainty, and Uncertainty in greater detail.

THE WORLD OF UNCERTAINTY

Ours is an especially uncertain world. In addition to wondering about the usual array of big questions (Where do we come from? Where are we going? What does it all mean?) questions that have vexed humanity since it became aware of its awareness of its existence (and its nonexistence)—we face the additionally vexing questions that advances in medicine and medical technology have created. Whether the question is about frozen embryos, which concerns only a few of us directly, or decision making at the end of life, which eventually will confront each of us quite directly, there is no end to the thorny questions that medicine and medical technology throw our way.

These questions differ, both in their nature and in their magnitude, from the questions that vexed bygone generations. In addition to wondering about the usual questions about the meaning of existence, we find ourselves having to wonder about the additional questions that technology, which supposedly enables us to master our existence, creates. We thus find ourselves in the ironic and not at all pleasant situation of having increased our mastery of the world only to find ourselves not relieved of the burden of decision, but even more burdened than before. Having set out to find that which is certain and eliminate that which is doubtful, we find our situation more ambivalent and more anxious than ever before.[1]

Our problem only begins here. Just as technology solves one problem by creating others, ethics seems to answer one question only to augur others into existence. Whether this occurs because philosophy undoes at night what it made during the day, or because the disenchantment of the world requires that ethics dunk itself in the acid-bath of reason, or because the commodification of ethics creates a kind of planned conceptual obsolescence, the result is the same—less instead of more certainty, and more instead of less anxiety.

Take, for example, decision making at the end of life. In the beginning, we wondered whether we might forgo life-sustaining treatment. We now know that we may do so. Having answered that general question, we now find ourselves wondering about the particular conditions under which we may do so. At first, when the world of patients consisted either of the clearly competent, terminally ill adult or the clearly incompetent, persistently vegetative adult, the answer seemed easy. We would trust that competent patients can and do know what they want, and that family members can and do know what other family members would want.

Over the years, what once seemed certain and uncontestable has become uncertain and more hotly contested. The confidence we derived from the competent, terminally ill adult has been cast into considerable doubt in the context of the less clearly competent (but clearly not incompetent), chronically ill patient. In the realm of surrogate decision making, perhaps owing to its origins in the subjunctive voice, matters have moved from more certain to increasingly less certain—in fact, if not in theory. Indeed, the more it has become clear that we may not know what we are doing when it comes to surrogate decision making, the greater the ardor of those who are certain that we can and do know what we are doing here.

This has left us with what amounts to three schools of thought about surrogate decision making, each answering in its own definitive, authoritative way what a patient would say if a patient could say something. These are: (1) that we can trust families to know what the patient would say even absent evidence that they do know; (2) that we must not trust families to know what patients would say absent evidence that they do know; and (3) that the only thing that matters is what seems to be in the patient's best interest right now, regardless of what the patient did or did not think at an earlier time. With each school of thought being as certain that it is right as it is that the others are wrong, these circles of perfect normative understanding have caught patients, families, and courts in something akin to a perfect storm of values. Having sought to increase our certainty and decrease our anxiety, we have produced the opposite result.

If this were all we had to deal with, we would have reason enough for being uneasy. But there is considerably more to our uneasiness than this. The questions we face about medicine, medical technology, and ethics arise within a haunted context that, when it does not occupy the foreground of our understanding, preoccupies the background of our understanding of medicine and ethics.[2] That haunting, of course, is the moral collapse whose depths were reached in Germany from 1933 to 1945, when ordinary and extraordinary individuals alike participated in morally unconscionable acts.

Whether we wonder, as others have, what it means for there to be poetry or education after Auschwitz, we do worry about what ethics means after Auschwitz.[3] And even if the rhetoric that those who hold certain views about the beginning and ending of life escalates (or deteriorates) into facile accusations that others think and act in ways that are consistent with what it "means" to be Nazi, the mere fact that we even use such language in reference to others bespeaks a deep, unresolved concern about what this all means to and about us[4]—an anxiety that is as manifest as the legacy that gives rise to it is suppressed. Enduring as this concern is, we find ourselves in the awkward situation of having to remind ourselves to take the lessons of Auschwitz more seriously than we have, which manifests itself as a series of reminders about the *Nuremberg Code* that amount to not much more than "Don't go to the lab without it!" Each time we pride ourselves on the fact that we have successfully avoided the abyss, we should wonder what it means that we skirt moral failure as often as we seem to do. After a while, so many close calls become more a source of discomfort than of anything else.

Within this context, the emergence of medical ethics consultation becomes an understandable phenomenon. We face tough choices, whose answers give rise to only more choices. And while we wish to be certain that we avoid the abyss, the fact that we even have to choose how we are to choose makes us less certain and more anxious about how we can and whether we will. No wonder we have medical ethics consultants. Thank goodness that we do. They are the answer to our prayers, a kind of moral sherpa that will show us the way without our running the risk of vanishing into thin air. They enable us to discern right from wrong, good from evil. Perhaps, but, given Uncertainty, perhaps not.

CREEPING ... ?

There may be less Certainty to ethics consultation than meets the eye, and more Uncertainty than ethicists can or will share with others. Some of the reasons for this are suggested, if not revealed, in Albert Jonsen's recent history of American bioethics.[5]

For as long as there have been philosophers, there has existed the tension between the timeless and the times, between philosophy and the real world. Socrates paid one price for bringing philosophy into the public place. Plato and Heidegger found somewhat different niches for themselves. That this tension exists means that the philosopher's relationship to the world is something that must be managed. One kind of risk attaches to remaining uninvolved; another kind of risk attaches to becoming involved. Consequences attach to how one chooses to emphasize the timeless or the times in the philosopher's life.

In ethics, this tension manifests itself in the relationship that exists between normative ethics (and applied normative ethics) and nonnormative ethics (including descriptive ethics and metaethics). As recently as 1959, Richard Brandt stated that normative ethics concerned itself with the truth of general ethical *statements,* and that it was no more concerned with whether the British were justified in seizing the Suez Canal, for example, than the field of physics might be with the size of the Rock of Gibraltar. Critical ethics, also known as metaethics, was to normative ethics what the philosophy of science was to science—challenging, questioning, wondering how true what passes for truth really is.[6] Whereas normative ethics had once been a central concern of moral philosophy, metaethics attained centrality and normative ethics was "spurned."[7]

Not satisfied with this state of affairs, some philosophers "struggled to keep normative ethics alive."[8] Eventually, these struggles led some to refurbish objective grounds for ethical judgments and to establish a basis and a method for making such judgments and believing in their validity. So did ethics begin to move once again from the timeless into the times, beginning the now familiar process of "saving" the life of ethics, through applied ethics, and then phronesis, and now ethnography.

Yet, the minute normative ethics manifested its belief in objectivism, it gave rise to its fear of relativism—which is simply another way of saying that an insistence on there being Certainty only makes what Uncertainty there is loom larger.[9] And, since uncertainty gives rise to anxiety, and eliminating doubt requires eliminating uncertainty, normative ethics and applied normative ethics must do something about Uncertainty.

The way that they have elected to combat Uncertainty is to assail relativism. Relativism seems to be the belief that anything goes, which makes a "relativist" about the worst thing one can call a philosopher or an ethicist. In philosophy and ethics, relativism is a four-letter word.

Once one examines relativism more closely, however, one both wonders and ceases to wonder what the problem is. Cultural relativism is not the issue; neither is ethical relativism. Nor, in fact, is "normative relativism," since there is not and cannot be such thing.[10] And, even if there were, it could not be a problem. In other words, if one looks for someone who supposedly believes that anything goes, one is not likely to find him or her; and if one does find such a person, the only following this individual is likely to have will consist of law enforcement.

The relativism that philosophers and ethicists do worry about is what is called epistemological relativism, which states that we lack criteria for judging, not right from wrong, but the validity of one view of right and wrong from another. Supposedly, there is something wrong with epistemological relativism, but what can that something be? If anything is true of philosophy it is that it lacks a method (that is a scientific method) for establishing what is true. That is what metaethics tells us. Thus, epistemological relativism only states something that is true, not false, about philosophy—a truth that manifests itself in the problem of incommensurability.

Can it be that the epistemological relativist is nothing other than a perspectivist, historicist, or some other-ist? It is difficult to see how this charge determines anything one way or the other. For if the problem with relativism is that it is time-bound instead of timeless, one can say that a belief in timelessness is also time-bound. Moreover, once normative ethics concerns itself not simply with the truth of general ethical statements, but also with whether the British were justified in seizing the Suez, the philosopher—by stepping from the timeless into the times—cannot say that historical, psychological, economic, and political features do not attach to his or her existence in the world.

There are a number of ways one could look at this problem. Following the lead Jay Katz has forged in how physicians deal with uncertainty, one could say that ethicists have a love-hate relationship with uncertainty, sharing uncertainty in order to get others to rely on them, and concealing Uncertainty for the same reason.[11] Or, if one were inclined to practice philosophy with a hammer (which means taking a hammer to what passes for philosophy), one could say that ethicists have succumbed to the knowledge-power syndrome, and that the manner in which they deal with uncertainty and Uncertainty has nothing to do with the search for truth and everything to do with preserving the privileged position that comes of their knowing something about knowing that no one else does. One might even argue that the misrecognition of Uncertainty results in a type of symbolic violence, in which ordinary persons become complicit in the denial of their moral autonomy. While one could make any of these arguments, there is no need to resort to what some would consider "ethics bashing" in order to flesh out the problem in a manner that meets ethicists where they are instead of where they are not.

What seems to be going on here is that normative ethicists would like to leave metaethics behind (and perhaps descriptive ethics as well). Why? Well, according to Jonsen, "metaethical discussion cut[s] at [the] very foundations" of normative ethics.[12] The "task of refuting or accommodating the metaethic critique" haunts those who work in the field of normative ethics. And what is that metaethical critique? It is the metaethical theory that conflicting ethical opinions are equally valid, in the sense that there is not and cannot be a method for deciding which is valid and which is not. The basis of this critique may be nonmethodological, as is the case in descriptive ethics (with its sociological and anthropological affinities), or methodological.[13] But, whatever the source of this critique, it serves to expose not uncertainty, but Uncertainty, that in some matters of conflict we do not and cannot know what the valid view may be. And if ethicists were to reveal that there is a body of thought that cuts at the very foundations of normative ethics, with respect to the belief that there are objective grounds for ethical judgments and some kind of method for resolving fundamental disputes, Uncertainty would rear its ugly head. Thus, the only way that ethicists can move from the timeless into the times is to leave metaethics behind (and descriptive ethics as well), which explains why these fields get such short shrift in biomedical texts.

THE WIZARDS OF OUGHTS?

To resort to the kind of analysis associated with poststructuralism, postmodernism not only serves to alienate some, it in fact constitutes a kind of overkill for assessing what amounts to nothing other than an internal dispute between those for whom normative ethics is dominant and those for whom metaethics is. One need not resort to a Continental critique to identify the flaw in how ethicists deal with Uncertainty (and, indeed, one should not if one hopes to get anyone to take such a critique seriously). Nor need one analyze facilitation and mediation in terms of linguistic exchanges of power, since what we know about genetic counseling establishes that nondirectiveness does not and cannot exist—which means that all ethics consultation risks being directive. Nor need one "prove" that there is more Uncertainty than justifies the enterprise of ethics consultation. Because applied ethics is a kind of technology; the burden of proof is on the proponents of ethics consultation to demonstrate that ethics consultation cannot and will not jeopardize the survival of human beings as moral beings.[14] Put another way, in the absence of a metaethical standard that can adjudicate whose system of belief is valid and whose is not (a process that would result in infinite regression), normative ethicists are making claims of expertise that cannot be founded.

To understand what is going on, one need only appreciate the history of the philosopher's struggle to bridge the timeless and the times. From that perspective, all we are witnessing is another instance in which the balance between the timeless and the times is playing itself out. It is only a matter of time before the effort to conceal Uncertainty's existence, by shielding ethics from Continental philosophy and the metaethical critique, falls apart. In short, this too shall pass.

And the manner of its passage is suggested (but not revealed) in Jonsen's history of American bioethics. He concedes that the efforts to find objective foundations and methods have largely failed, and observes that Europeans think that American bioethics is distinguished by the "relative poverty" of its theory (which presumably includes efforts to resuscitate phronesis as some kind of method, in the light of Gadamer's demonstration that phronesis is not a method). And Jonsen acknowledges that there has been (which presumably means there still is) a dispute internal to the community of philosophers about whether there is something or nothing to normative ethics.[15] In other words, American bioethics is protected against Uncertainty by the thin facade of the belief that we can shield normative ethics from descriptive and metaethical critique (and from Continental thought as well, but that is a separate issue).

Given what gave rise to American bioethics, and the ethos that we can "do something" about Uncertainty, how will Uncertainty be revealed? In keeping with ethos of American bioethics, the image that comes to my mind is that of the Wizard of Oz. One merely needs to think of ethicists as the Wizards of Oughts. They and we want and need to believe that they possess some special insight, knowledge, and wisdom. This is the quaint belief that is typical of American exceptionalism and pragmatism—the belief that our "can do" attitude means that we can do something about uncertainty without getting "burned," just like the Doughboys thought before they hit the trenches in World War I. All we need do is follow the yellow brick road to the Emerald City, where all will be revealed by the one who remains concealed—The Wizard of Oughts.

Of course, this view of ethics consultation will likely find no more adherents than would a post-Nietzschean analysis. But, if ethics consultation is the product of the American ethos, and if the American ethos is embodied in Disney World—a kind of never-never land in which no one ages, no one suffers, and every death is a good one—one should expect ethics consultation to be imbued with the naïve belief that we can do what no one else can do: bridge the gap that separates the timeless from the times. Just because Plato kept the company of tyrants, Heidegger erred in joining the Nazis, and Dewey was wrong to preach peace after Pearl Harbor, doesn't mean that the rest of us will not or cannot get it right. In short, when the issue is American exceptionalism, who needs Nietzsche when Toto will do?

In truth, the Wizard of Oughts cannot pull it off, since what he or she really knows (if reminded of what one was taught in the metaethics lecture and what one reads in sociology and anthropology), is that he or she does not know (and perhaps cannot know). The fear, of course, is that once the metaethical critique undercuts the foundations of bioethics—once the truth is out—Uncertainty will stand between the Wizard of Oughts and others.

In fact, the opposite is more likely the case. What stands between the Wizard and others is the belief that Uncertainty does not exist; it is the denial of this reality and the suppression of the metaethical critique that separates us from one another. In the Wizard of Oz, disappointment and anger yield to a genuine sharing of wisdom. In the same vein, we know that when physicians share uncertainty their patients tend to think more highly of them, not less so. It stands to reason, therefore, that if ethicists could reveal Uncertainty in a manner that demonstrates to others that it is not and need not be a destabilizing influence, they would perform a more valuable service than they do by suggesting that they know instead of that they do not.

BACK TO CASES (AND KANSAS)

For now, we can only say that Uncertainty is not the problem, even though it is problematic. The problem lies in how we respond and react to Uncertainty. Our inability to manage our fallibility is connected to the manifestation of the evil that comes of a zeal to eliminate this reminder of the fact that we are not infallible.[16] To the extent that ethics consultation masks this fact, ethicists are not so much doing this to us as they are doing this for and with us, with the result that we become increasingly alienated from ourselves and from one another. Until now Uncertainty has served only to separate us from one another, and even to alienate us from ourselves. Were we to see common ground around the fact that there is no ground, we might understand that, at bottom, what we share is our perplexity in the face of Uncertainty.[17] And that, no matter what else we have, we have one another; and that this may be all we want and need. Ill-prepared though we may think we are to live with the "daily throbbing pain that no sacral opiate can blot out," the fact remains that "we are destined to live openly in the anguish from which the gods [have] spared us since the beginning of the human venture."[18] By coming to terms with Uncertainty, through humility, we can embrace the kind of humanism that humanizes instead of dehumanizes our existence, and thereby one another as well. While I know that we can and believe that we should learn to share Uncertainty, I continue to wonder whether and when we will.

NOTES

1. Z. Bauman, *Modernity and Ambivalence* (Ithaca, N.Y.: Cornell University Press, 1991); A. Giddens, *The Consequences of Modernity* (Palo Alto, Calif.: Stanford University Press, 1990).

2. R.A. Burt, "The Suppressed Legacy of Nuremberg," *Hastings Center Report* 25, no. 5 (1996): 30-6; R. Primus, "A Brooding Presence: Totalitarianism in Postwar Constitutional Thought," *Yale Law Journal* 106 (1996): 423-57.

3. T.W. Adorno, *Negative Dialectics* (New York: Continuum, 1994), 361-8; T.W. Adorno,

"Education after Auschwitz," in *Critical Models,* ed. T.W. Adorno (New York: Columbia University Press, 1998), 123-40.

4. R. Wuthnow, *Meaning and Moral Order* (Berkeley: University of California Press, 1987), 123-40.

5. A.R. Jonsen, *The Birth of Bioethics* (New York: Oxford University Press, 1998).

6. R.B. Brandt, *Ethical Theory* (Englewood Cliffs, N.J.: Prentice-Hall, 1959), 4-10.

7. See note 5 above, p. 73.

8. Ibid.

9. R.J. Bernstein, *Beyond Objectivism and Relativism: Hermeneutics, Science, and Praxis* (Philadelphia: University of Pennsylvania, 1983).

10. L. Bell, "Does Ethical Relativism Destroy Morality?" *Man and World* 8 (1975): 415-33.

11. J. Katz, *The Silent World of Doctor and Patient* (New York: Free Press, 1984).

12. See note 5 above, p. 73.

13. See note 6 above, pp. 271-94.

14. H. Jonas, *The Imperative of Responsibility* (Chicago: University of Chicago Press, 1984).

15. A. Baier, "Some Thoughts on How We Moral Philosophers Live Now," *Monist* 67 (1984): 490; A. Macintyre, "Does Applied Ethics Rest on a Mistake?" *Monist* 67 (1984): 498.

16. P. Ricoeur, *Symbolism of Evil* (Boston: Beacon Press, 1969); P. Ricoeur, *Fallible Man* (New York: Fordham University Press, 1986).

17. R.L. Logan and P.J. Scott, "Uncertainty in Clinical Practice: Implications for Quality and Costs of Health Care," *Lancet* 347 (1996): 595-8.

18. M. Gauchet, *The Disenchantment of the World* (Princeton, N.J.: Princeton University Press, 1997), 207.

21

Errors in Healthcare Ethics Consultation

John C. Fletcher, Robert J. Boyle, and Edward M. Spencer

INTRODUCTION

This chapter, in five parts, discusses errors in ethics consultation. The first section briefly surveys the history of ethics consultation. Next the chapter discusses the findings of a national task force that defined standards for education and training of consultants and for the process of consultation. The third section describes the most prevalent error in ethics consultation—the conscious or unconscious efforts of consultants to be "morally proactive" and control the outcome of decision making. As examples, two cases and several lawsuits involving committees or consultants are discussed. The fourth section concerns errors in the process of ethics consultations, and the final section proposes a resolution for consultants' conflicts of loyalty and ways to protect the freedom of ethics committees and consultants to work without intimidation.

HISTORY OF ETHICS CONSULTATION

Healthcare ethics consultation is a service by an individual or group to assist with ethical problems. Such problems frequently arise in patient care and in governing or managing the institution and its relations with third parties.[1] In addition, an ethics committee or program can offer three other services: staff and community education in healthcare ethics and relevant health law, policy development, and research aimed to prevent or moderate frequent ethical problems.

OVERVIEW OF HISTORY

There are several accounts of the history of ethics consultation.[2] A brief overview of this history may be helpful for readers unfamiliar with the subject.

In the 1960s, a diverse social movement galvanized largely by values of democracy, respect for persons, and moral pluralism slowly reformed the closed traditional social arrangements of biomedical research. Prior group review of proposals for research involving human subjects and voluntary informed consent became the two main ways to respect these values. In the 1970s, the movement focused on traditional practices in clinical medicine. Reforms in traditional medical ethics were much more diffused, but real changes in practices of informed consent did occur. The contemporary fields of bioethics and medical humanities, along with ethics committees, evolved from this movement.

In the United States and Canada, ethics consultation first emerged in the work of ethics committees, medical humanists, and bioethicists in the early 1970s.[3] Ethics committees were created to meet two needs. The first was the new ethical complexity of innovative life-sustaining treatments. Such complexity required deeper resources than traditional medical and nursing ethics could offer. For example, life-and-death decisions in organ transplantation and kidney dialysis required fresh responses (that is, a "new medical ethics")[4] that were more open to the values of democracy and interdisciplinary cooperation than the traditions of medical or nursing ethics, which were burdened by paternalism and academic isolation. Ethics committees provided a forum for multidisciplinary debate and perspectives on these issues.

The erosion of medical paternalism created a second need. Until this period, physicians gave directive moral advice to patients and "protected" them, for example, by nondisclosure of a cancer diagnosis. Paternalistic practices were criticized by civil rights and consumer movements. New legal requirements for informed consent assumed the equality of patient and physician. As paternalism receded, the role of individual and family decision making was increasingly emphasized. Needs arose within hospitals, nursing homes, and other healthcare settings to assist decision makers who were unfamiliar with their rights and roles. A national commission on ethics in medicine, created by the President and Congress, affirmed shared decision making and recommended that ethics committees be resources for consultation.[5] Clinicians began to turn to the founders of medical humanities programs[6] and members of new ethics committees[7] for advice, especially about patients' refusal of treatment or surrogate decisions to forgo all treatments (including ventilation and food and fluids) when the patient was incapacitated.[8]

EARLY PROBLEMS AND RESPONSES

At first, either whole ethics committees or single consultants provided consultation. There were no clear-cut definitions or models of ethics consultation. The first generation had to learn by trial and error to distinguish their services from a prevailing model of medical consultation.[9] Soon, the prevalent modes of consultation came under sharp criticism for the following reasons:

- inadequate education and training of committee members and consultants in ethics, healthcare law, clinical medicine, and skills in the process of consultation[10]

- decisions made "behind closed doors" to side with clinicians' desires and the exclusion of patients or surrogates from decision making[11]
- neglect of process issues and protection of patient confidentiality[12]
- lack of empirical evidence of benefits of consultation, especially to patients, family, or surrogates[13]
- lack of institutional and financial support for ethics committees[14]
- displacement of the committee's mission in ethics by concerns to protect the institution's risks of liability[15]
- concern about the moral bias of a single consultant dominating the decision-making process[16]

These criticisms resulted in some internal reforms. By the early 1990s, many institutions had replaced ethics consultation by a committee or an individual, with an ethics consultation service or a team.[17] Today, in most hospitals, a consultation service or team is still accountable to a multidisciplinary ethics committee with one or more community members. In smaller hospitals, one still finds a variety of modes of consultation, such as a committee, individual consultants, or teams. Ethics consultation is less prevalent in long-term care facilities, hospice programs, and home health agencies than it is in hospitals.

Responding to the great need for education and training, the newly formed Society for Bioethics Consultation (SBC) convened a special conference in 1988.[18] Participants identified the following areas of knowledge and skill required for consultants: (1) biomedical ethics, (2) healthcare law and public policy, (3) clinical medicine and decision making, (4) cultural and religious traditions and their effects on healthcare decisions, and (5) training in psychological and interpersonal knowledge and skills. The conference also recommended the formation of a joint task force with the Society for Health and Human Values (SHHV) to define these areas more carefully and to study the pros and cons of various approaches to standards for ethics consultation (such as certification of consultants, accreditation of training programs, and other alternatives). The spirit of the conference was that the time had come to consider the need for standards for ethics consultation.[19]

In planning the task force's work, its leaders were united by two convictions. First, when ethics consultation is requested by clinicians, patients, or family members, consultants who respond are obliged to be competent in knowledge and skill to carry out this task. Second, healthcare institutions are obliged to support the training of consultants financially and to maintain a climate of freedom for ethics consultation. In the interim before the task force began its work, the Virginia Bioethics Network adopted voluntary standards for ethics services that included education and training for ethics consultants.[20]

THE JOINT TASK FORCE

By 1995 the Joint Task Force on Standards for Bioethics Consultation of the SBC and SHHV was funded and began to work[21] with a mandate to describe the knowledge, skills, and character traits required for ethics consultation and to make recommendations on approaches to the issue of standards. These two societies (SHHV and SBC) merged in 1997 with the American Association of Bioethics (AAB) to become the new American Society for Bioethics and the Humanities (ASBH). The new ASBH board officially approved and adopted the SHHV-SBC Task Force Report, *Core Competencies for Health Care Ethics Consultation*, in 1998.[22]

One of us (JCF) served as a member of the task force. The arguments in this chapter often reflect the content of its report. We (JCF, RJB, and EMS) collaborated to shape an ethics consultation service for an academic medical center and an approach to recruitment, education, and training of new members of the service.[23] Our reflections on errors in ethics consultation arise from having made most of them ourselves. Also, having led bi-annual, six-day intensive conferences since 1990 to strengthen ethics programs in hospitals in and beyond Virginia, we have seen firsthand the most frequent and troubling errors in consultation.

TWO SPECIAL CONTRIBUTIONS

Two contributions to the history of ethics consultation deserve special mention. The Joint Commission on Accreditation of Healthcare Organizations (JCAHO) accredits at least 80 percent of the nation's hospitals,[24] which admit 96 percent of all inpatients. A hospital's eligibility to receive Medicare and Medicaid payments depends on JCAHO approval. In 1990, JCAHO required its members to have a process to address ethical issues in patient care, which propelled the growth of ethics committees and consultation. In 1995, JCAHO added a requirement in "organization ethics." This rule responded to members' concerns that the ascendancy of market forces in the reimbursement and delivery of healthcare seriously threatened the integrity of the patient-centered ethics of medicine and nursing.

Second, Ellen Fox and James Tulsky organized an important conference in Chicago in 1995 on evaluation of ethics consultation.[25] The conference made two advances: (1) participants reached consensus on goals for ethics consultation,[26] and (2) participants formed the Consortium for Evaluation of Ethics Case Consultation, to develop instruments for evaluation and seek support for empirical research on the benefits and risks of ethics consultation for all parties.[27]

ETHICS CONSULTATION:
GOALS AND ROLE OF CONSULTANTS

This section contains our full discussion of errors in ethics consultation. To frame the discussion of errors, we briefly review the SHHV-SBC Task Force's main finding, as well as the goals and the role of the ethics consultant.

THE "ETHICS FACILITATION" APPROACH

The SHHV-SBC Task Force document, *Core Competencies*, recommends an approach to ethics consultation it describes as "ethics facilitation"[28] as a middle ground between extremes of "authoritarian" and "pure facilitation" approaches. In a key passage, the report describes two main features of this approach, which it desires to keep in balance:

1.   Those doing the consultation should help to identify and analyze the value uncertainty or conflict underlying the consultation. This requires:
   - gathering relevant data (e.g., through discussion with involved parties, examination of medical records or other relevant documents);
   - clarifying relevant concepts (e.g., "confidentiality," "privacy," "informed consent," "best interest");
   - clarifying relevant normative issues (e.g., the implications of societal values, law, ethics, and institutional policy for the case); and
   - helping to identify a range of morally acceptable options within the context.

2.   Those doing the consultation should help to address the value uncertainty or conflict by facilitating the building of consensus (i.e., agreement by all involved parties) among involved parties (e.g., patients, families, surrogates, healthcare providers). This requires:
   - ensuring that involved parties have their voices heard;
   - assisting involved individuals in clarifying their own values; and
   - helping to facilitate the building of morally acceptable shared commitments or understandings within the context.[29]

The *Core Competencies* document views authoritarian and pure facilitation approaches as sources of errors. The report criticizes the former for violating the process requirements in item 2 and the latter for neglecting to meet the normative requirements of item 1. The report places great emphasis on respect for the "rights of individuals to live by their own moral values" and "not misplacing decision-making authority or privileging the personal moral views of the consultant(s)."[30]

We share and support the *Core Competencies* document's basic understanding of ethics consultation and its criticism of any approach where consultants dominate decision making or have a privileged place within it. However, we believe its portrayal of the two extreme and erroneous approaches is overidealized. In actuality, these extremes are not the main cause of error in consultation.

GOALS, ROLE ELEMENTS, AND EVALUATION

As a preface to understanding error, we will discuss three other topics. First, we will build on the work of the Chicago conference and the *Core Competencies* to offer a unified statement of the goals of consultation, the elements of the role of ethics consultant, and end points for evaluation of consultations (either as single events or in an aggregate number).

The role of an ethics consultant has four elements: moral diagnostician, educator, facilitator and/or mediator, and bridge to authority. The goals are stated below with the role elements and end points for evaluation at the appropriate places. As stated by the *Core Competencies*, the general goal of ethics consultation is to:

- "improve the provision of healthcare and its outcome through the identification, analysis, and resolution of ethical issues as they emerge in consultation regarding particular clinical cases in healthcare institutions" (*all four role elements*)
- evaluate the level of satisfaction among all participants in ethics consultation.

This general goal is more likely to be achieved if consultation accomplishes the intermediary goals of helping to:
- identify and analyze the nature of the value uncertainty or conflict (i.e., ethical problem) that underlies the consultation" (*moral diagnostician and educator*)
- "facilitate resolution of conflicts in a respectful atmosphere with attention to the interests, rights, and responsibilities of those involved" (*facilitator or mediator*)
- "assist individuals in handling current and future ethical problems by providing education in healthcare ethics" (*educator*)
- "inform institutional efforts at policy development, quality improvement, and appropriate utilization of resources by identifying the causes of ethical problems and to promote practices consistent with ethical norms and standards" (*bridge to authority*)
- *evaluate these end-points*: (1) Was a moral consensus among decision makers facilitated by the consultant(s)? (2) Was the consensus within morally acceptable boundaries? (3) Did others—those with moral and legal standing to do so—actually make the decisions that promoted resolution? (4) If there was an absence of moral consensus, did the consultant(s) continue to help to seek a resolution that was nonetheless morally acceptable? (5) What evidence is there that consultant(s) bridge between experience in consultation and efforts to improve policies, quality of care, and prevention of frequent ethical problems?[31]

Core Competencies serve as a framework within which to begin to discern error in ethics consultation.

WHAT SOURCES OF ETHICS?

A second topic concerns the normative work of consultants. What sources of ethics ought to be used to define the boundaries for acceptable moral options? Four sources will be described in this section: (1) the law and institutional policy, (2) the values and moral beliefs of the adult patient or surrogate, (3) consensus positions and recommendations of national bioethics bodies, and (4) ethical considerations inferred from the peer-reviewed and published literature in bioethics and medical humanities, as well as the many disciplines that inform these fields. Three of these sources are briefly discussed in the *Core Competencies*.[32] A full defense of these sources requires more argument than space allows.

Law is a "floor" of morality in any society and presumably expresses the voluntary will of the majority about the moral content of the law. However, a majority can be morally wrong or ambivalent on a legal issue. Also, simply invoking the law as the source of morality can end conversation and deter creative moral debate. Nonetheless, because law exists on almost every ethical issue in patient care, the moral content of the law is relevant to and barely sufficient for adequate moral choices, which may exceed what is required by law. In an impasse in finding moral consensus, consultants can point out who the legally authorized decision makers are. Institutional policies do not have the moral weight of law, but, if well designed, policies translate laws and legal opinions into useful guidance for clinicians and other decision makers on a variety of issues.

The values and moral beliefs of patients and surrogates are a second source of ethical guidance that has been traditionally overlooked. It requires special skill to elicit these values and beliefs from ill persons and their anxious relatives.

The *Core Competencies* did not identify a third source of ethical guidance: the consensus positions or recommendations of official bodies in public bioethics.[33] The President's Commission on Ethical Problems in Medicine and Biomedical and Behavioral Research (1978 to 1983) issued groundbreaking reports, widely cited by legislatures and courts, especially about forgoing life-sustaining treatment, diagnosing brain death, and clarifying informed consent. This source is certainly relevant to framing moral options and weighing them, and an aspect of the mission of such bodies is to inform the work of local ethics committees and consultants.

A fourth source is ethical considerations inferred from the peer-reviewed literature published in bioethics and medical humanities. This literature includes clinical and organizational ethics, as well as works in philosophical and religious ethics. Examples of such considerations for clinical ethics include balancing benefits and harms in the care of patients; disclosure, informed consent, and shared decision making; the norms of family life; the responsibilities of physicians and nurses in the context of relationships with patients; professional integrity; societal norms of cost-effectiveness and allocation; cultural and religious variations; and considerations of power.

The *Core Competencies* describe the level of knowledge required to discern and use these considerations as "advanced."[34] Assessing the degree of consensus and variation on a particular issue in this body of literature and offering an authoritative opinion in a consultation or consult report is a complex task.

THE MORAL VIEWS OF THE CONSULTANT

A third topic concerns the consultant's role in discussion of the range of morally acceptable options in cases. The *Core Competencies* report does address the issue of the consultant's moral views and how these should be expressed in discussing options.[35] The report makes the distinction between a consultant's "guiding" the discussion in a way that favors an option that appears best for a patient, and "driving" the discussion in a controlling way. We believe that the choice of the term "guiding" in this context is incompatible with the ethics facilitation approach. Participants in consultations are seldom so morally lost that they need a guide. The issue at stake is whether and how the moral views of the consultant should support the moral consensus that is the goal of the discussion. A pure facilitation model would call for the consultant to be neutral or unwilling to be part of the moral consensus that emerges among the decision makers. This approach negates the value of the consultant's education in ethics and the consultant's role of educator about the moral options. However, if the consultant actively guides discussion to favor an option, manipulation and pressure can easily occur. The way through this problem is for the consultant, at this stage of a consultation, to educate others about morally acceptable options without expressing a preference. Rather than guide the discussion toward a preferred outcome, the consultant ought to help those parties who favor one option over another to persuade those who disagree. The skill involved is one of facilitating moral deliberation, but those who deliberate are the participants, with the consultant's help rather than guidance. The main benefit of this approach is that the consultant does not dominate the process of moral deliberation. The participants can persuade and argue in their own words, if they are helped to do so. If a consensus forms among the parties and is within morally acceptable boundaries, the consultant may say that he or she can support it. However, the evidence should be that the consultant facilitated a consensus rather than guided the group to it. If an option is morally controversial but constitutionally protected (for example, a reproductive choice such as abortion), the consultant should make that point clear. If a class of cases (such as some reproductive or end-of-life choices) is legally protected but at odds with the consultant's particular moral views, a prior decision is indicated about whether or how the consultant should participate in such cases. Society and the law support some choices with which consultants of good will morally disagree. Should they avoid participation in such cases at all? We hope that the discussion of conflicts of loyalty later in this chapter will alleviate, if not resolve, this question.

On the other hand, some consultants' moral views favor debatable options that are, at present, morally unacceptable, without exception, in this society. Two examples are performing voluntary euthanasia of competent, terminally ill patients and transplanting the organs of anencephalic infants, with parental permission, without waiting until whole brain death is determined. In spite of their views, consultants in these situations should clearly inform decision makers that such options are unacceptable. It is appropriate on such occasions to teach about the moral boundaries of the case, but the consultant's role does not permit supporting deliberate violations of morality while in that role. For this reason, the consultant should actively discourage decision makers who are considering such directions or actions. Consultants with ethical perspectives that are critical of a culturally or legally permissible option (such as abortion) may refer the case to others or may participate, prepared to give equal time to the pros and cons of all permissible options.

ERRORS IN ETHICS CONSULTATION

MORAL PROACTIVISM

The most common error in ethics consultation occurs when consultants who see themselves as neither authoritarian nor pure facilitators nonetheless take a morally proactive approach to a case. Typically, they enter a case having made a moral judgment about the problem at hand and consciously or unconsciously attempt to guide or manipulate the process to achieve the outcome that is most compatible with their judgment. The error does not lie in making a moral judgment about the problem at hand, which is to be expected. Even very experienced consultants commonly err by trying to control an outcome or by taking sides in a dispute where more than one moral option is acceptable. The error's main effects displace the moral authority of the key decision makers and bias the normative information that they are due.

We observe that moral proactivism is much more prevalent in ethics consultation than true moral authoritarianism is. Authoritarianism is found in distinctively religious clinical settings—but not only there. Any consultant can absolutize a source of ethics and communicate in an authoritarian manner. Consultants who mainly rely on the four sources of ethics described above tend to have a morally pluralistic perspective. However, our hypothesis is that a morally proactive approach prevails among them as well. This hypothesis could be confirmed or disproved by empirical studies.

CAUSES OF MORAL PROACTIVISM

Moral proactivism among ethics consultants has at least three causes. The first cause is lack of exposure to external scrutiny of current practices or training in process-centered ethics consultation. Consultants who have never seen themselves practice in training sessions or have others watch them do consultations can be quite unaware of their moral proactivism.

The second cause is loyalty to a specific model of consultation that requires moral proactivism and presumes expertise in medicine and ethics. For example, La Puma and Scheidermeyer recommend that ethics consultants should examine patients (on the premise that consultants are physicians) and also emphasize that "attempting to effect an ethical outcome in a case is a central goal of consultation."[36]

The need for approval by clinicians is a third cause of moral proactivism. Many committees and consultants believe that clinicians would be disappointed if they are not directive with their moral advice, as in a medical consultation. A good example arose recently. A consultant in a large medical center criticized the *Core Competencies* report as overly concerned with "moral consensus." The critic said that his consultation service was constantly involved in disagreements and disputes. Asked to explain, the consultant said that clinicians expected their ethics service to give advice and to argue for it. The team went into each case with a prepared point of view as to the preferable option, as if it were the goal of the consult was to cause conflict. Too much identification with the medical model of consultation is a source of moral proactivism.

TWO CASES OF MORAL PROACTIVISM

Case 1

We offer two cases to illustrate error due to moral proactivism. In Case 1, one of us (JCF) was the solo consultant.

In October 1987, J.P., a 36-year-old single male accidentally caught the sleeve of his jacket in a mechanically driven post-hole digger. His body went through the machine, which tore off his arms. J.P. and his arms were immediately flown by helicopter to the University of Virginia Medical Center (UVa) in the hope of possible reattachment. On the flight, J.P. made clear to the members of the response team that he was a Jehovah's Witness and refused any blood products.

On admission to the emergency room, he refused blood products and said, "I would rather die first." A nurse, acting as proxy, signed a form used by the emergency room for Jehovah's Witness patients who refused blood products. This form was put into his medical record.

A plastic surgeon attempted microsurgical reattachment of his least damaged arm for several hours. J.P's lost blood was replaced with artificial volume expanders. The surgeon halted efforts due to blood loss and a dangerously low hematocrit. The shoulder stumps were surgically closed. J.P. was admitted to the surgical intensive care unit (SICU) in critical condition, where he remained intubated and on mechanical ventilation. His very survival was tenuous. His hematocrit (an indicator of the amount of hemoglobin available to carry oxygen to cells) was 16 percent (normal is 35 to 47 percent). During the night, his hematocrit dropped to a low of 8 percent. He continued to refuse blood transfusions and was informed of his likely death.

Aiming to save his life, J.P.'s father (a retired member of the UVa medical faculty) and the plastic surgeon sought and obtained a judge's authorization that allowed them, but did not order them, to give blood products to J.P. The judicial ruling was obtained by phone between 1:00 and 2:00 a.m. The judge did not come to the hospital to speak with J.P. The surgeon called the SICU and ordered that blood be given to J.P. After intense discussion with J.P. (who at this point indicated assent or dissent by gesture and by nodding his head), the resident and nurses decided not to give blood, even though a court order permitting it had been issued.

The resident telephoned the surgeon and informed him of the staff's decision. The surgeon responded angrily: "I'll come in and hang the blood myself! I'm on my way!" The resident then called the ethics consultant at 3:00 a.m., described the problem, and defined the situation as an emergency. The consultant explored options (and consequences) with the resident, ranking them as: (1) to respect the patient's wishes and risk his death; or (2) to acquiesce to J.P.'s father's wishes, save the patient's life, and also risk adverse legal action brought by J.P. and the Jehovah's Witnesses for violating the patient's constitutional rights. The resident's preference was for a plan of care for the patient that included his remaining in intensive care, medicated for pain, fully hydrated and fed, but without blood transfusions under any circumstances.

The consultant then prepared the resident for a possible confrontation with the surgeon. The consultant proposed that, if the surgeon was resolute in his intent, the resident should place his body between J.P. and the surgeon. The consultant instructed the resident to tell the surgeon that if he touched the resident, it would be a case of assault and battery. Further, if he touched J.P. against his will, it would be a more serious case of assault and battery, even with the court order. The consultant also predicted that if the surgeon proceeded to give a transfusion, another court would later void the court order because the judge did not come to the hospital to see the patient.

The consultant urged the resident to ask the surgeon to telephone the consultant as soon as possible. He also suggested that if an agreement were reached both physicians should cosign a note in the chart with instructions. Shortly, the surgeon called the consultant, and a three-way discussion began. The surgeon had already begun to rethink his position, which he said had been taken earlier with considerable emotion. He said, "I may have gone too far, but I do not know if I can live with myself if the patient dies and I could have prevented it." He also noted the strong influence that J.P.'s grieving father had in the case. He reluctantly reversed his position, seeing that the patient's wishes were clear and his right to refuse was protected by society. Both physicians signed a chart note to the effect that transfusions would not be given, in respect for J.P.'s informed refusal of blood transfusions, based on religious principles. The consultant asked if he could accompany the surgeon the next morning on his rounds at the bedside, stating that "We need to sure that J.P. understands the complete situation." The surgeon and the resident agreed.

The next morning, the consultant attended rounds with the surgeon and SICU staff to evaluate the intervention of the previous evening. J.P. was awake but too weak to speak. The consultant reviewed the case step by step, asking J.P. at each point if he understood. At each point, the patient nodded in the affirmative. The consultant asked the patient, "Do you agree with what has happened?" J.P. nodded with even more vigor. The consultant wrote a chart note describing the case as one involving the right to refuse treatment by a capable patient, widely supported in clinical ethics and the law. He noted the prior disagreement and its resolution, along with the continued informed refusal of J.P.

J.P. survived his ordeal, largely due to his good state of health prior to the accident, and continues to live in Blacksburg, Virginia. He is active in his congregation, has learned to drive an automobile, and he regularly returns to UVa with an elder in the congregation to discuss this case with medical students in a course on clinical ethics.[37]

Ethics consultation admittedly was far less developed when this case occurred in 1987. Errors in the J.P. case were identified through collegial critique of the consultant's approach and insight gained in mock consultations. The consultant failed to facilitate a process allowing all participants to seek a moral consensus after examining all options fairly.

Three errors stand out. First, the consultant did not go to the SICU to gather data and have a face-to-face meeting with the two physicians, nurses, J.P., his father, and an elder from the Jehovah's Witness congregation. The consultant defined the situation as an "emergency" that had to be dealt with on the telephone, which radically limited dialogue. The consultant could have told the resident to inform the surgeon that he had requested an ethics consultation and that the consultant would meet them to help with the decision making. Second, the consultant excluded the participation of J.P. and others. J.P.'s condition permitted him to communicate with signs as he did the next morning. Third, education about the moral options was deficient. The option to respect J.P.'s wishes received the most attention and the consultant's support, and it prevailed. The option of treatment with blood products over the patient's objection was not given the time and respect that it deserved. The court order and the physician's values created an acceptable (however debatable) moral option for treatment. At the time of this case, it was not unusual to override the requests of adult Jehovah's Witnesses, although it would have been morally and legally controversial. In teaching about the options, the consultant could have (1) been more reserved about his moral judgment or (2) could have stated that, while respect for J.P.'s wishes had strong ethical reasons to support it, treatment could also be ethically defended. Treatment with blood was not a morally unacceptable option. The consultant could have engaged the disputants in trying to persuade one another. The elder could have spoken for J.P. If a consensus had been reached on either option, today the consultant could say that he would support it. If consensus could not have been reached, the outcome that occurred would have probably been the same, but the process would have been much fairer to all concerned. The consultant's influence on the outcome of the case was far too strong. The surgeon clearly retreated from his moral position because of opposition from the resident, backed by the consultant, rather than because he was morally persuaded to do so.

Case 2

Case 2 occurred in 1990 and has been reported in the literature.[38] The authors, physicians who provide ethics consultation within their hospital, report on why they decided to act in place of others to disconnect a ventilator from a patient. In doing so, they performed what is now called "terminal sedation."[39]

The patient, Mr. L., was a 67-year-old, obese man with post-polio syndrome. He was ventilator dependent with a tracheostomy and could not be weaned. The patient requested that the ventilator be discontinued, realizing that he would die as a result. Following psychiatric evaluation of his capacity and situational depression and a very thorough ethics consultation about the validity of his refusal of treatment, all concerned supported the patient's wishes. The patient's sedation to unconsciousness and ventilator removal were scheduled three days later, to enable his family to be with him. The attending physician, to be assisted by a pulmonary consultant, was to do the procedures.

Half an hour before the appointed time, the ethics consultants received a call from a distraught intern, who said that 13 family members were present, the attending physician could not be present until five hours later, and that the pulmonologist's availability had not been verified. The attending physician had "been called away unexpectedly" and had delegated the task to the intern. The ethics consultants were in a dilemma. They were qualified medically to perform the disconnection, yet they were aware that so to act was "beyond our role as ethics consultants." They also were unwilling to allow an inexperienced intern to proceed alone.

They decided to undertake the task themselves, because the patient had waited a week since his original request and the family was present. They discussed this choice with the patient, who strongly desired them to act. The authors did not report communicating with the chair of the clinical department, authorities in the hospital, or the ethics committee prior to their decision. The remainder of their report details their actions, their guilty feelings as physicians for actively killing the patient, and their subsequent ethical justification of their actions as physicians in respecting the patient's autonomy and request. The authors conclude: "It is beyond the usual role of ethics consultants to take over patient care responsibilities and actually perform ventilator withdrawal. We do not intend to make it our practice to do this because it is really the appropriate role of the care-providers, who should enlist the support of a pulmonary-intensivist."[40]

The authors are to be commended for reporting this case. They made no critique of their decision from the perspective of ethics consultation, noting only that it was "beyond the usual role." In our view, while their decision was emotionally understandable, it seriously violated the role of an ethics consultant. If ethics consultants do not have societal authority to "take over" decision making from those with legal and moral standing, then it surely follows that *to act* in the place of the physician is far outside the boundaries of the role.

The consultants had several options that fit the role element of bridge to authority. They could have (1) advised the intern to contact the chair of the department, inform him or her of the crisis, and recommend prompt action; (2) acted for the intern in this capacity; or (3) located another physician. A fourth, more drastic option, was for the most technically qualified of the two to resign from the consultation service before asking the patient's permission to proceed. The approval of hospital authorities and the ethics committee, even after the fact, would have also shown accountability. Paternalistic actions can be justified if they are of the last resort and a way to avoid great harm. This action did avoid the harm of delay, but the consultants did not truly know that it was an act of last resort. They failed to pursue real options.

Several letters to the editor about the report showed only sympathy for the authors as sensitive and caring physicians.[41] None of these letters addressed the authors' role conflict as ethics consultants. Probably few readers even understood the role. A letter from New Zealand recommended that a hospital ethics committee oversee such patient refusals.[42] The authors rightly rejected giving such power to a committee, when a capable patient's autonomy is ethically sufficient for a valid refusal.[43] The authors did not mention their own ethics committee or that they had consulted it afterwards.

The consultants in case 2 did superbly up to the resolution stage of the case. Then, in a crisis they did not create, their familiar role as physicians overwhelmed their newer role as ethics consultants. Could one recommend that others do likewise in similar situations to case 1 and the resolution stage of case 2? If not, the basic flaw in these cases is clear. Namely, unjustified paternalism by ethics consultants is just as indefensible as the old medical paternalism.

These two cases illustrate that moral proactivism, whatever its cause, violates the goals of the enterprise and the role of the consultant. Ethics consultants are not the agents of a higher societal power authorized to take over disputes, make decisions, or act. They are facilitators of moral consensus among all of the key decision makers who ought to resist pressures from within self or others to act otherwise.

LEGAL CASES INVOLVING ETHICS COMMITTEES OR CONSULTANTS

Some critics of ethics consultants and committees observe that they provide cover for the institution and are easily co-opted.[44] Unfortunately, some court cases confirm this criticism. To date, we are aware that committees or consultants have been named in five lawsuits and criticized by a federal judge in a sixth. Below, we discuss these six cases in chronological order. The third case, *Bryan*, is only summarized because errors in ethics consultation were not a causative factor.

Bouvia v. Superior Court (Glenchur), United States

Beginning in 1983 at the age of 25, Elizabeth Bouvia, a quadriplegic, refused feeding by artificial means. Legal proceedings upheld physicians' forcefully feeding her. She became a patient at Los Angeles County High Desert Hospital in 1985. The ethics committee, apparently without dissent, supported her physicians' decision to force feed her by a nasogastric tube. Her physicians believed that her failure to eat more was a suicidal attempt to starve herself to death. She claimed that she was eating as much as she could. Bouvia had been examined by a psychiatrist and found to be a capable decision maker. In 1986, a California court of appeals overturned an earlier court decision siding with her physician and the hospital, stating: "Bouvia's decision to forego medical treatment or life-support through a mechanical means belongs to her. It is not a medical decision. . . . Neither is it a legal question. . . . It is not a conditional right subject to approval by ethics committees or courts of law. It is a moral and philosophical decision that, being a competent adult, is hers alone."[45]

After the tube was removed, Bouvia and her attorney sued the hospital and the physicians for money damages. Learning that her physicians had stated that the ethics committee was as responsible as the physicians were, she filed an amended complaint against each member of the committee as a defendant.[46] Ms. Bouvia never served the members and voluntarily dropped the suit to avoid publicity.[47]

Bouvia is an early example of the pitfalls to which some committees might succumb and the error of strongly taking sides. The committee was co-opted by physicians and was tribunal-like. No process of ethics consultation was offered involving the patient, nor was education or mediation about all morally acceptable options. In *Bouvia,* the court had to force physicians to face the moral acceptability of the competent patient's right to refuse all treatments. Clearly, the committee's role should have been more mediatory and educational. Moral support for Bouvia's refusal and questions about the moral acceptability of coercive treatment were both appropriate, given the clear consensus in the literature well in advance of the time of this case.[48]

In Re Baby K

In 1992, an ethics consultation team at Fairfax Hospital in Virginia had a role in the *Baby K* case. A federal court judge criticized its participation. The critique doubtless alerted plaintiff's attorneys and other interested parties to the errors of ethics committees and consultants.

At physicians' request, a team of the ethics committee met with Baby K's mother, who demanded life-sustaining measures for a newborn with anencephaly. The staff of the neonatal intensive care unit viewed these measures as futile and violations of their professional integrity. A three-person team (family practitioner, psychiatrist, and minister) was unsuccessful in resolving the dispute. The team's chart note stated that care was "futile" and advised that the hospital "attempt to resolve this through our legal system" if, after a waiting period, no change occurred in the mother's position. Judge Hilton wrote in his opinion that her "treating physicians requested the assistance of the Hospital's 'Ethics Committee' in overriding the mother's wishes."[49]

Our interpretation is that the judge put quotation marks around the committee's name to deride their taking sides and their failure to give due attention to the moral arguments for Baby K's mother's position.

Judge Hilton's ruling that the Emergency Medical Treatment and Active Labor Act (EMTALA) required the hospital to provide emergency ventilatory treatment for Baby K's periodic apnea (by then, Baby K was residing in a nearby nursing home) was upheld by the Fourth Circuit Court of Appeals.[50] The U.S. Supreme Court declined to hear an appeal by the hospital, Baby K's father, and the guardian *ad litem.*

Again, the main lesson for consultants is to avoid strongly taking sides in a morally complex case. In this case, there were also errors and omissions of process, (such as not including Baby K's father or a clergyperson of the mother's faith) that are discussed elsewhere.[51]

Bryan v. Stone et al. and Bryan v. Rector and Visitors of the University of Virginia et al.

Bryan, the executrix of the estate of a 53-year-old patient who died at the University of Virginia (UVa) Hospital on 25 February 1993, brought two lawsuits that named the ethics committee chair and an ethics consultant (JCF), among others. The suits alleged violation of the federal EMTALA and the Virginia Health Care Decisions Act due to use of the hospital's do-not-resuscitate (DNR) policy, which permits physicians to write a DNR order over objections of surrogates in futility disputes. The suits were decided in the university's favor. The federal suit resulted in an important appellate-level ruling about EMTALA in the wake of the *Baby K* case.[52] Ethics consultation was refused by the family early in the case and was not a precipitating cause of the suits. The case is fully reported elsewhere.[53]

The family was aggrieved because of physicians' refusals to "do everything" including vigorous resuscitation for a hopelessly ill patient. An *ad hoc* committee, headed by the chair of the ethics committee, reviewed the case and concurred with physicians that the DNR order was appropriate. The report of this committee was entered into the medical record. The patient died eight days after the DNR order was written. Later, a dispute arose between the hospital's billing department and the family. The family turned over a "final notice" to their attorneys, whose medical record review found the committee's report.

Gilgunn v. Massachusetts General Hospital

A 71-year-old woman in very poor health broke her hip in a fall. Before she underwent orthopedic surgery, she suffered seizures followed by brain damage and coma. Her daughter, the surrogate of choice, informed physicians that her mother would have "wanted everything done." After several weeks, the medical team desired to stop treatment that they considered futile. The hospital's optimum care committee was one of the earliest types of patient care ethics committees in the nation, a small group that confined its scope mainly to intensive care. The committee's chair is a psychiatrist with a long-standing practice of advocating DNR when incapacitated and hopelessly ill patients have lengthy ICU stays and families demand that "everything be done."[54] The chair persuaded the attending physician to write a DNR order, which the attending physician later revoked when the daughter protested. The chair then supported a subsequent attending physician's decision to write a DNR order. The chairman and ethics committee did not meet with the surrogate. After a DNR order was written, the attending physician gradually extubated the patient over the surrogate's objections. The patient died, and her daughter sued for violations of her own, rather than the patient's rights. A trial court jury sided with the hospital.[55] The decision was on appeal, but the plaintiff withdrew the appeal shortly before trial.[56]

Capron discussed the ethical and legal significance of this important case.[57] He was correct, in our view, to criticize the intervention of the chair of the optimal care committee, who acted not like an ethics consultant but, in Capron's words, "in the style of a medical consultant." The mediational and educational benefits of ethics consultation were not evident in the process used in this case.

Estate of James David Bland v. Cigna Healthplan of Texas et al.

The family of a patient with AIDS sued for intentional infliction of emotional harm as a result of decisions made by the chair of the ethics committee, who was also a pulmonologist, linked to the manner of the patient's death.[58] The case was fully reported in a 1995 article about managed care and medicine in Texas.[59]

The patient was a registered nurse who understood that he had a terminal illness and would die soon. In July 1993, he was admitted to Houston's Park Plaza Hospital's ICU and placed on a respirator. He was given a paralytic drug to make him comfortable, and the respirator took over his breathing function. Afraid of suffocating if he was taken off the respirator, he asked his physician to allow him to die peacefully while being ventilated. His physician agreed, and the patient soon lapsed into a coma.

The physician explained his plan to the family, who understood and agreed to a DNR order on the condition that the patient remain on the respirator. Bland's physician then withdrew from the case and turned over care to a Cigna primary-care physician. After a few days, the medical director of Cigna contacted the chair of the ethics committee, a pulmonologist in charge of the unit in question. The Cigna official raised questions about the patient's stay in the ICU and whether he could be moved. The chair of the ethics committee went to the unit, presumably in the role of a physician—but not the patient's physician—without consulting the patient's family or the original physician with whom the comfort care plan was made. He did discuss the care plan with the Cigna primary-care physician. As a result of the intervention, the patient was removed from the respirator by a respiratory therapist and died shortly thereafter.[60] The circumstances of Bland's death and the involvement of the pulmonologist were not discussed with the family. They learned the facts from documents prepared for another lawsuit brought the patient's original physician against Cigna. The family's suit was settled out of court for an undisclosed amount.

The Cigna official's contact raises an issue of organizational ethics. However, the main error is that this contact should have prompted an ethics consultation better provided by someone other than the chairman, who had a conflict of interest. There was a failure of moral diagnosis and education. The ethics committee chair failed to gather data on the prior history of the patient. He also failed to convert this request into an ethics consultation that could have been led by other consultants who could educate about the options with all parties present. There was a serious ethical problem—namely, the promise made to the patient and family regarding how death would occur was being infringed by the financial interests of the managed-care company. The Cigna primary-care physician also abdicated his role by permitting the pulmonologist to go to the patient's room and initiate a process leading to removal of the ventilator with no discussion with the family. If the act occurred as alleged in the suit, it favored a morally unacceptable option—that is, a physician's unilateral decision making at the end of life. It is a well-established moral practice that physicians share such crucial decisions with surrogates. To make such decisions without consulting surrogates likely violates the Texas Natural Death Act.[61]

Bland is an example of two serious errors by the ethics committee chairperson. The first was failure to seek information relevant to the ethical history of the case, resulting in a flawed moral diagnosis. The second was engagement in such a direct action while in two roles—pulmonologist and ethics committee chair. The *Core Competencies* report takes a strong position that "an individual should never serve as an ethics consultant on a case in which he/she has clinical or administrative responsibility."[62]

Rideout v. Hershey Medical Center

Brianne Rideout, a two-year-old patient with a brainstem glioblastoma (a malignant tumor), had undergone neurosurgery at the Johns Hopkins University Hospital. She was admitted to the emergency department of the Hershey Medical Center on 6 April 1992. While at Hershey, she lapsed into a stupor and required assistance to breathe. By 13 April, she had a tracheostomy and was placed on a ventilator. Physicians regarded her condition as incurable, but her parents favored aggressive treatment.

The family and physicians began a period of negotiation regarding home care or hospital care. Home care was ruled out due to inadequate wiring for a ventilator. By 20 May, the patient's parents learned that her insurance coverage would soon be depleted and Medicaid would have to cover costs. The next day, the ethics committee met at the request of the patient's physician (without the parents present) to discuss the case, and the committee supported a decision to write a DNR order. On 22 May, when the Rideouts were informed of this decision, they stated that they were opposed, because it meant giving up on the child's life. They began to search for an appropriate alternate site without success. On 12 July, the child's pupils became fixed and dilated for the first time. On 13 July, her physician decided, based on discussions with the ethics committee and in the light of the child's deteriorating condition, to remove the ventilator.

On 14 July, the physician informed the Rideouts that he would withdraw the ventilator that day. The chair of the ethics committee met with the parents to confirm the decision. Following this meeting, the parents complained to the patient advocate, who persuaded the physician and ethics committee chair to delay to allow legal consultation. Nonetheless, the removal was scheduled for 11:00 a.m. on 15 July. The parents secured the services of an attorney and sought a judicial order to stop the action. The hospital had asked local police to be present to prevent disorder. While the parents were in the office of the patient advocate speaking with their attorney by phone, the physician removed the ventilator. The hospital's chaplain communicated the action to the Rideouts. Hearing this, they rushed to her room. They were described in their complaint as hysterical and crying that their daughter was being murdered. They requested that the ventilator be reconnected, but the physician declined to do so. Mr. Rideout reportedly had an acute asthma attack. The patient died two days later, in the presence of her parents.

The Rideout's 11-count complaint raised common law, statutory, and constitutional claims, each of which the hospital contested.[63] On 29 December 1995, a three-judge panel overruled the medical center's challenge to claims that by stopping the ventilator over the parents' wishes, the hospital committed an assault and battery on the child, negligently and intentionally inflicted emotional distress on the parents, and impinged parental rights rooted in the free exercise of religion.[64] The panel refused to rule out punitive damages. The hospital won arguments that it did not violate constitutional privacy and liberty interests and that EMTALA was not violated. The panel's decision meant that the parents were free to continue their lawsuit in a jury trial. The hospital eventually settled the case before it went to trial.[65]

The Hershey ethics committee and its chairperson may have erred in the process of the case in two respects. First, was it good practice to meet originally with the physician without notifying and inviting the parents? An opportunity to involve them was missed. Second, later in the case, was it good practice for the chairperson to meet with the parents for the purpose of notifying them that the decision to withdraw would be carried out? Closing out morally acceptable options is not the role of a committee. There were two other options available, even at that point: (1) transferring the patient to an alternate site or, failing that, (2) seeking a court's concurrence with the decision to withdraw.

The hospital's ethics committee appears to have strongly taken sides with the physician and hospital authorities against the patient's parents. The alternative stance is only to offer consultation, education, and mediation about the morally acceptable options. Also, the committee appears to have been a party to a unilateral decision to remove a ventilator over the parents' objections. In such a situation, the ethics committee's role should be confined only to searching for other morally acceptable alternatives to such a morally dubious action. If that search fails, then the physician and hospital should seek the help of a court in resolving the dispute. Physicians and ethics committees are not the final arbiters of futility disputes until our society works out fairer approaches to allocation of expensive healthcare resources. The institutions of law must be involved to ensure the highest standards of impartiality.

Some of these cases—especially *Baby K, Bland,* and *Rideout*—raise serious legal questions about some actions of committees or their consultants. Ethics consultation is coming to the attention of the legal system. Sooner or later, a court will ask: "For what exactly is an ethics consultant (or a team acting for a committee) responsible and accountable? Is there a standard of care for ethics consultation?"

ERRORS IN PROCESS AND POLICY

This section indentifies some common errors and omissions in the consultative process or in institutional policy about consultation. The *Core Competencies* report addresses some of these issues.[66]

ACCESS TO CONSULTATION

Some institutions erroneously limit access to ethics consultation to attending physicians. Such a practice stems from fear and misunderstanding and displays disrespect for the rights of patients, families, and other clinicians. The *Core Competencies* report supports a general policy of open access and states, "requests for consultation by patients, families, or surrogates must be honored without restriction."[67] Intimidation or veiled threats (usually by physicians) against other clinicians (usually nurses) who request or desire to request an ethics consultation are a violation of open access.

NOTIFICATION AND PARTICIPATION

Good practice in medicine is to inform patients or surrogates, except in emergencies, of any and all requests for medical and other consultations. This standard is frequently breached in practice. We believe that careful study of ethics consultation would find that many capable patients or their surrogates were unaware that an ethics consultation affecting the patient's care had even occurred. This omission is especially grievous when the patient's or surrogate's participation is ethically required for shared decision making but the patient or surrogate is shut out of the process. *Bouvia, Gilgunn, Bland,* and *Rideout* illustrate this error. The *Gilgunn* and *Rideout* suits may have been unpreventable, but it is an open question as to whether notification and participation could have contributed to a different outcome.

Not all consultations require notification. For example, when two healthcare providers morally disagree and request help to sort out the issues to find a unified approach, it is not necessary to notify patients or their surrogates. Consultants must use judgment as to when to notify patients or surrogates about a request for ethics consultation and advise clinicians when this ground rule is in effect. The most obvious thresholds are when consultants must review a patient's chart and medical record to gather data and when participation of the patient or surrogate in decision making is required to seek a moral consensus. Notification is not required until a request for a full consultation has been made.

The aims of notification are to respect the privacy of patients and surrogates and to increase the chances of their participation in the process of consultation. If the patient's or surrogate's participation is ethically indicated and the consultation proceeds without them, there is clearly a significant process error. As the *Bland* and *Rideout* cases show, exclusion of one or more key decision makers is a fundamental error that can violate their rights.

If the medical record is reviewed by consultants who have no direct health-care responsibility, without the knowledge of the patient or family, there is a serious and legally actionable breach of the patient's privacy. The information in the medical record belongs to the patient. The patient or surrogate should know that a consultation has been requested and that the consultants will review the record in advance of any discussions. To fail to notify the attending physician that a consultation has been requested by another party is also a serious process error. This error surely occurs less frequently than failure to notify patients or surrogates.

Anyone may refuse to participate in an ethics consultation. If a patient or surrogate refuses, the consultation does not proceed, but the consultants may continue to support the healthcare team and discuss issues with them in a general manner. There needs to be a reliable process to address an attending physician's refusal of ethics consultation. One approach is to avoid direct conflict between the attending physician and the consultant(s) by a requirement to refer the issue to the chairperson of the ethics committee. The chairperson is authorized to discuss the reasons for the refusal with the attending physician and make a decision about whether the consultation should go forward. Only a patient or the patient's legally authorized representative ought to be able to veto an ethics consultation.

DOCUMENTATION AND EVALUATION

Failure to document any consultation in the patient's medical record is an error, including an ethics consultation. We differ with the *Core Competencies* report, which recommends documentation in the medical record or "in some other permanent record."[68] The latter alternative usually means an account of the consultation written for an ethics committee that may or may not be distributed to the parties to the consultation. These accounts may be filed in the records of the committee. This reflects an attempt to be flexible in the face of a variety of practices of documentation.

A better approach to documentation is a "both-and" rather than the "either-or" option of the task force. Good documentation requires an appropriate note in the medical record and a longer, detailed account of the case suitable for evaluation and review. The goals of documentation are (1) to inform all hospital staff caring for the patient of the issues and important details of the consultation, (2) to have an accurate history of all phases of the patient's care, (3) to aid in education in clinical ethics and healthcare law, and (4) to aid in the task of quality assurance. To omit documentation in the medical record is to fail to seek these goals. To write only a chart note but no consultation report prevents good education and reduces quality assurance.

Hesitancy to document in the medical record usually arises from one of the following three causes: (1) fears of subsequent lawsuits in which the record would be discoverable, (2) lack of consultant training in writing appropriate notes, or (3) the marginality of consultants or the committee to clinical decision making in the institution. If such factors are evident, the remedies are to strengthen the ethics program and to educate and train consultants or the committee in better practices of documentation.

Documentation ought to serve quality assurance. Exhibit 21-1 lists the recommended elements in an adequate chart note that would be relevant to end points for evaluation provided earlier in this chapter.

Exhibit 21-2 presents a format for a consultation report that can be adapted to particular cases. In our view, an adequate consultation report includes the four major parts presented in the exhibit—the consultant's assessment; the consultant's moral diagnosis and educational aims; goals, decision making, and implementation; and evaluation—and all lettered topic headings. Some numbered items are relevant to each case and some would not be relevant. The format is worded so that parts I and II could be a consultant's work up for key participants to use in a meeting to seek moral consensus. Parts III and IV are worded retrospectively after such a meeting to complete a full consultation report. The full report could be for committee review or to share with participants and the administration when the case raises policy issues.

The information in Exhibits 21-1 and 21-2 would presumably be useful for quality assurance and for evaluation of particular consultations. For more systematic evaluation of particular consultations or an aggregate number of consultations, instruments can be designed from the end points provided earlier in this chapter.

LACK OF INSTITUTIONAL POLICY ON ETHICS CONSULTATION

We assume that most healthcare institutions have a policy statement on the mission and functions of the ethics committee. Such policies typically state that ethics consultation is a committee function, but are vague about standards for consultation. All institutions that offer ethics consultation have a duty to clarify standards for ethics consultation in terms of competence, fairness, and accountability. Exhibit 21-3 outlines the elements of an adequate policy statement.

The policy may also recognize a place for ethics conversations preliminary to formal consultations or alongside the practice. Ethical concerns of importance to clinical staff arise that may or may not require a full consultation to explore and resolve. Institutions ought to have high standards for the consulta-

---

Exhibit 21-1
An Adequate Chart Note

- Requester and time of request
- Requester's stated concern or ethical problem(s)
- Who notified patient/surrogate and attending physician
- Consultant's view of the ethical problem(s) in the case
- Capacity of patient and whether advance directives exist
- Decision makers with legal and moral standing and, if needed, efforts to involve them
- If a meeting was required, date/time and participants
- Moral options considered and whether consensus was achieved
- If no consensus, did decision makers with legal standing resolve the question? If not, why not?
- Further recommendations of consultants as to the process of resolution

Exhibit 21-2
Elements of a Consultation Report

I.   Consultant's assessment
    A.   What is the patient's medical condition?
        1.   Identification of medical problems
        2.   Diagnosis/diagnostic hypotheses
        3.   Predictions and uncertainties regarding prognosis
            a.   Prospects for full or partial recovery
            b.   Is the patient terminally ill?
    B.   What are the goals of treatment and care?
        1.   Any reasonable alternatives
    C.   What are the relevant contextual factors?
        1.   Demographic facts: age, gender, education
        2.   Life situation and lifestyle of patient
        3.   Family relationships
        4.   Setting of care: home or institution
        5.   Socioeconomic facts (e.g., insurance coverage)
        6.   Language spoken
        7.   Cultural factors
        8.   Religion
    D.   Is the patient capable of decision making?
        1.   Legally incompetent (e.g., child, court determination of incompetence)
        2.   Clearly incapacitated (e.g, unconscious)
        3.   Diminished capacity (e.g., depression or other mental disorder interfering with understanding or judgment)
        4.   Fluctuating capacity
        5.   Prospects for enhancing capacity
    E.   What are the patient's preferences?
        1.   Understanding of condition
        2.   Views on quality of life
        3.   Values relevant to decision making about treatment
        4.   Current wishes for treatment
        5.   Advance directives
        6.   Any reasons for seeking treatment regarded as medically inappropriate or refusing treatment regarded as medically indicated
    F.   What are the needs of the patient as a person?
        1.   Psychic suffering and possible interventions for relief
        2.   Interpersonal dynamics
        3.   Resources and strategies for helping patient cope
        4.   Adequacy of home environment for care of patient
        5.   Preparation for dying
    G.   What are the preferences of family/surrogate decision makers?
        1.   Competence as surrogate decision maker

   2. Knowledge of relevant patient preferences

   3. Opinions on quality of life of patient

   4. Opinions on best interest of patient

   5. Reasons for seeking treatment regarded as medically inappropriate or refusing treatment regarded as medically indicated

  H. Are there interests other than, and potentially competing with, those of the patient?

   1. Interests of family (e.g., concerns about burdens of caring for patient, disagreements with preferences of patient)

   2. Interests of a fetus

   3. Scarce resources and competing needs for their use

   4. Interests of healthcare providers (e.g., professional integrity)

   5. Interests of healthcare organization

  I. Are there issues of power or conflict in the interactions of the key actors in the case that need to be addressed?

   1. Between clinicians and patient/family

   2. Between patient and family

   3. Between family members/surrogates

   4. Between members of the healthcare team (e.g., attendings and house staff, physicians and nurses)

  J. Have all the parties involved in the case had an opportunity to be heard?

  K. Are there institutional factors contributing to moral problems posed by case?

   1. Work routines

   2. Fears of malpractice/defensive medicine

   3. Biases favoring disproportionately aggressive treatment or neglect of treatable conditions

   4. Cost constraints/economic incentives

II. Consultant's moral diagnosis and educational aims

  A. How is the moral problem in this case being framed by the participants? Does this need to be reconsidered and replaced by an alternative understanding?

  B. Identify and rank the range of relevant moral considerations

  C. Are there relevant institutional policies pertaining to the case?

  D. Consider ethical standards and guidelines, drawing on consensus statements of commissions and interdisciplinary or specialty groups

  E. Consider similar cases and discussions in the literature that might shed light on the analysis and resolution of moral problems in the case

  F. What are the morally acceptable options for resolving the moral problem(s) posed by the case?

III. Goals, decision making, and implementation

  A. Key decision makers' considerations of the goals of treatment and care for the patient

  B. Ideas for possible interventions to meet the needs of the patient and resolve moral problems

  C. Deliberations about merits of alternative options for resolving the moral problem

  D. Was a moral consensus achieved? Was it within morally acceptable boundaries?

E.   Was an acceptable plan of action negotiated and implemented?

F.   If consensus was not achieved, what did the consultant do to seek resolution? (e.g., decision makers with legal authority encouraged to resolve the issue)

IV. Evaluation

A.   Current

1.   Is the plan of action working? If not, why not?

2.   Have conditions changed in a way that suggests the need to rethink the plan?

3.   Are interactions between clinicians and the patient or surrogate helping to meet the needs of the patient, to respect the patient as a person, and to serve the goals of the plan of care?

4.   Are there relevant interests, institutional factors, or normative considerations that have not been adequately addressed in planning for the care of the patient?

B.   Retrospective

1.   What opportunities for resolving the moral problem(s) were missed?

2.   How did the care received by the patient match up to standards of good practice?

3.   What factors contributed to a less than optimal resolution of the problems posed by the case?

4.   Was the process of problem solving satisfactory in this case?

5.   What might have been done to improve the care of the patient?

6.   Are there desirable changes in institutional policy, feasible changes in the clinical environment, or educational interventions that might help in preventing or better resolving the moral problems posed by similar cases?

---

tion arm of their ethics programs. Clinicians ought not to face barriers when they ask for information or reassurance from their ethics service. Also, ethics conversations frequently lead to full consultations and should not end without the consultant exploring the need for a consultation. Consultants can make mistakes in ethics conversations and use them as substitutes for a full consultation. Patient privacy can also be easily breached. To guard the privacy of the patient, it is best to avoid using the patient's name in the conversation or to access the patient's chart. Consultants should keep notes about their ethics conversations and report them routinely to the ethics committee.

ISSUES OF LOYALTY AND FREEDOM

THE LOYALTY OF ETHICS CONSULTANTS

To whom or what should ethics consultants be primarily loyal and accountable? Claims on consultants' loyalties are made by patients and surrogates, the institution that employs them, clinicians whose approval they need, the fields of bioethics and medical humanities, and particular moral traditions.

Misplaced loyalty leads to errors, and clarification of this issue may help to prevent errors and lawsuits. In case 1, the consultant erred due to excessive loyalty to the patient and his clearly valid refusal of blood transfusion. In case 2, loyalty to the patient and family caused the consultants to violate the role of ethics consultant by disconnecting a respirator. In the legal cases of *Bouvia, Baby K, Gilgunn,* and *Rideout,* loyalty to medical colleagues and professional integrity were causative. In *Bland,* the ethics committee chair was more responsive, if not loyal, to the interests of an important third-party payer than to others in the case.

The problem of conflicting loyalties is real, but it can be resolved by taking the position that consultants owe primary loyalty to the process of ethics consultation in their institution and the role of a consultant as defined by that process. This view is compatible with the SHHV-SBC Task Force's position that the *Core Competencies* document be used as "voluntary guidelines."

We take this position with a condition and a recommendation. First, any process of ethics consultation worthy of the name ought to be open to evaluation, constructive criticism, and improvement. No aspect of healthcare ought escape the scrutiny of quality assurance, including ethics consultation. Institutions have a duty to support and improve this service. Our recommendation is that the institutional policy statement on ethics consultation include a statement of support for the education and training of those who provide it, as shown in Exhibit 21-3. It should not be optional to have a written policy or to support education and training of consultants, because of the risks involved in neglecting these issues. It is optional to cite the *Core Competencies* report as the source of standards that the institution voluntarily accepts for education and training and for the process of consultation.

We freely admit that our view permits several types and models for ethics consultation, including those that are authoritarian or morally proactive. In a morally pluralistic society, there will never be uniformity or consistency in ethics consultation. For example, it is not an error to be authoritarian as a consultant in a religious setting where theological traditions limit some but not all options. Consultants in these settings must be loyal to their process and its values.

Exhibit 21-3
Elements of a Policy on Ethics Consultation

---

1. Philosophy that informed clinicians are primary resources—with patients and families—to identify and resolve ethical problems
2. Educational program in clinical ethics and healthcare law to support this philosophy
3. Institutional support for education and training of ethics consultants in competencies and skills (option: cite the *Core Competencies* report)
4. An open policy on who may request consultation
5. Notification of the attending physician
6. Notification of the patient or surrogate if, ethically, the consultation requires their participation
7. A process to address physician's objections to a consultation
8. Institutional protection for the requester
9. A protocol specifying that ethics consultations will be documented in the patient's chart
10. A statement about no charges or billing for consultation
11. Outline of accountability structure
12. Provision for evaluation of consultation and a process for complaints

Our view places responsibility for standards for ethics consultation on institutions, rather than on the fields of bioethics and medical humanities or an idea of a profession for ethics consultants. In the strict sense of the term, there is no profession of ethics consultation that admits new members, trains them, transmits a tradition, and commands loyalty of its members. Concerns about professionalization of ethics consultants, long alleged in Scofield's writings, are firmly set to rest by the *Core Competencies* report.[69] Consultants who view themselves as agents of bioethics and medical humanities misunderstand their role. Ethics consultants are surely not the agents of society, like judges and juries, with authority to take over disputes and resolve them. They can only serve a process and role located in institutions that appoint them to provide this service. It follows that their authority to be consultants flows from the institution, rather than from society, a profession, or an academic field.

When this view of the locus of consultants' loyalty is joined with the *Core Competencies* report's conclusion that its findings be regarded as voluntary guidelines, two crucial questions can be resolved: (1) Should consultants be certified? (2) Is there a standard of care (in the legal sense) for ethics consultation?

The SHHV-SBC Task Force studied the question of whether certification of individual consultants or accreditation of training programs was advisable. To approve either of these models would have located the source of authority for standards in ethics consultation in the interdependent fields of bioethics and medical humanities or in an agency that these fields designated to certify or accredit programs. The Task Force also stated that these models would tend to displace the moral standing of key decision makers, be divisive within interdisciplinary fields, and promote ideas of moral expertise that were incompatible with the approach of ethics facilitation. The *Core Competencies* report rejected both of these approaches, leaving the operational choice about standards for consultation to each institution that offers this service.

What is the place of ethics consultation in the fields of bioethics and medical humanities? These fields are most certainly sources of bodies of knowledge required for the normative work of ethics consultation. The *Core Competencies* report now emanates from these fields as a new increment of knowledge about the competencies and skills required for ethics consultation.

But are these fields more than sources of authoritative knowledge? Should the locus of accountability for standards of ethics consultation be located in these fields? All arguments for this direction tend to increase the degree of professionalization of consultants, elevate their role as moral experts, and diminish the role of patients and providers as key decision makers at the bedside. The Task Force does not have any evidence (nor do we) that leaders in these fields desire either a significant degree of professionalization for consultants or the financial and legal responsibility to certify individuals or accredit training programs. Leaders in these fields should be concerned with reviewing their graduate study and fellowship programs in the light of the Task Force's recommendations and with creating regional programs for education and training wherever these do not exist.

LEGAL RISKS OF COMMITTEES AND CONSULTANTS

It is reasonable to expect lawsuits, probably small in number, due to decisions and actions of ethics committees and consultants. Some suits will be brought due to errors in consultation. Other suits, like *Bryan*, will occur because of the need for judicial review of federal or state laws and their interface with institutional policy. Consultants who adhere to the model of ethics facilitation and who resist moral proactivism need not be concerned about precipitating lawsuits. There is always a risk in healthcare settings, however, that one will be named in a suit. The institution's liability policy ought to cover the legal costs of any committee member or consultant so named.

We do not believe that ethics committees or consultants ought to have legal immunity from civil or criminal liability, and we agree with Wilson's lucid analysis of this issue.[70] Four states (Arizona, Hawaii, Maryland, and Montana) immunize committees and their consultants as well as healthcare providers who rely on their advice. We believe that immunity is a mistake that can wrongly shield errors in consultation that may violate patients' or surrogates' rights. Leaders in these states ought to rescind the immunity provision of these laws. Any decision or action of a committee or a consultant ought to be open to legal scrutiny.

If and when lawsuits arise because consultants' or committees' actions are the source of the complaint, it would not be reasonable for a court to regard the *Core Competencies* as a legal standard of care from which to scrutinize actions central to the dispute. There is a standard of care in the practice of medicine or nursing because there are ways to measure efficacy and safety, and these professions have the power and authority to articulate such standards. There is nothing comparable for ethics consultation except the standards of the institution for this activity. It is proper for a court to determine whether a consultant's actions were in keeping with the institution's own guidelines for consultation. Institutions that adopt and cite the *Core Competencies* report as guidelines for their own protocol could have some protection by showing that consultants' actions were within these boundaries. Institutions lacking a policy or a protocol for consultation may be at a higher risk of liability for ethics consultants' mistakes that violate a patient's or surrogate's rights or inflict emotional harm.

SOURCES OF PROTECTION OF THE FREEDOM OF ETHICS CONSULTANTS

Can committee members or consultants whose livelihood depends on a healthcare organization be sufficiently free and critical to do their work? If the source of authority for ethics consultation resides in the institution, the burden of protecting this freedom falls directly on the institution. Healthcare institutions have a duty to protect the freedom of ethics consultants just as academic and scientific institutions protect academic and scientific freedom. Consultants should not be pressured by administrators to compromise the process or content of consultations. As stated below, the institutional policy on consultation can also be brought to bear on the issue of intimidation of those who request ethics consultations. If violations of such freedoms were serious, it would be appropriate to complain to JCAHO. In the light of its rules, JCAHO could discipline a member institution where repeated intimidation of ethics consultants occurred.

We also find five main sources of protection of the freedom of consultants and committees: (1) an open policy on who may request consultation, (2) a policy statement that intimidation of those who request ethics consultation violates institutional policy and can warrant discipline, (3) effective community members of the ethics committee, (4) assurance of the committee's authority to initiate discussion or study of any policy question relevant to its mission, and (5) evaluation of ethics consultation that gathers data from all participants and invites scrutiny by external auditors.

CONCLUSION

This chapter introduces readers to ethics consultation in healthcare and the sources and range of errors in providing this service. The initiative to implement the work of the *Core Competencies* report, aimed to raise standards in ethics consultation but stop short of providing a standard of care, now clearly rests with the many thousands of persons who provide this service and with those who govern healthcare organizations.

NOTES

1. Ethics consultation for problems in governing or managing healthcare organizations is very new and far less developed than ethics consultation provided in the clinical setting.

2. J.C. Fletcher, N. Quist, and A.R. Jonsen, ed., *Ethics Consultation in Health Care* (Ann Arbor, Mich.: Health Administration Press, 1989): 8-13; A.R. Jonsen, *The Birth of Bioethics* (New York: Oxford University Press, 1998), 3-33; J.D. Moreno, "Ethics Committees and Ethics Consultants," in *Companion to Bioethics*, ed. H. Kuhse and P. Singer (Malden, Mass.: Blackwell, 1998), 475-84.

3. An important Canadian project to clarify the role of the ethics consultants was reported in F. Baylis, ed., *The Health Care Ethics Consultant* (Totowa, N.J.: Humana, 1989).

4. R.R. Faden and T.L. Beauchamp, *A History and Theory of Informed Consent* (New York: Oxford University Press, 1986), 91-3.

5. President's Commission for the Study of Ethical Problems in Medicine and Biomedical and Behavioral Research, *Decisions to Forego Life-Sustaining Treatment* (Washington, D.C.: U.S. Government Printing Office, 1983): 153-60.

6. A.R. Jonsen, "Can an Ethicist Be a Consultant?" in *Frontiers in Medical Ethics*, ed. V. Abernethy (Cambridge, Mass.: Ballinger, 1980).

7. R.E. Cranford and E.A. Doudera, *Institutional Ethics Committees and Health Care Decision Making* (Ann Arbor, Mich.: Health Administration Press, 1984).

8. See note 4 above.

9. R.B. Purtilo, "A Comment on the Concept of Consultation," in *Ethics Consultation in Health Care*, see note 2 above, pp. 99-108.

10. D.E. Hoffman, "Evaluating Ethics Committees: A View from the Outside," *Milbank Quarterly* 71, no. 4 (1993): 677-701.

11. B. Lo, "Behind Closed Doors: Promises and Pitfalls of Ethics Committees," *New England Journal of Medicine* 317 (1987): 46-50.

12. S. Fry-Revere, "Some Suggestions for Holding Bioethics Committees and Consultants Accountable," *Cambridge Quarterly of Healthcare Ethics* 2 (1993): 449-55; S.M. Wolf, "Ethics Committees and Due Process: Nesting Rights in a Community of Caring," *Maryland Law Review* 50 (1991): 798-858.

13. J.A. Tulsky and B. Lo, "Ethics Consultation: Time to Focus on Patients," *American Journal of Medicine* 92 (1992): 343-5.

14. D.E. Hoffman, "Regulating Ethics Committees: Is It Time?" *Maryland Law Review* 50 (1991): 746-97.

15. G.J. Annas, "Ethics Committees: From Ethical Comfort to Ethical Cover," *Hastings Center Report* 21, no. 3 (1991): 18-21.

16. G.R. Scofield, "Ethics Consultation: The Least Dangerous Profession," *Cambridge Quarterly of Healthcare Ethics* 2 (1993): 417-25.

17. J.C. La Puma et al., "An Ethics Consultation Service in a Teaching Hospital: Utilization and Evaluation," *Journal of the American Medical Association* 260 (1988): 808-11; S. Wear et al., "The Development of an Ethics Consultation Service," *HEC Forum* 2, no. 2 (1990): 75-87; K.H. Simpson, "The Development of a Clinical Ethics Consultation Service in a Community Hospital," *The Journal of Clinical Ethics* 3, no. 2 (Summer 1992): 124-30.

18. Society for Bioethics Consultation, Special Conference on Ethics Consultation, St. Louis, Mo., 26-28 May 1988.

19. J.C. Fletcher and D.E. Hoffman, "Ethics Committees: Time to Experiment with Standards," *Annals of Internal Medicine* 120, no. 4 (1994): 335-8.

20. C.P. Leeman et al., "Quality Control for Hospitals' Clinical Ethics Services: Proposed Standards," *Cambridge Quarterly of Healthcare Ethics* 6 (1997): 257-68.

21. Funding largely was by the Greenwall Foundation; however, financial contributions were made to the project by 37 bioethics organizations and the Soros Foundation.

22. Society for Health and Human Values-Society for Bioethics Consultation Task Force on Standards for Bioethics Consultation, *Core Competencies for Health Care Ethics Consultation* (Glenview, Ill.: American Society for Bioethics and the Humanities, 1998).

23. J.C. Fletcher, "Needed: A Broader View of Ethics Consultation," *Quality Review Bulletin* 18, no. 1 (1992): 12-4; J.C. Fletcher and E.M. Spencer, "Ethics Services in Health Care Organizations," in *Introduction to Clinical Ethics,* 2nd ed., ed. J.C. Fletcher et al. (Hagerstown, Md.: University Publishing Group, 1997): 258-85.

24. Joint Commission on Accreditation of Healthcare Organizations (JCAHO), *Hospital Accreditation: What It Means and How It Works* (Oakbrook Terrace, Ill.: JCAHO, April 1998): 3.

25. E. Fox and J.A. Tulsky, "Evaluation Research and the Future of Ethics Consultation," *The Journal of Clinical Ethics* 7, no. 2 (Summer 1996): 146-49.

26. J.C. Fletcher and M. Siegler, "What Are the Goals of Ethics Consultation? A Consensus Statement," *The Journal of Clinical Ethics* 7, no. 2 (Summer 1996): 122-26.

27. E. Fox, "Concepts in Evaluation Applied to Ethics Consultation Research," *The Journal of Clinical Ethics* 7, no. 2 (Summer 1996): 116-21.

28. See note 22 above, pp. 6-7.

29. Ibid., 13-15.

30. Ibid., 7.

31. The *Core Competencies* report on goals was a more concise summary of the statement accepted by the Chicago conference. See note 22 above, p. 9, and note 26 above.

32. See note 22 above, p. 5.

33. J.C. Fletcher and F.G. Miller, "The Promise and Perils of Public Bioethics," in *The Ethics of Research Involving Human Subjects: Facing the 21st Century,* ed. H.Y. Vanderpool (Hagerstown, Md.: University Publishing Group, 1996): 155-84.

34. See note 22 above, p. 17.

35. Ibid., 8.

36. J. La Puma and D. Schiedermayer, *Ethics Consultation: A Practical Guide* (Boston: Jones & Bartlett, 1994), 35.

37. A somewhat different version of this case was previously published in F.G. Miller, J.C. Fletcher, and J.J. Fins, "Clinical Pragmatism: A Case Method of Moral Problem Solving," in *Introduction to Clinical Ethics,* see note 23 above, pp. 21-38.

38. M.J. Edwards and S.W. Tolle, "Disconnecting a Ventilator at the Request of a Patient Who Knows He Will Then Die: The Doctor's Anguish," *Annals of Internal Medicine* 117, no. 3 (1992): 254-56.

39. D. Orentlicher, "The Supreme Court and Physician-Assisted Suicide: Rejecting Assisted Suicide but Embracing Euthanasia," *New England Journal of Medicine* 337, no. 17 (1997): 1236-9; "Terminal Sedation" (letters), *New England Journal of Medicine* 338, no. 17 (1998): 1230-1.

40. See note 38 above, p. 256.

41. "Reflections on the Doctor's Anguish" (letters), *Annals of Internal Medicine* 118, no. 1 (1993): 78-80.

42. A.B. Baker, J. Stokes, and D.R. Bowie, Letter to the Editor, *Annals of Internal Medicine* 118, no. 1 (1993): 78.

43. M.J. Edwards and S.W. Tolle, Letter to the Editor, *Annals of Internal Medicine* 118, no. 1 (1993): 80.

44. See note 15 above.

45. *Bouvia v. Superior Court* (Glenchur), 19 Cal. App. 3d 1127, 225 Cal. Rptr. 297, 1986. The entire *Bouvia* case is well reported, except for the involvement and suit against the committee, in G.E. Pence, *Classic Cases in Medical Ethics*, 2nd ed. (New York: McGraw-Hill, 1995), 41-7.

46. "Bouvia Sues Hospital Ethics Committee," *Hospital Ethics* 3, no. 1 (1987): 13-4; L.J. Nelson, "Legal Liability of Institutional Ethics Committees to Patients," *Clinical Ethics Report* 6, no. 4 (1992): 1-8.

47. C. Blades and M. Curreri, "Law, Ethics, and Health Care: An Analysis of the Potential Legal Liability of Institutional Ethics Committees," *BioLaw* 2, no. 33 (1989): S317-26. Nelson, in "Legal Liability" (see note 46 above), also cites a personal communication with the late Richard Scott, Bouvia's attorney at the time.

48. A.M. Capron, "Right to Refuse Medical Care," in *Encyclopedia of Bioethics*, ed. W.T. Reich (New York: Free Press, 1978): 1501.

49. *In Re Baby K*, 832 F. Supp. 1022 (E.D. Va. 1993). This case and the ethics committee's role is discussed at length in J.C. Fletcher, "Bioethics in a Legal Forum: Confessions of an 'Expert Witness,' " *Journal of Philosophy and Medicine* 22 (1997): 297-324.

50. *In Re Baby K*, 16 F. 3d 590 (4th Cir. 1994).

51. Fletcher, "Bioethics in a Legal Forum," see note 49 above, pp. 319-20.

52. *Bryan v. Rector and Visitors of the University of Virginia*, 95 F.3d 349 (1996).

53. J.C. Fletcher and E.M. Spencer, "Ethics Services in Health Care Organizations," in *Introduction to Clinical Ethics*, see note 23 above, pp. 271-2.

54. T.A. Brennan, "Incompetent Patients with Limited Care in the Absence of Family Consent," *Annals of Internal Medicine* 109 (1988): 819-25.

55. Super. Ct. Civ. Action No. 92-4820, Suffolk Co., Mass., verdict 21 April 1995; G. Kolata, "Court Ruling Limits Rights of Patients," *New York Times*, 22 April 1995, A1.

56. J. Paris, Professor of Law at Boston College, personal communication with J.C. Fletcher, 4 May 1998.

57. A.M. Capron, "Abandoning a Waning Life," *Hastings Center Report* 25 no. 4 (1995): 24-6.

58. *Estate of James Davis Bland v. Cigna Healthplan of Texas; Kenneth Lawrence Toppell, M.D., Milton Thomas, MD, and Park Plaza Hospital*, District Court of Harris County, Tex., 11th Dist., No. 93-52630 (1995).

59. M. Swartz, "Not What the Doctor Ordered," *Texas Monthly* (March 1995): 86-9, 115-32.

60. According to the pulmonologist's deposition, he went to the room and changed the settings on the patient's ventilator, observed him breathing on his own, and then returned to the previous settings. The pulmonologist testified that a respiratory therapist was called who "put him on a T-tube . . . on twenty-eight percent oxygen." See note 58 above.

61. Natural Death Act, *Vernon's Texas Codes Annotated* 672.001 (1992).

62. See note 22 above, p. 30.

63. *Marlene and Tyrone Rideout v. Hershey Medical Center*, No. 96-5260, Court of Common Pleas, Dauphin County, Pa. (1995).

64. Ibid. The court decision is discussed in W.P. Murphy, "Hospital Faces Liability for Cutting Life Support," *Pennsylvania Law Weekly* 19, no. 3 (15 January 1996): 1, 22.

65. See note 56 above.

66. See note 22 above, p. 9.

67. Ibid., 10.

68. Ibid.

69. See note 16 above.

70. R.F. Wilson, "Hospital Ethics Committees as the Forum of Last Resort: An Idea Whose Time Has Not Come," *North Carolina Law Review* 76, no. 2 (1998): 353-406.

Contributors

JUDITH ANDRE, PHD, is a Professor in the Center for Ethics and Humanities in the Life Sciences Department of Philosophy at Michigan State University in East Lansing.

FRANÇOISE E. BAYLIS, PHD, is an Associate Professor in the Department of Philosophy, Bioethics Education and Research, Faculty of Medicine at Dalhousie University in Halifax, Nova Scotia, Canada.

ELLEN W. BERNAL, PHD, is an Ethicist at St. Vincent Mercy Medical Center in Toledo, Ohio.

CHARLES L. BOSK, PHD, is a Professor in the Department of Sociology at the University of Pennsylvania in Philadelphia.

ROBERT J. BOYLE, MD, is a Professor of Pediatrics at the University of Virginia School of Medicine in Charlottesville and is the Director of the Ethics Consultation Service at the University of Virginia Medical Center.

TOD CHAMBERS, PHD, is an Assistant Professor in the Medical Ethics and Humanities Program at Northwestern University Medical School in Chicago.

RITA CHARON, MD, is an Associate Professor of Clinical Medicine in the Division of General Medicine at the College of Physicians and Surgeons of Columbia University in New York.

KENNETH DE VILLE, PHD, JD, is an Associate Professor in the Department of Medical Humanities in the School of Medicine at East Carolina University in Greenville, North Carolina.

CARL ELLIOTT, MD, PHD, is an Associate Professor in the Center for Bioethics at the University of Minnesota in Minneapolis.

JOHN C. FLETCHER, PHD, is a Professor of Biomedical Ethics (Emeritus) at the University of Virginia School of Medicine in Charlottesville.

JOEL E. FRADER, MD, is an Associate Professor of Pediatrics and an Associate Professor of Medical Ethics and Humanities at Northwestern University Medical School and Children's Memorial Hospital in Chicago.

DAVID HILFIKER, MD, is a physician practicing in Washington, D.C.

EDMUND G. HOWE, MD, JD, is a Professor of Psychiatry and Director of Programs in Medical Ethics at the Uniformed Services University of the Health Sciences in Bethesda, Maryland.

JOHN D. LANTOS, MD, is an Associate Professor and Section Chief of General Pediatrics in the Department of Pediatrics at the University of Chicago Pritzker School of Medicine.

LUCIAN L. LEAPE, MD, is in the Department of Health Policy and Management at the Harvard School of Public Health in Boston.

WILLIAM MAY, PHD, is an Associate Professor of Religion in the School of Religion at the University of Southern California in Los Angeles.

MARTHA MONTELLO, PHD, is an Assistant Professor in Department of History and Philosophy of Medicine at the University of Kansas School of Medicine in Kansas City.

JAMES LINDEMANN NELSON, PHD, is a Professor in the Department of Philosophy at the University of Tennessee in Knoxville.

ROBERT S. OLICK, JD, PHD, is an Associate Professor in the Program in Biomedical Ethics and Medical Humanities and in the Department of Family Medicine at the University of Iowa in Iowa City.

ROSA LYNN PINKUS, PHD, is Associate Director of the Center for Bioethics and Health Law and Associate Professor of Medicine/Neurology at the University of Pittsburgh.

PAUL J. REITEMEIER, PHD, is a consulting ethicist for Healthcare Ethics Integration in Rockford, Michigan, and holds faculty appointments in the Department of Preventive and Societal Medicine at the University of Nebraska Medical Center in Omaha, Nebraska.

SUSAN B. RUBIN, PHD, is Co-Founder of The Ethics Practice in Berkeley, California.

GILES R. SCOFIELD, JD, is a Visiting Professor in the Department of Social Medicine at the University of North Carolina in Chapel Hill.

VIRGINIA A. SHARPE, PHD, is an Associate for Biomedical and Environmental Ethics at the Hastings Center in Garrison, New York.

EDWARD M. SPENCER, MD, is an Assistant Professor of Biomedical Ethics at the University of Virginia School of Medicine in Charlottesville and is a Senior Consultant in the Virginia Bioethics Network.

GEORGE C. WEBSTER, DMIN, is a Clinical Ethicist in the Health Care Ethics Service at St. Boniface General Hospital in Winnipeg, Manitoba, and is an Assistant Professor in the Faculty of Medicine and Adjunct Professor in the Department of Philosophy at the University of Manitoba, Canada.

BRUCE E. ZAWACKI, MA, MD, is Associate Director for Education at the Pacific Center for Health Policy and Ethics, and is an Emeritus Associate Professor of Surgery and of Religion at the University of Southern California-Los Angeles.

LAURIE ZOLOTH, PHD, is Co-Founder of The Ethics Practice in Berkeley, California and is an Associate Professor and Chair of the Jewish Studies Program at San Francisco State University in San Francisco.